The Color Diagrammatic Atlas of
Congenital Heart Disease

Edited by
Bülent Oran

Pediatric Cardiology, İzmir, *Turkey*

MEDICANA
HEALTH GROUP

The Color Diagrammatic Atlas of Congenital Heart Disease

Bülent Oran M.D.

Prof. of Pediatric Cardiology
Former head of Pediatrics Department
Selçuk University, Medical School, Konya.
Department of Pediatric Cardiology,
MEDICANA International Hospital,
İzmir-Turkey

ISBN 978-1-949872-39-2

CONTENT

*Corresponding author Oran B: Medicana International Hospital, Department of Pediatric Cardiology, İzmir, Turkey
E-mail:boran@medicana.com.tr and bulentoran@hotmail.com

*Corresponding author Oran B: Medicana International Hospital, Department of Pediatric Cardiology, İzmir, Turkey
E-mail:boran@medicana.com.tr and bulentoran@hotmail.com

*Corresponding author Oran B: Medicana International Hospital, Department of Pediatric Cardiology, İzmir, Turkey
E-mail:boran@medicana.com.tr and bulentoran@hotmail.com

*Corresponding author Oran B: Medicana International Hospital, Department of Pediatric Cardiology, İzmir, Turkey
E-mail:boran@medicana.com.tr and bulentoran@hotmail.com

*Corresponding author Oran B: Medicana International Hospital, Department of Pediatric Cardiology, İzmir, Turkey
E-mail:boran@medicana.com.tr and bulentoran@hotmail.com

CHAPTER 10

*Corresponding author Oran B: Medicana International Hospital, Department of Pediatric Cardiology, İzmir, Turkey
E-mail:boran@medicana.com.tr and bulentoran@hotmail.com

*Corresponding author Oran B: Medicana International Hospital, Department of Pediatric Cardiology, İzmir, Turkey
E-mail:boran@medicana.com.tr and bulentoran@hotmail.com

*Corresponding author Oran B: Medicana International Hospital, Department of Pediatric Cardiology, İzmir, Turkey
E-mail:boran@medicana.com.tr and bulentoran@hotmail.com

FOREWORD

I would like to congratulate my colleague Dr. Bülent Oran on his outstanding work "The Color Diagrammatic Atlas of Congenital Heart Disease". This work has taken many years, all for the benefits of patients and their providers. This book will be an important supplement to medical students, nurses, pediatric and adult cardiologists (established or trainees), and anyone who has an interest in this important field. Currently and at least in the USA, there are more adults with congenital heart diseases than children. This atlas with its simple diagrams explains very well the lesion and its basic physiology and anatomy. Every unit that deals with such patients should have access to this atlas. Again, congratulations to outstanding work.

Ziyad M. Hijazi, MD

*Corresponding author Oran B: Medicana International Hospital, Department of Pediatric Cardiology, İzmir, Turkey
E-mail:boran@medicana.com.tr and bulentoran@hotmail.com

*Corresponding author Oran B: Medicana International Hospital, Department of Pediatric Cardiology, İzmir, Turkey
E-mail:boran@medicana.com.tr and bulentoran@hotmail.com

"A picture is worth a thousand words"

PREFACE

Rapid developments in congenital heart disease diagnosis and treatment have allowed children with congenital heart disease to survive to adulthood. In particular, advances in pediatric cardiology during the 2000s have shifted the majority of congenital heart disease-related mortalities to adulthood. Consequently, there are now hundreds of thousands of adults with congenital heart defects worldwide. In the near future, cardiologists are expected to encounter a steady increase in patients at grown-up congenital heart centers.

This atlas includes representations of common congenital heart defects and complete sets of surgical or transcatheter interventions with the most recent acquisitions. Diagrams will serve clinicians as well as provide information for patients. The atlas also provides a selection of diagrams (more than 200 diagrammatic heart figures) from the cardiac catheterization laboratory of a pediatric or grown-up cardiology unit that can be easily modified by various software programs. Simple line or symbol-based drawings, rather than artistic illustrations, have been used in figures to facilitate sharing and customization. The European Paediatric Cardiac Codes (EPCC), The International Paediatric and Congenital Cardiac Code (IPCCC) and the Eleventh Iteration of the International Classification of Diseases (ICD-11) were used for nomenclature of congenital cardiac disease.

In conclusion, I believe that this atlas is a necessary reference with great utility for cardiologists, heart surgeons, radiologists, clinical staff, medical students, nursing personnel, patients and their families. A further advantage of this type of publication is the potential for inexpensive and rapid distribution online.

Bülent Oran

*Corresponding author Oran B: Medicana International Hospital, Department of Pediatric Cardiology, İzmir, Turkey
E-mail:boran@medicana.com.tr and bulentoran@hotmail.com

*Corresponding author Oran B: Medicana International Hospital, Department of Pediatric Cardiology, İzmir, Turkey
E-mail:boran@medicana.com.tr and bulentoran@hotmail.com

CHAPTER 1

Lesions with Left-Right Shunt

Oran B.

Medicana International Hospital, Department of Pediatric Cardiology, İzmir, Turkey

*Corresponding author Oran B: Medicana International Hospital, Department of Pediatric Cardiology, İzmir, Turkey
E-mail:boran@medicana.com.tr and bulentoran@hotmail.com

Normal Heart

In this atlas, all congenital heart defects were prepared by modifying this normal heart diagram. To facilitate adaptation of the diagrams by different catheter laboratories, simple line or symbol-based drawings were displayed, rather than artistic illustrations.

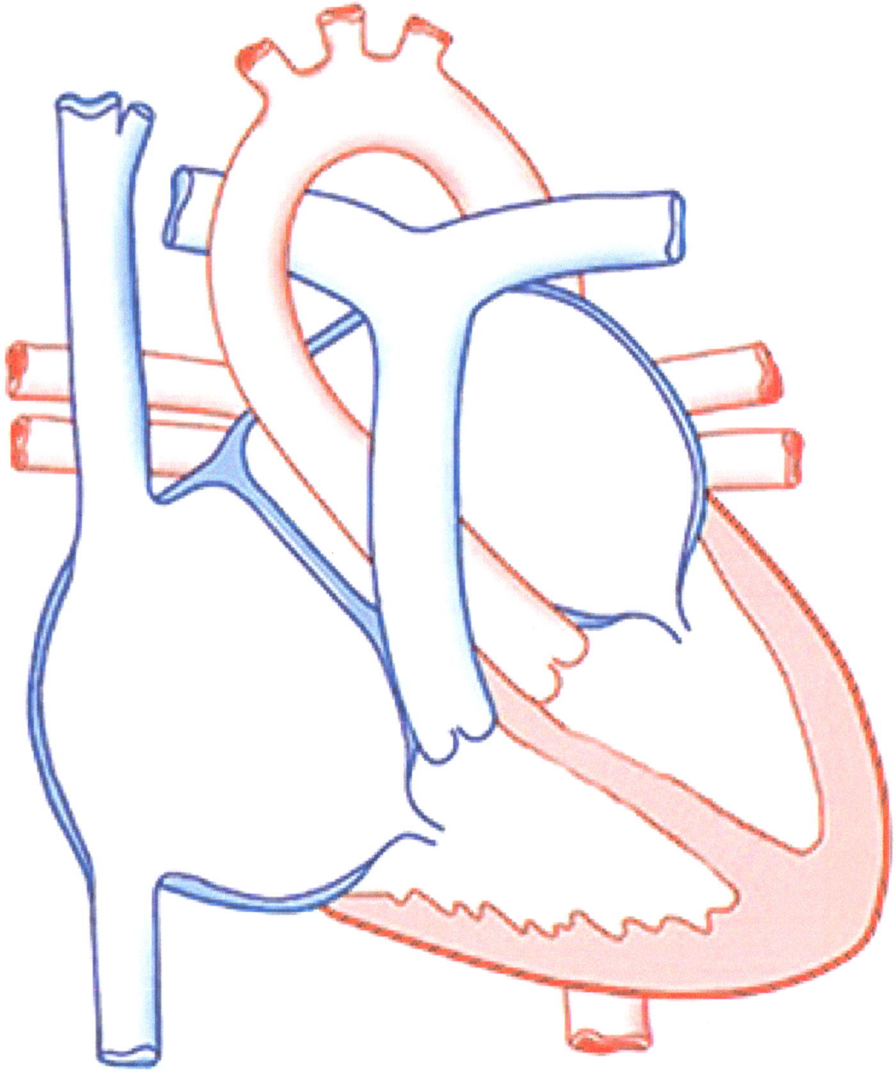

Figure 1: Normal heart.

*Corresponding author Oran B: Medicana International Hospital, Department of Pediatric Cardiology, İzmir, Turkey
E-mail:boran@medicana.com.tr and bulentoran@hotmail.com

Patent Foramen Ovale

One quarter of adults have a patent foramen ovale without clinical symptoms. This small defect results from the failed fusion of the septum primum and secundum after birth.

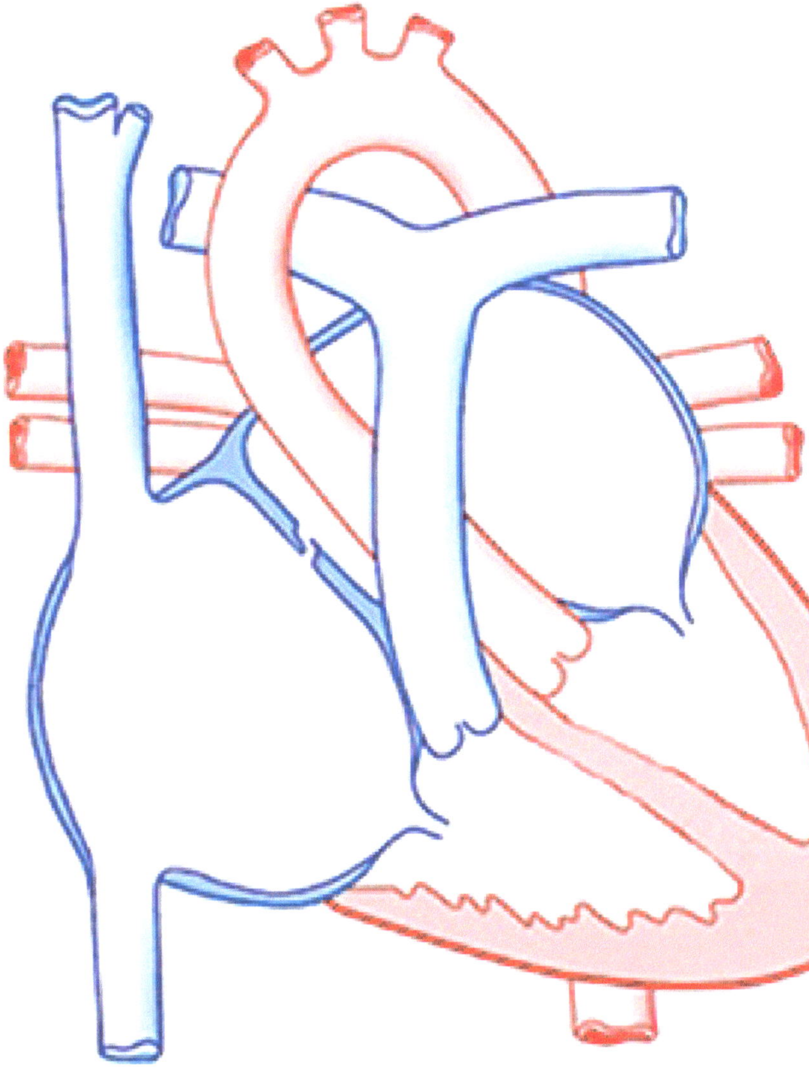

Figure 2: Patent Foramen Ovale, PFO, Patent oval foramen.

*Corresponding author Oran B: Medicana International Hospital, Department of Pediatric Cardiology, İzmir, Turkey
E-mail:boran@medicana.com.tr and bulentoran@hotmail.com

Ostium Secundum Atrial Septal Defects

The secundum atrial septal defect (ASD) is a common malformation that causes shunting of blood between the pulmonary and systemic circulation and is characterized by deficient septum secundum tissue. An oval fossa defect allows direct communication between atrial chambers. These defects are associated with Holt-Oram syndrome, trisomy 21, pulmonary valvar stenosis, ventricular septal defect (VSD), patent ductus arteriosus (PDA), coarctation of aorta, tetralogy of Fallot, and partial anomalous pulmonary venous connection.

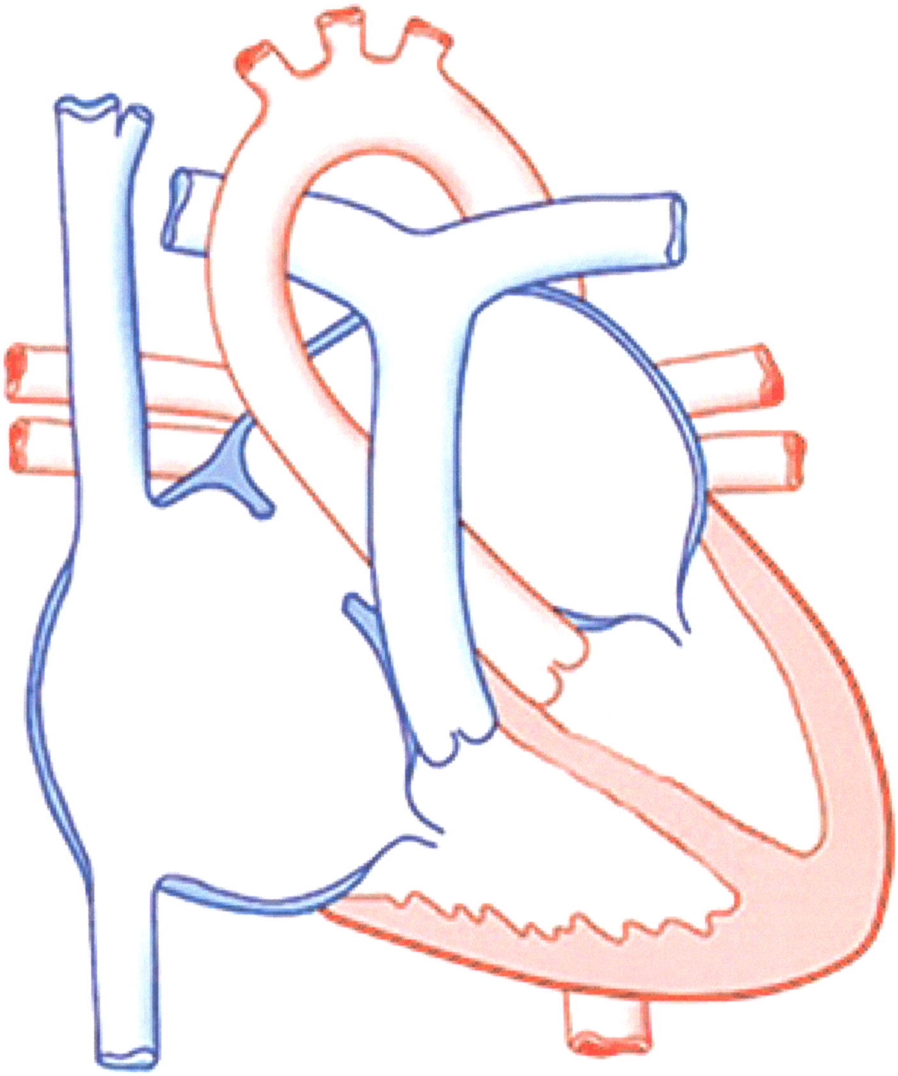

Figure 3: Atrial septal defects within oval fossa (secundum), Atrial septal defects, secundum.

*Corresponding author Oran B: Medicana International Hospital, Department of Pediatric Cardiology, İzmir, Turkey
E-mail:boran@medicana.com.tr and bulentoran@hotmail.com

Ostium Primum Atrial Septal Defects

Septum primum defects are the atrial component of atrioventricular septal defects (AVSDs) and are often associated with trisomy 21.

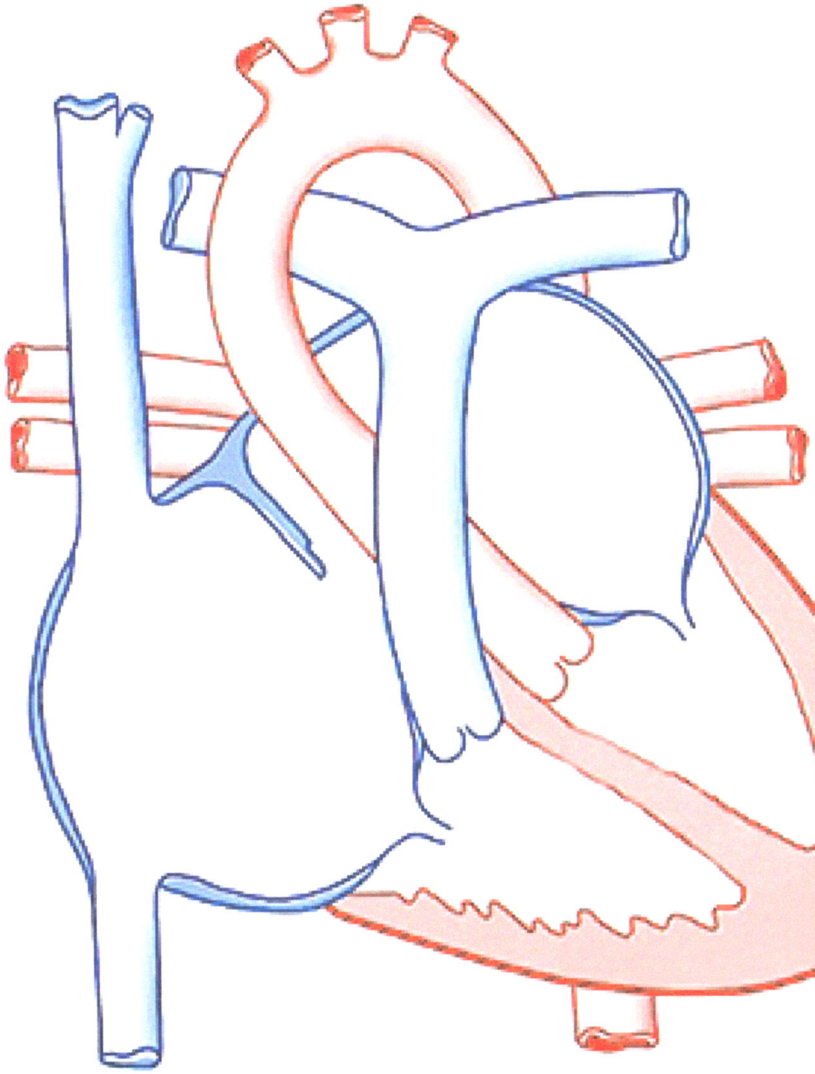

Figure 4: Isolated atrial component (primum ASD), Atrioventricular septal defects with communication at the atrial level only. (Interatrial communication).

*Corresponding author Oran B: Medicana International Hospital, Department of Pediatric Cardiology, İzmir, Turkey
E-mail:boran@medicana.com.tr and bulentoran@hotmail.com

Sinus Venosus Atrial Septal Defects

Sinus venosus ASDs can occur near the superior vena cava or inferior vena cava, but are most common near the superior vena cava. These defects impair the folding of the superior vena cava of the atrial wall. Sinus venous ASDs are associated with partial anomalous pulmonary venous drainage and ectopic atrial pacemakers (in sinoatrial node defects).

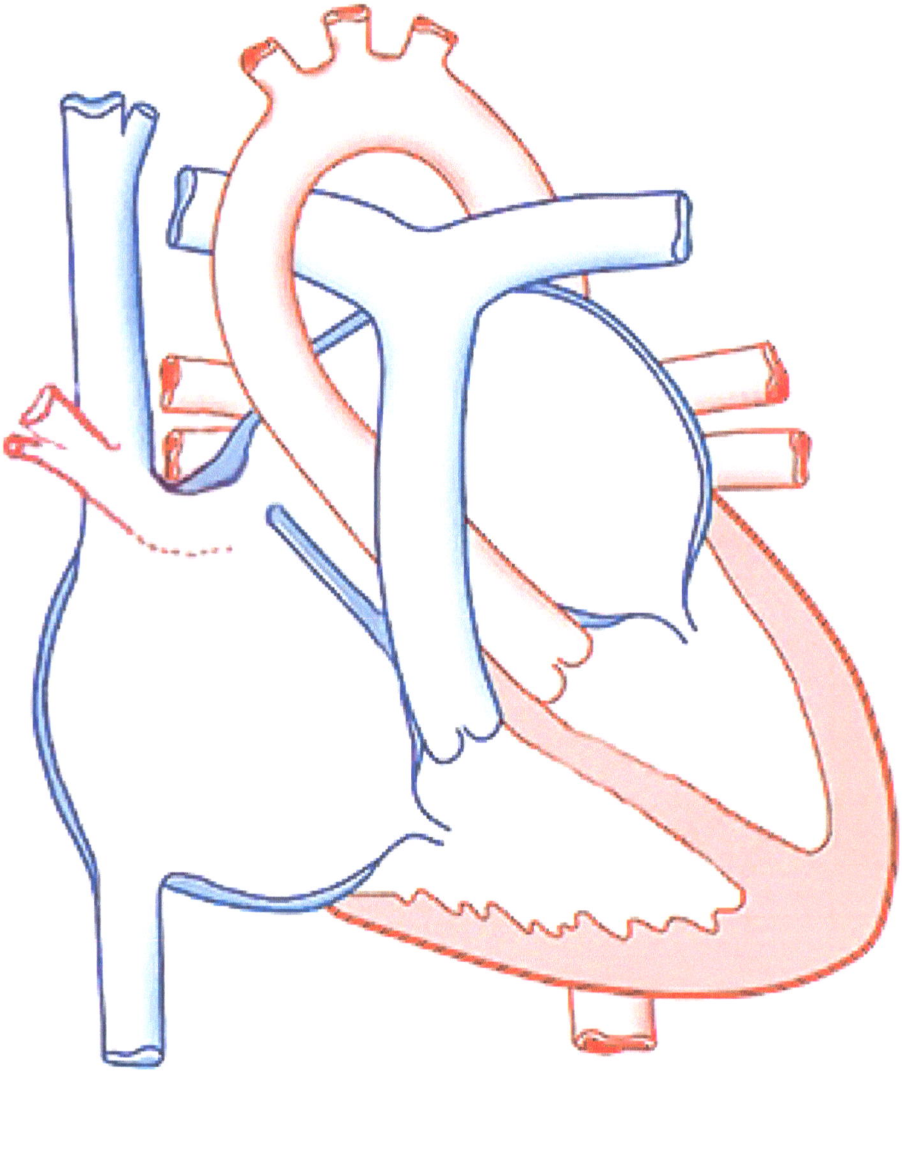

Figure 5: Sinus venosus atrial septal defect, (Sinus venosus defect) superior vena cava type with parsiel anomalous pulmonary venous return.

*Corresponding author Oran B: Medicana International Hospital, Department of Pediatric Cardiology, İzmir, Turkey
E-mail:boran@medicana.com.tr and bulentoran@hotmail.com

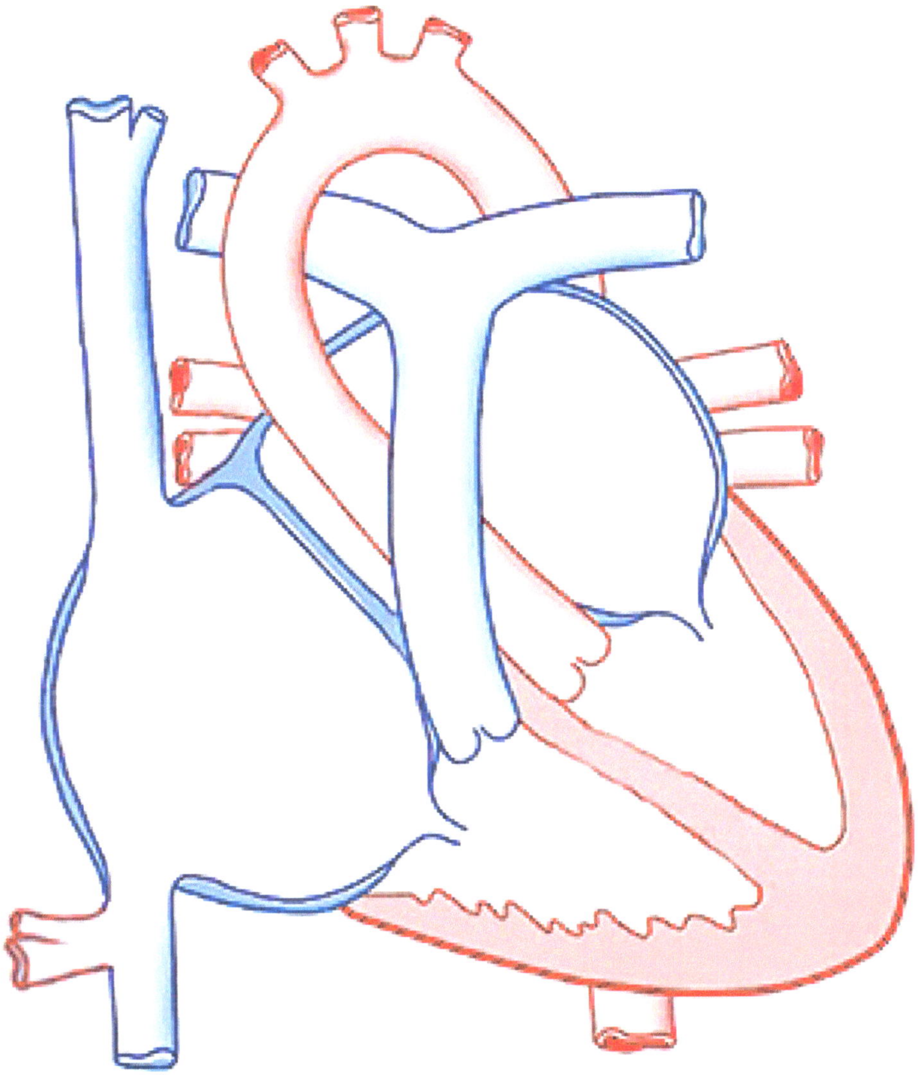

Figure 6: Sinus venosus atrial septal defect, (Sinus venosus defect) inferior vena cava type with parsiel anomalous pulmonary venous return.

*Corresponding author Oran B: Medicana International Hospital, Department of Pediatric Cardiology, İzmir, Turkey
E-mail:boran@medicana.com.tr and bulentoran@hotmail.com

Coronary Sinus Defect

Coronary sinus defects are rare and involve malformation of the entry site of the coronary sinus to the left atrium. The roof separating the coronary sinus from the left atrium is also absent (unroofed coronary sinus). Persistent left superior vena cava drainage to the coronary sinus is a typical result, which causes right-to-left shunting and cyanosis.

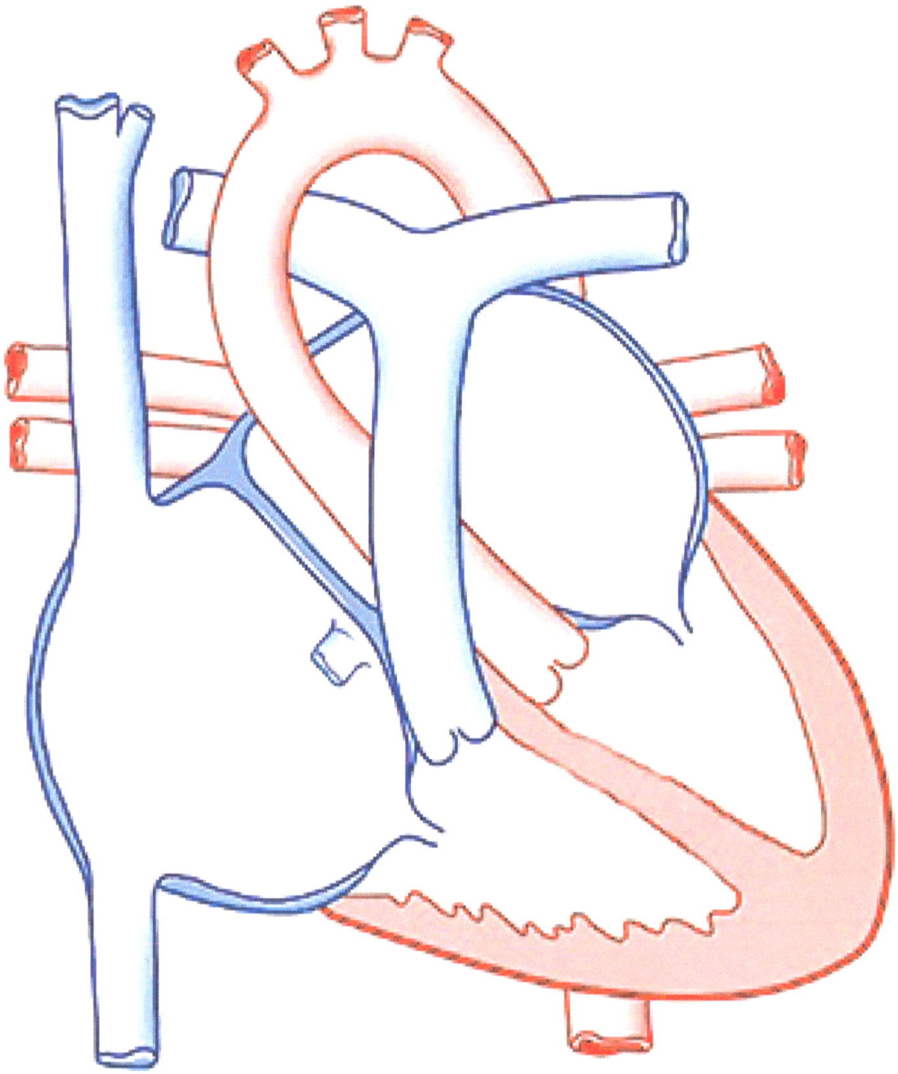

Figure 7: Interatrial communication (ASD) through coronary sinus orifice, Coronary sinus type defect.

*Corresponding author Oran B: Medicana International Hospital, Department of Pediatric Cardiology, İzmir, Turkey
E-mail:boran@medicana.com.tr and bulentoran@hotmail.com

Common Atrium

Common atrium is a rare congenital condition characterized by the absence of atrial septal tissue. It is typically diagnosed in childhood and is associated with serious symptoms. It may occur on its own or as a component of Ellis van Creveld Syndrome.

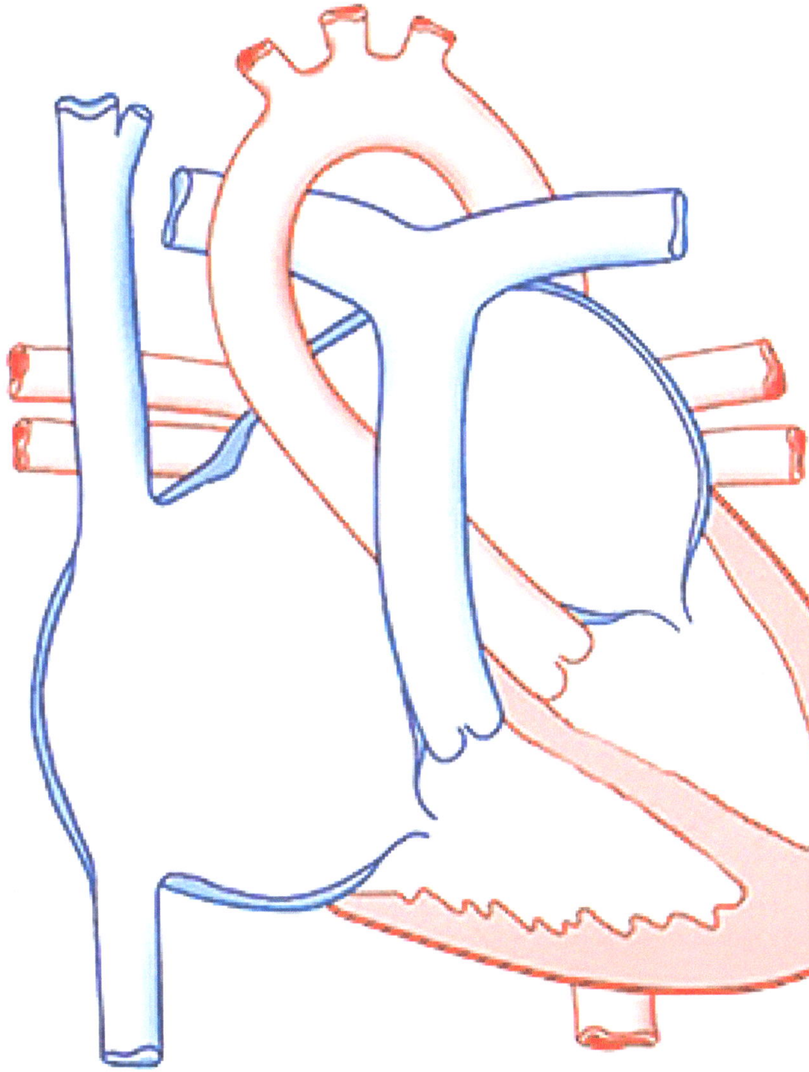

Figure 8: Common atrium (virtual absence of atrial septum), Common atrium with separate atrioventricular junctions.

*Corresponding author Oran B: Medicana International Hospital, Department of Pediatric Cardiology, İzmir, Turkey
E-mail:boran@medicana.com.tr and bulentoran@hotmail.com

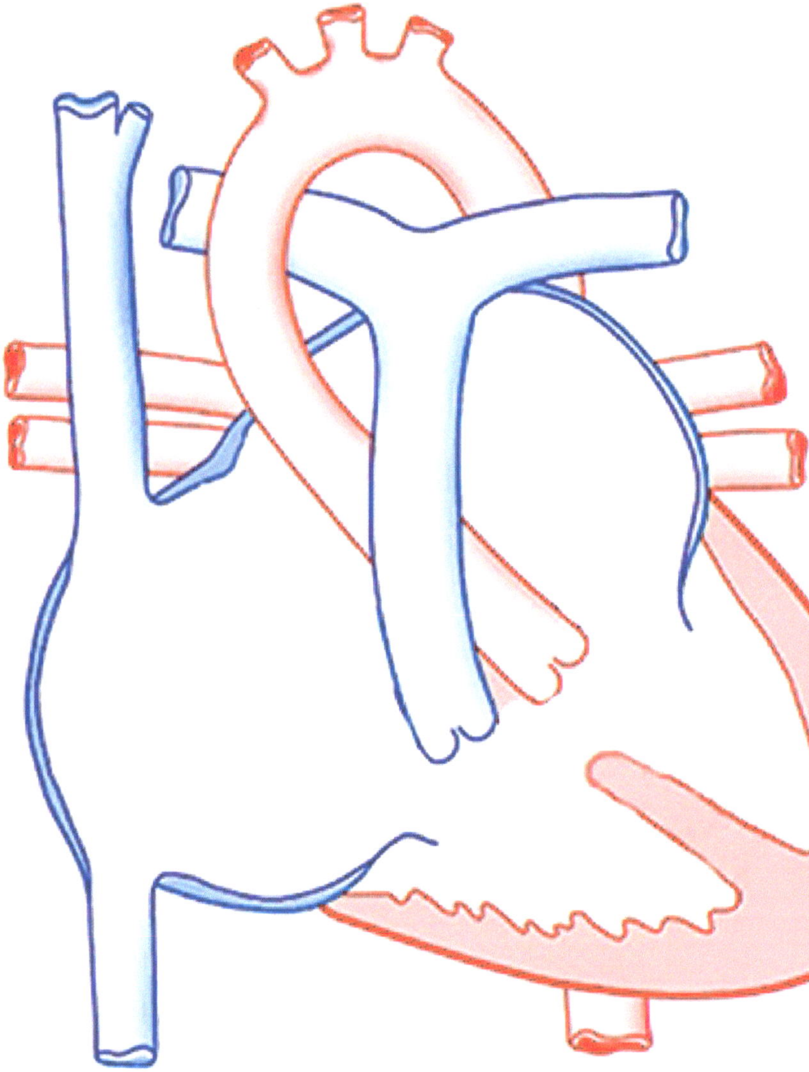

Figure 9: Common atrium (virtual absence of atrial septum), Common atrium with common atrioventricular junctions.

*Corresponding author Oran B: Medicana International Hospital, Department of Pediatric Cardiology, İzmir, Turkey
E-mail:boran@medicana.com.tr and bulentoran@hotmail.com

Ventricular Septal Defects

Ventricular septal defects (VSDs) result from developmental failure of the interventricular inlet septum, muscular trabeculated septum, outlet septum, or perimembranous septum. VSDs are classified by their location within the septum and by their borders (viewed from the right ventricle). Membranous VSDs occur with inlet, outlet, or trabecular extension and are bordered in part by fibrous continuity between the leaflets of the atrioventricular and arterial valves. Doubly committed subarterial VSDs are situated in the outlet septum and are bordered by fibrous continuity between the aortic and pulmonary valves. Aortic regurgitation may develop in perimembranous and doubly committed subarterial type VSDs. VSDs are associated with coarctation of aorta and tetralogy of Fallot.

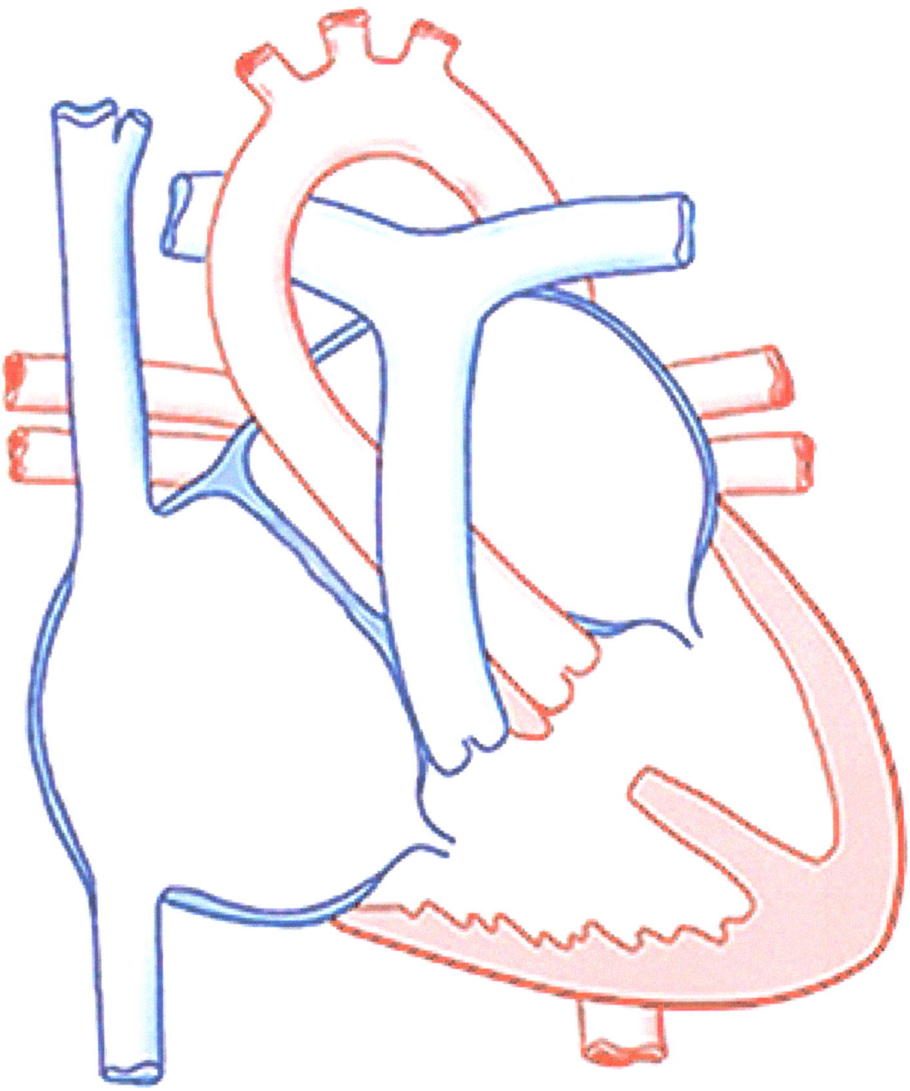

Figure 10: Ventricular Septal Defect (VSD).

*Corresponding author Oran B: Medicana International Hospital, Department of Pediatric Cardiology, İzmir, Turkey
E-mail:boran@medicana.com.tr and bulentoran@hotmail.com

Muscular Ventricular Septal Defects

Muscular VSDs are bordered entirely by myocardium and their locations may be trabecular, inlet, or outlet.

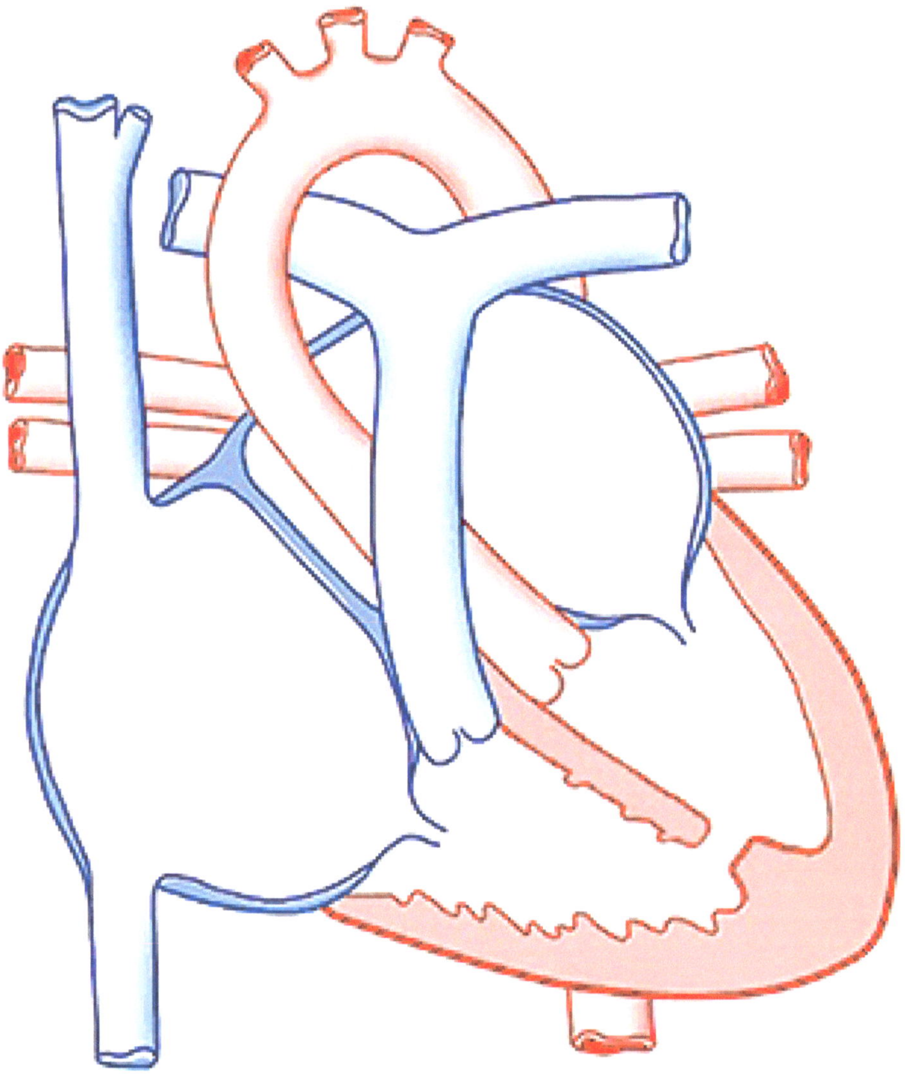

Figure 11: Muscular ventricular septal defect, VSD (Muscular).

*Corresponding author Oran B: Medicana International Hospital, Department of Pediatric Cardiology, İzmir, Turkey
E-mail:boran@medicana.com.tr and bulentoran@hotmail.com

Multiple Ventricular Septal Defects

The interventricular septum contains two or more septal defects.

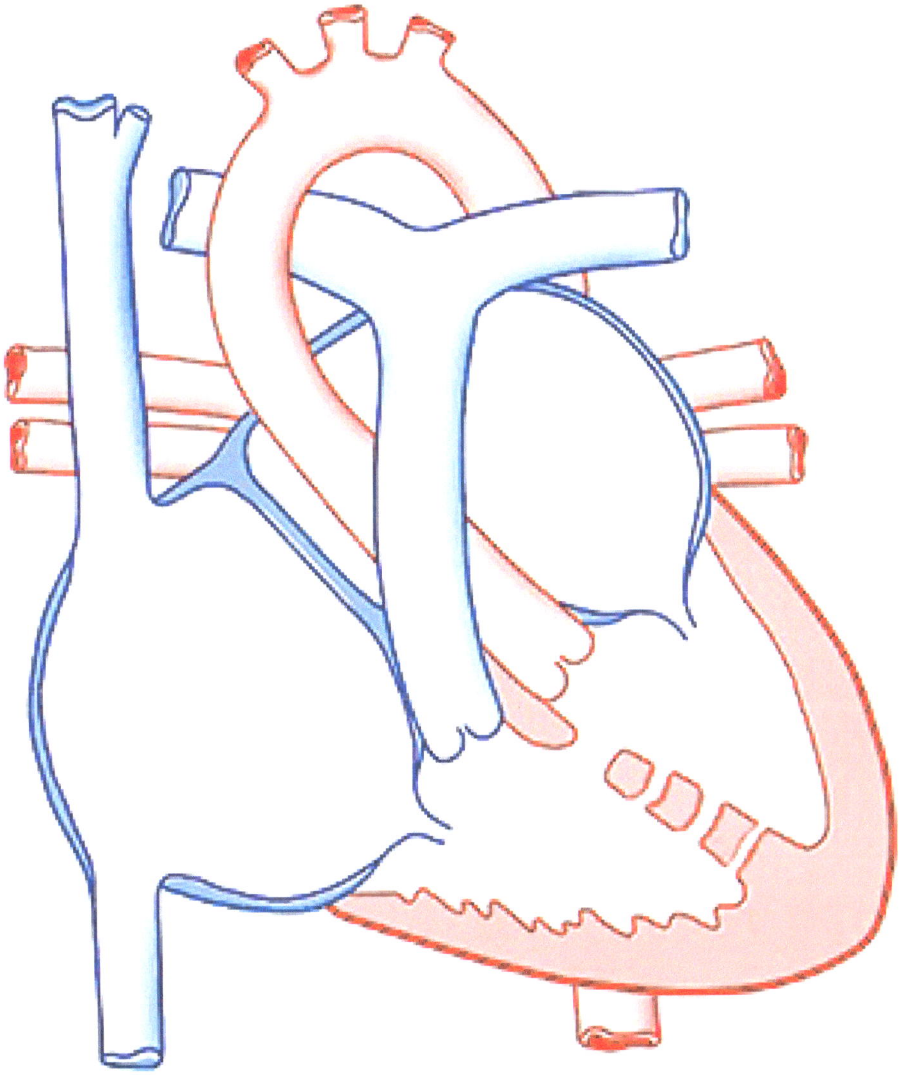

Figure 12: Multiple ventricular septal defect (VSD).

*Corresponding author Oran B: Medicana International Hospital, Department of Pediatric Cardiology, İzmir, Turkey
E-mail:boran@medicana.com.tr and bulentoran@hotmail.com

Gerbode-type Ventricular Septal Defects

These rare VSDs involve left ventricular to right atrial communication. The blood in the left ventricle flows through the small area of the membranous septum, above the tricuspid valve.

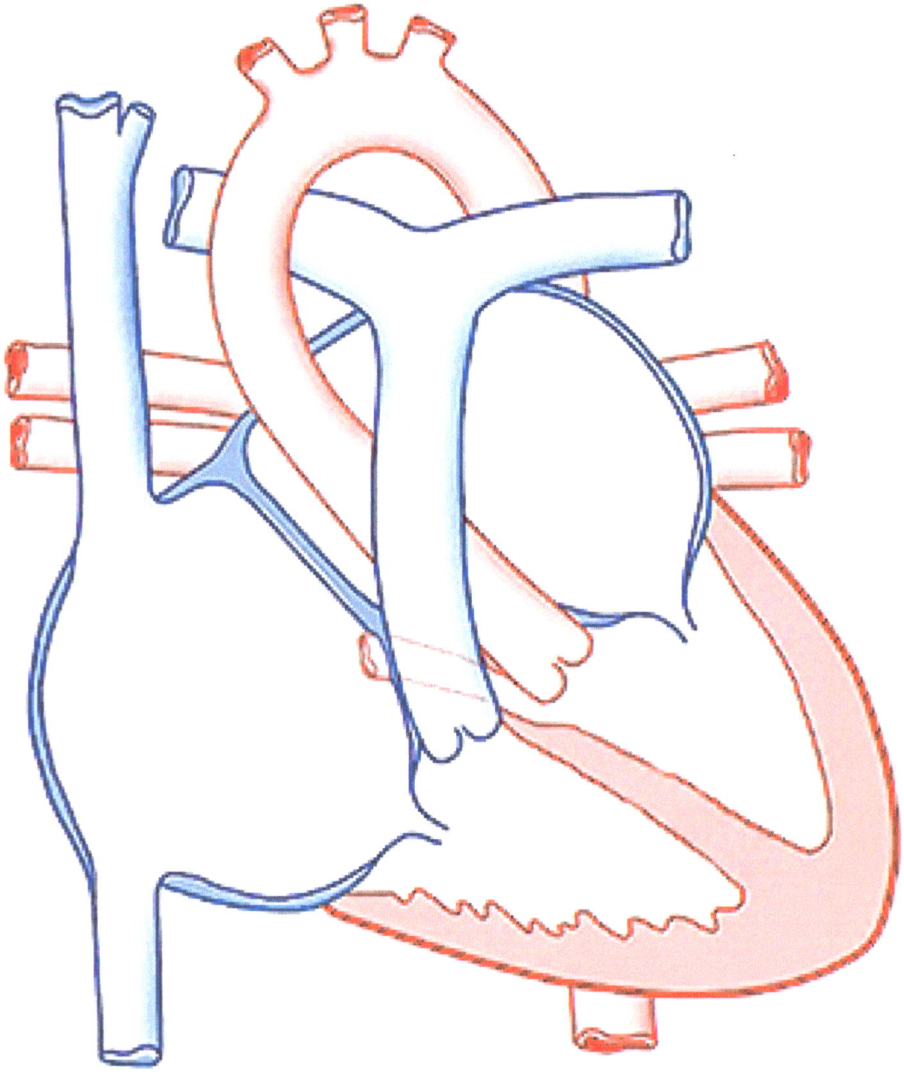

Figure 13: Communication between LV-RA (Gerbode defect), Gerbode-type ventricular septal defect (Communication between left ventricle and right atrium - Gerbode defect)

*Corresponding author Oran B: Medicana International Hospital, Department of Pediatric Cardiology, İzmir, Turkey
E-mail:boran@medicana.com.tr and bulentoran@hotmail.com

Atrioventricular Septal Defects

AVSDs comprise a spectrum of anomalies. The atrial component of an AVSD is an ostium primum type defect. The defect causes both atrioventricular valves to be located on the same plane. The atrioventricular valves are not true mitral and tricuspid valves; they are termed "left" and "right" atrioventricular valves. There are three types of AVSDs: partial, intermediate, or complete.

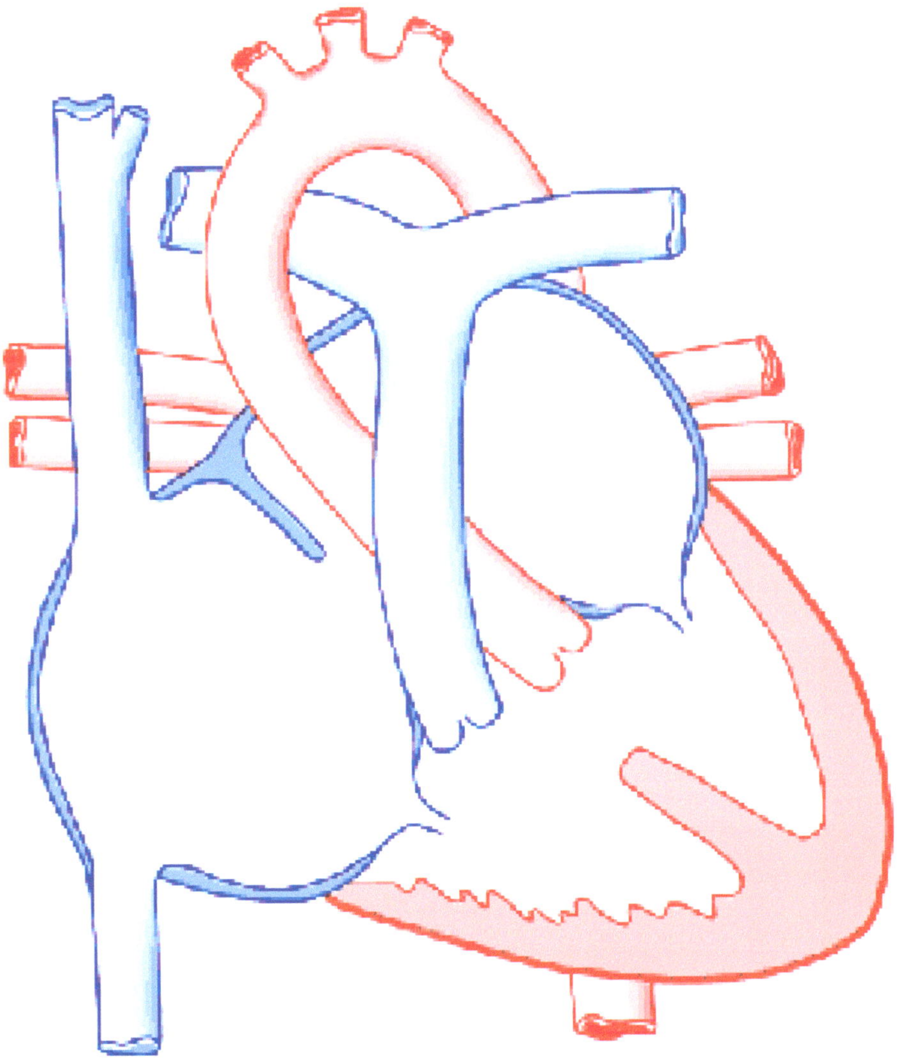

Figure 14: Atrioventricular septal defect (general), Atrioventricular septal defect with balanced ventricles.

*Corresponding author Oran B: Medicana International Hospital, Department of Pediatric Cardiology, İzmir, Turkey
E-mail:boran@medicana.com.tr and bulentoran@hotmail.com

Partial Atrioventricular Septal Defect

Partial AVSDs are characterized by a cleft in the adjoining leaflet of the left or right atrioventricular valve and an intact ventricular septum.

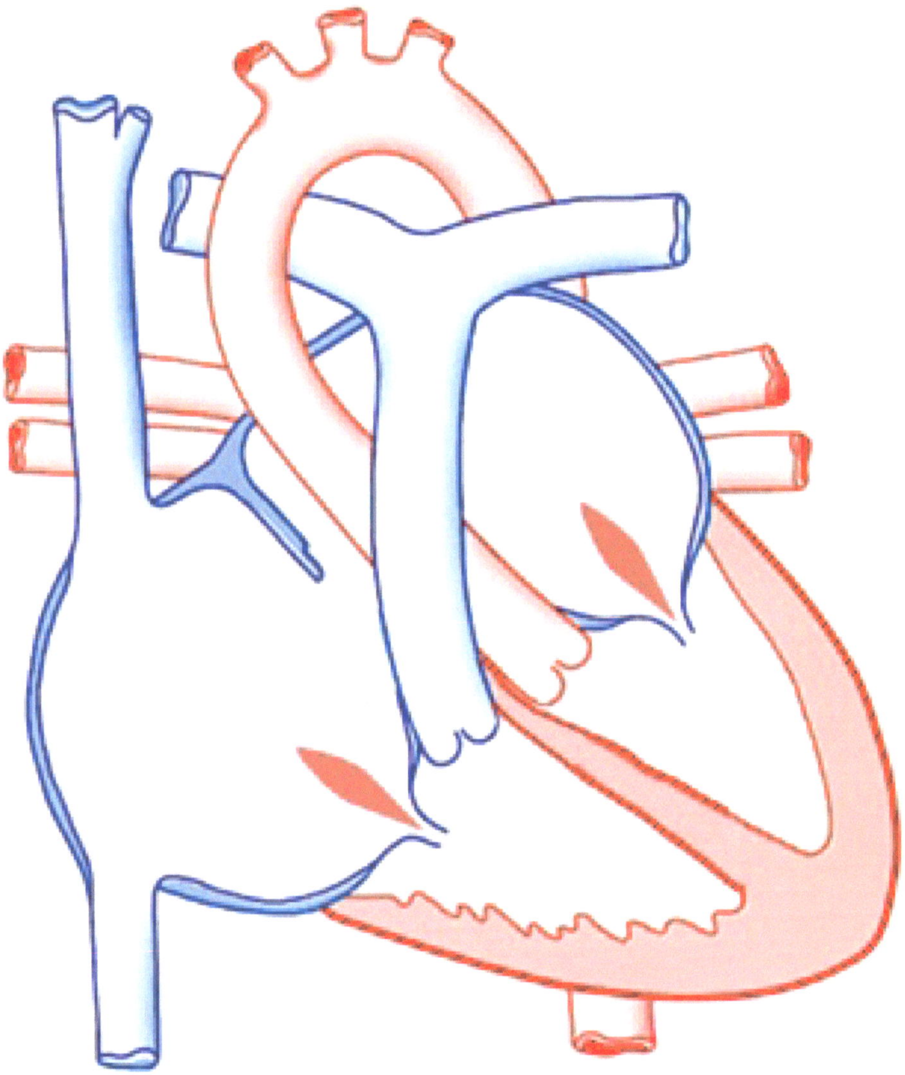

Figure 15: Partial atrioventricular septal defect, Atrioventricular septal defect with communication at the ventricular level only.

*Corresponding author Oran B: Medicana International Hospital, Department of Pediatric Cardiology, İzmir, Turkey
E-mail:boran@medicana.com.tr and bulentoran@hotmail.com

Intermediate Atrioventricular Septal Defects

Intermediate AVSDs are primum ASDs with a restrictive ventricular septal abnormality and two separate atrioventricular valves.

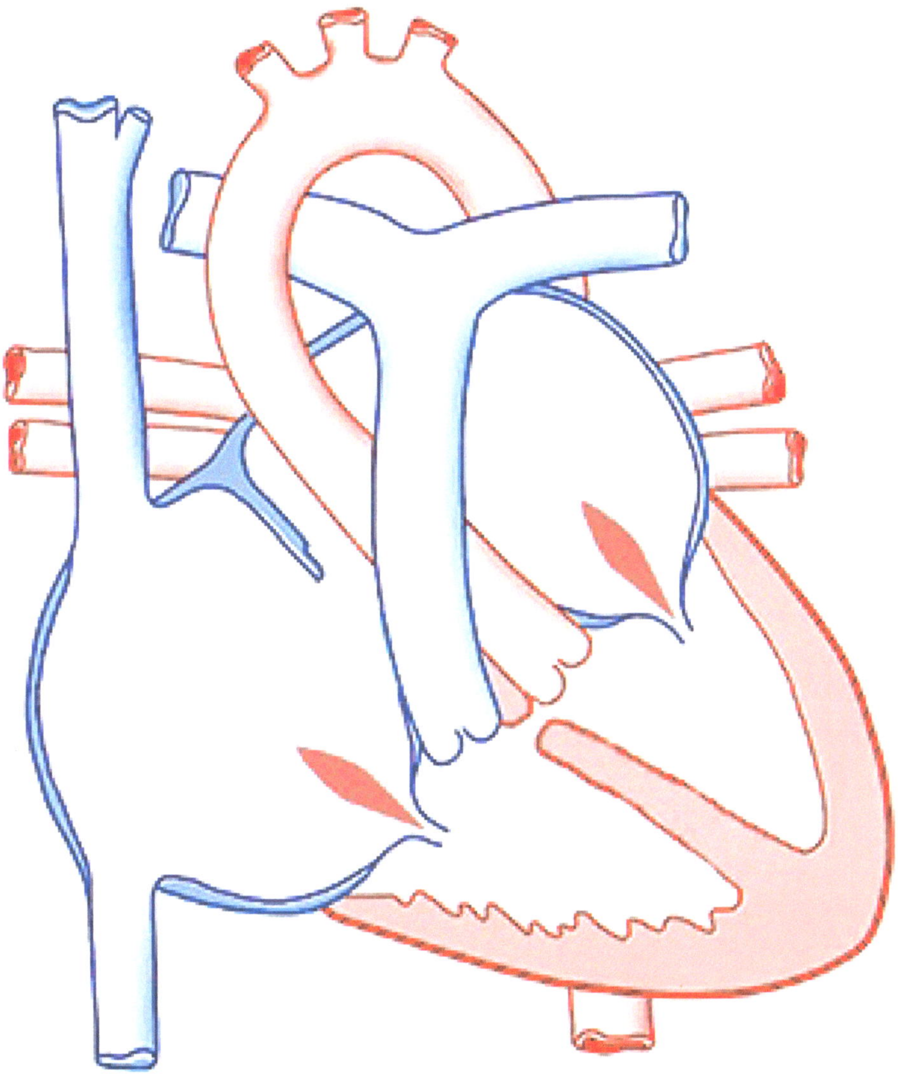

Figure 16: AVSD: atrial & ventricular components + separate AV valves ('intermediate'), Intermediated atrioventricular septal defect (Atrioventricular septal defect with communication at atrial level and restrictive communication at ventricular level) (Common atrioventricular valvar regurgitation)

*Corresponding author Oran B: Medicana International Hospital, Department of Pediatric Cardiology, İzmir, Turkey
E-mail:boran@medicana.com.tr and bulentoran@hotmail.com

Complete Atrioventricular Septal Defects

Complete AVSDs are characterized by a nonrestrictive VSD, a common atrioventricular valve, and a five-leaflet atrioventricular valve that may be regurgitant. It is rare for these patients to survive into adulthood without interventional procedures or surgery. Complete AVSDs are associated with trisomy 21, tetralogy of Fallot, and double-outlet right ventricle.

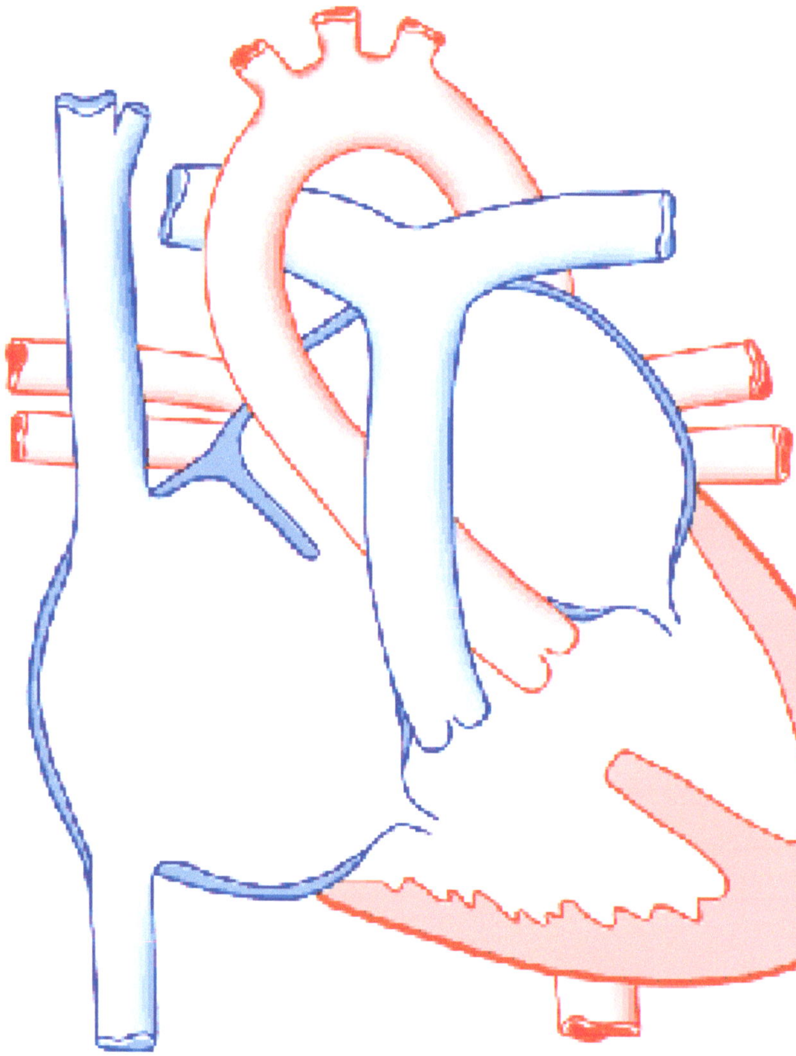

Figure 17: AVSD: atrial & ventricular components (complete) + separate AV valves, Complet atrioventricular septal defect (Atrioventricular septal defect with communication at atrial level and unrestrictive communication at ventricular level).

*Corresponding author Oran B: Medicana International Hospital, Department of Pediatric Cardiology, İzmir, Turkey
E-mail:boran@medicana.com.tr and bulentoran@hotmail.com

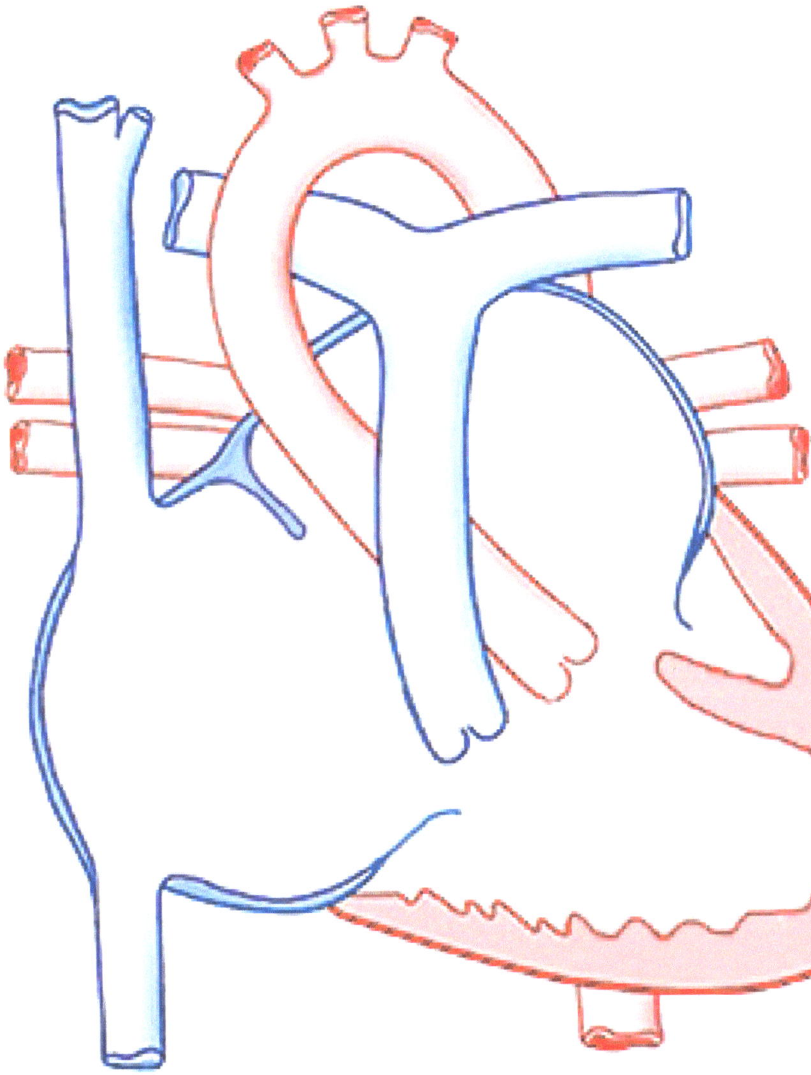

Figure 18: Complet AVSD: atrial & ventricular components (complete) with hypoplastic left ventricle. Complet atrioventricular septal defect, hypoplastic left ventricle with ventricular imbalance.

*Corresponding author Oran B: Medicana International Hospital, Department of Pediatric Cardiology, İzmir, Turkey
E-mail:boran@medicana.com.tr and bulentoran@hotmail.com

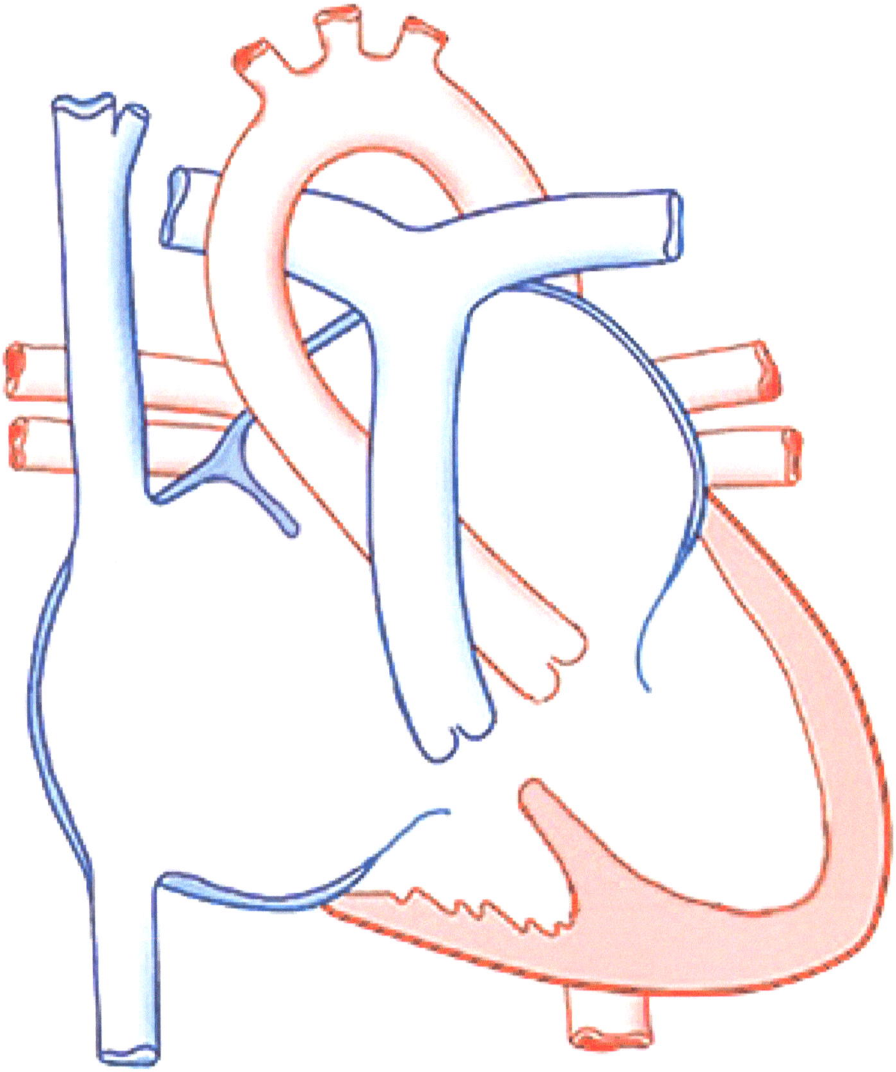

Figure 19: Complet AVSD: atrial & ventricular components (complete) with hypoplastic right ventricle. Complet atrioventricular septal defect, hypoplastic right ventricle with ventricular imbalance.

*Corresponding author Oran B: Medicana International Hospital, Department of Pediatric Cardiology, İzmir, Turkey
E-mail:boran@medicana.com.tr and bulentoran@hotmail.com

Patent Ductus Arteriosus

Patent ductus arteriosus (PDA) is a hole in the vessel connecting the pulmonary artery to the aorta. This structure is vital during fetal heart development. The size and shape of the PDA varies greatly. From a clinical perspective, PDA is graded as (1) silent: tiny defect without audible heart murmurs; (2) small: no hemodynamic significance, normal left atrial and left ventricular sizes without pulmonary hypertension; (3) moderate: enlargement of the left atrium and left ventricle, with some degree of pulmonary hypertension; or (4) large: typically observed in adults with Eisenmenger physiology and signs of pulmonary hypertension. This malformation is associated with coarctation of the aorta, VSDs, and vascular ring anomalies.

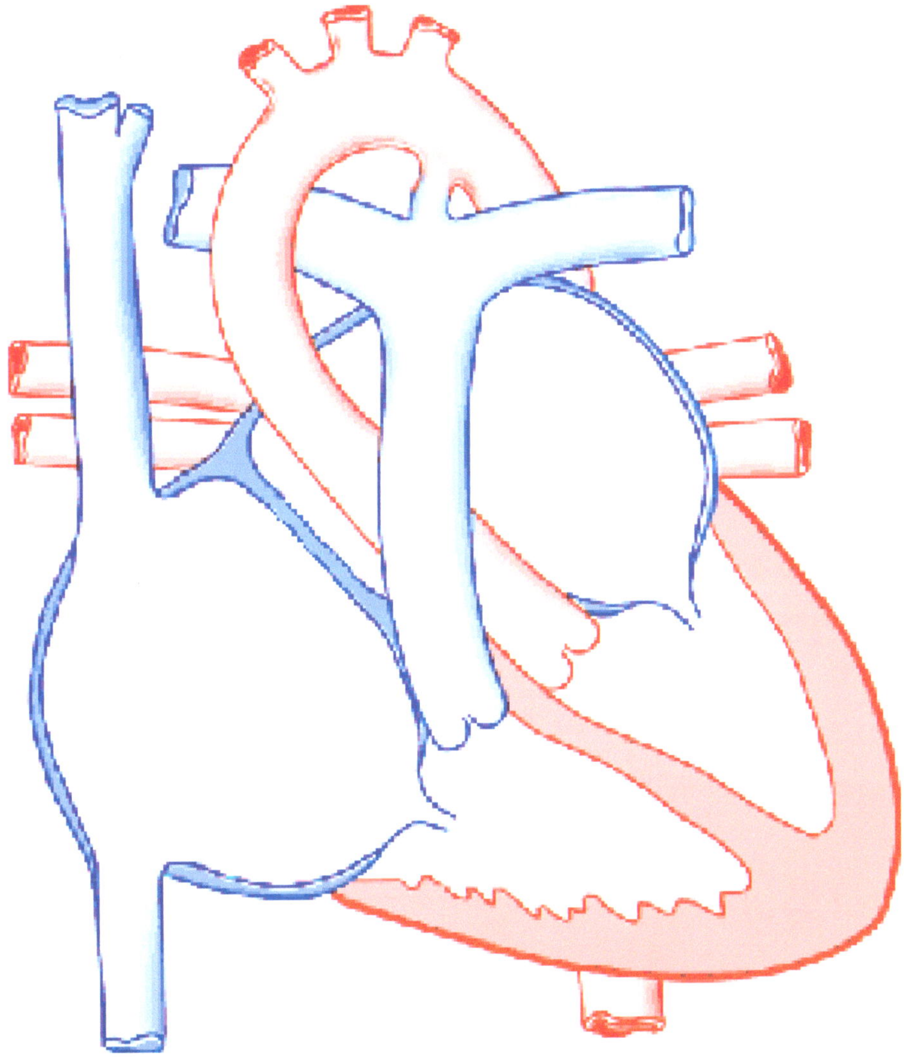

Figure 20: Patent ductus arteriosus. Patent arterial duct (PDA).

*Corresponding author Oran B: Medicana International Hospital, Department of Pediatric Cardiology, İzmir, Turkey
E-mail:boran@medicana.com.tr and bulentoran@hotmail.com

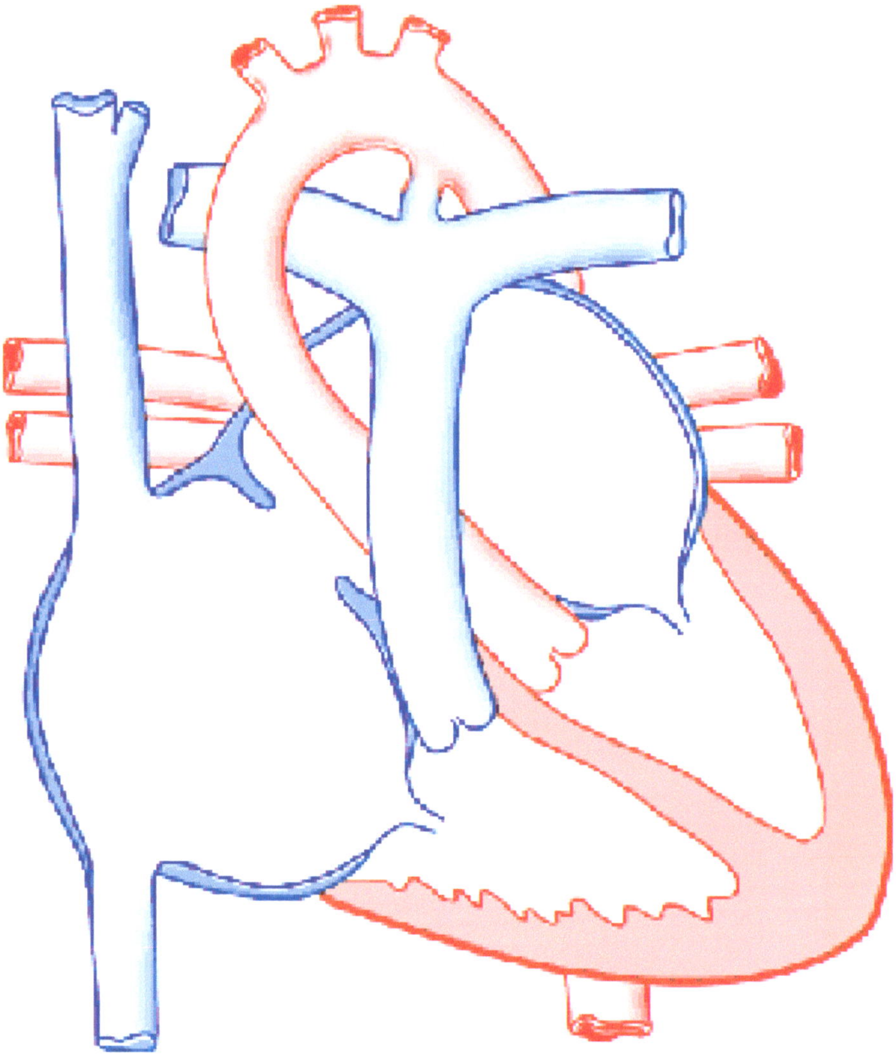

Figure 21: Patent ductus arteriosus with secundum atrial septal defect. Patent arterial duct (PDA) with atrial septal defect, secundum.

*Corresponding author Oran B: Medicana International Hospital, Department of Pediatric Cardiology, İzmir, Turkey
E-mail:boran@medicana.com.tr and bulentoran@hotmail.com

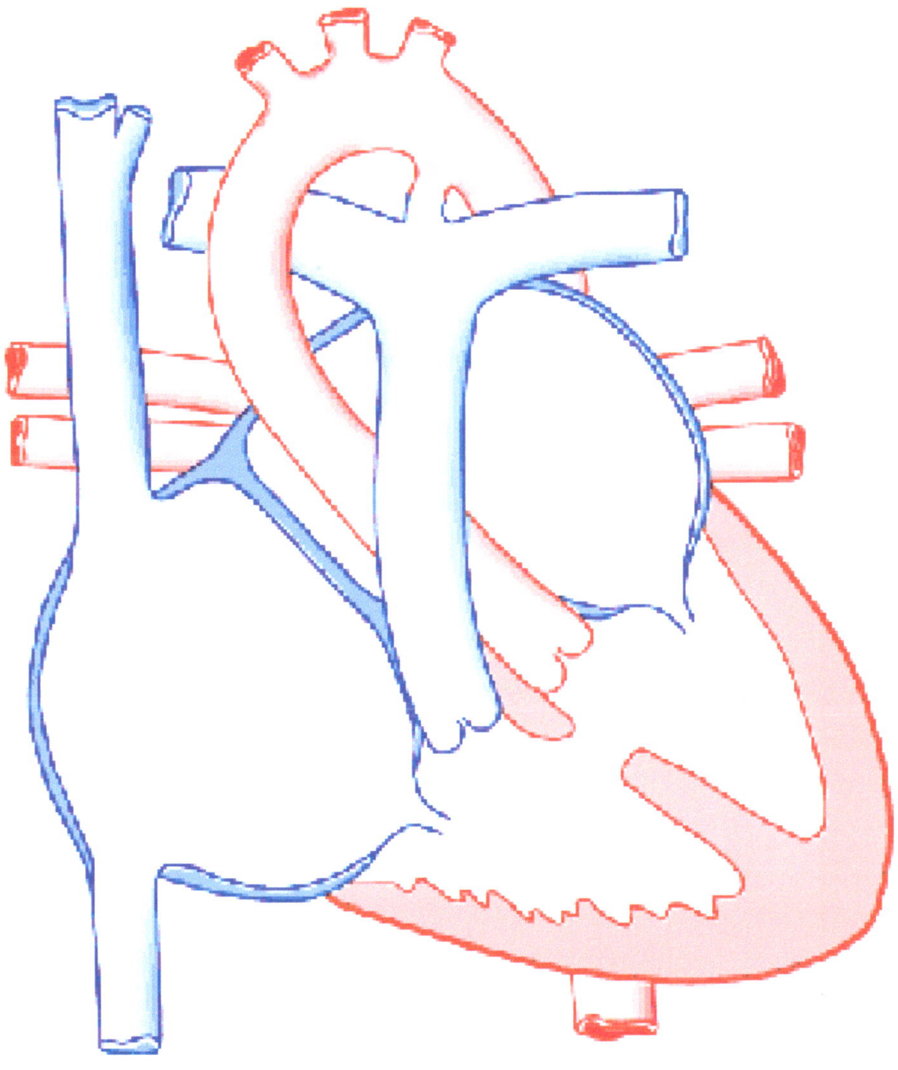

Figure 22: Patent ductus arteriosus with ventricular septal defect. Patent arterial duct (PDA) with ventricular septal defect.

*Corresponding author Oran B: Medicana International Hospital, Department of Pediatric Cardiology, İzmir, Turkey
E-mail:boran@medicana.com.tr and bulentoran@hotmail.com

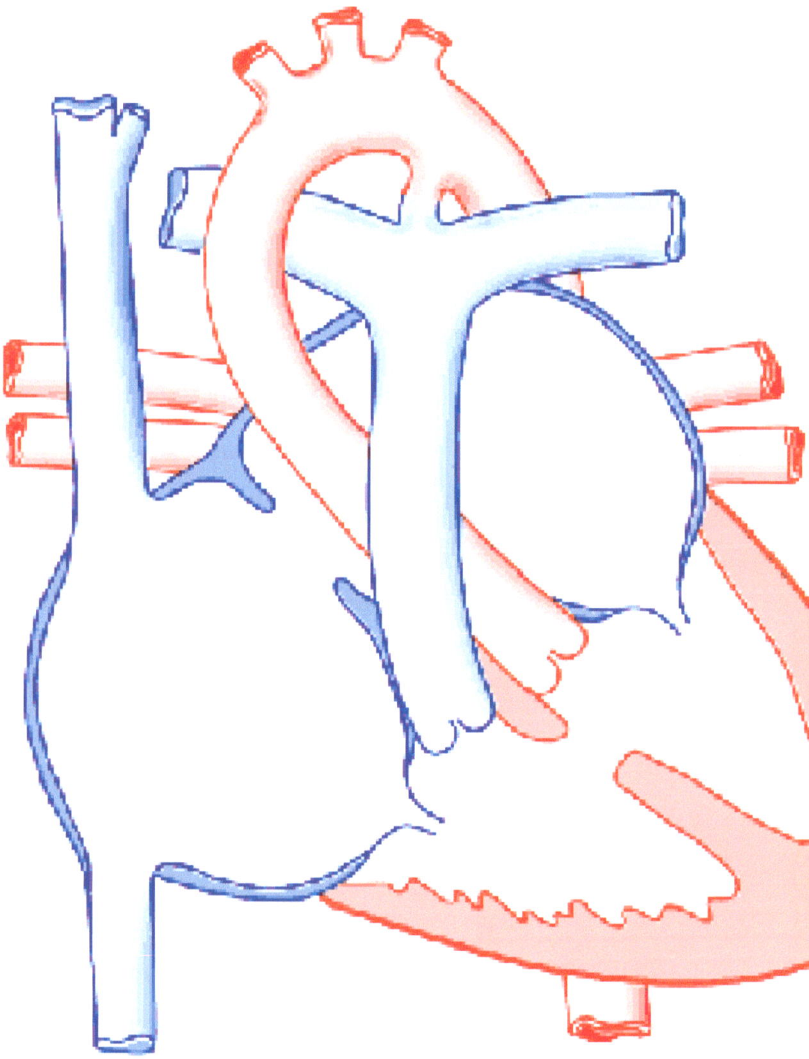

Figure 23: Patent ductus arteriosus, atrial septal defect, and ventricular septal defect. Patent arterial duct (PDA).

*Corresponding author Oran B: Medicana International Hospital, Department of Pediatric Cardiology, İzmir, Turkey
E-mail:boran@medicana.com.tr and bulentoran@hotmail.com

CHAPTER 2

Aorta Anomalies

Oran B.

Medicana International Hospital, Department of Pediatric Cardiology, İzmir, Turkey

*Corresponding author Oran B: Medicana International Hospital, Department of Pediatric Cardiology, İzmir, Turkey
E-mail:boran@medicana.com.tr and bulentoran@hotmail.com

*Corresponding author Oran B: Medicana International Hospital, Department of Pediatric Cardiology, İzmir, Turkey
E-mail:boran@medicana.com.tr and bulentoran@hotmail.com

Congenital Aorto-Pulmonary Window

The aorto-pulmonary window is a rare lesion that can mimic patent arterial duct defects. It involves a direct communication between the ascending aorta and pulmonary artery. Because affected patients are likely to develop Eisenmenger syndrome, it is rare for these patients to survive into adulthood without surgery. This defect is typically large; therefore, there is a high likelihood of pulmonary hypertension in adult patients, unless closure was performed early in childhood. Aorto-pulmonary windows are commonly associated with other cardiac lesions, such as VSDs, tetralogy of Fallot, subaortic stenosis, and ASDs.

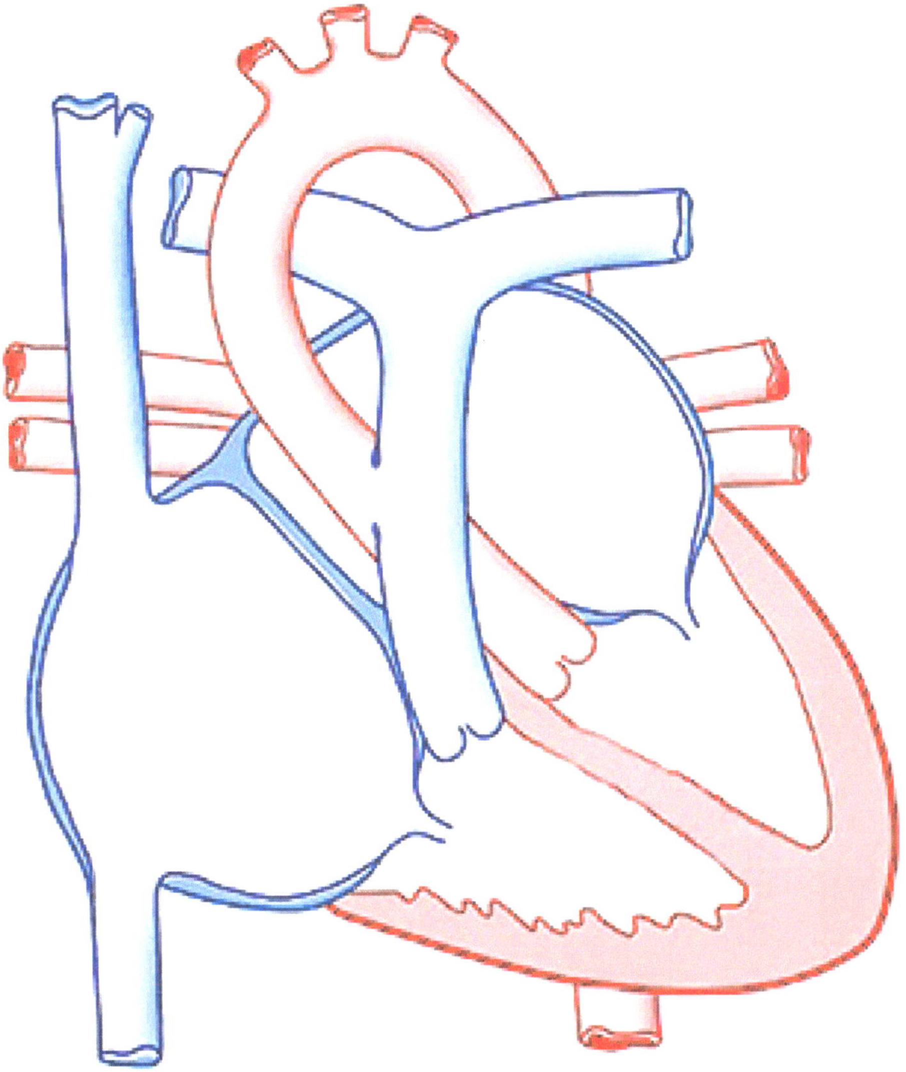

Figure 1: Congenital aortopulmonary window, Congenital aortopulmonary window.

*Corresponding author Oran B: Medicana International Hospital, Department of Pediatric Cardiology, İzmir, Turkey
E-mail:boran@medicana.com.tr and bulentoran@hotmail.com

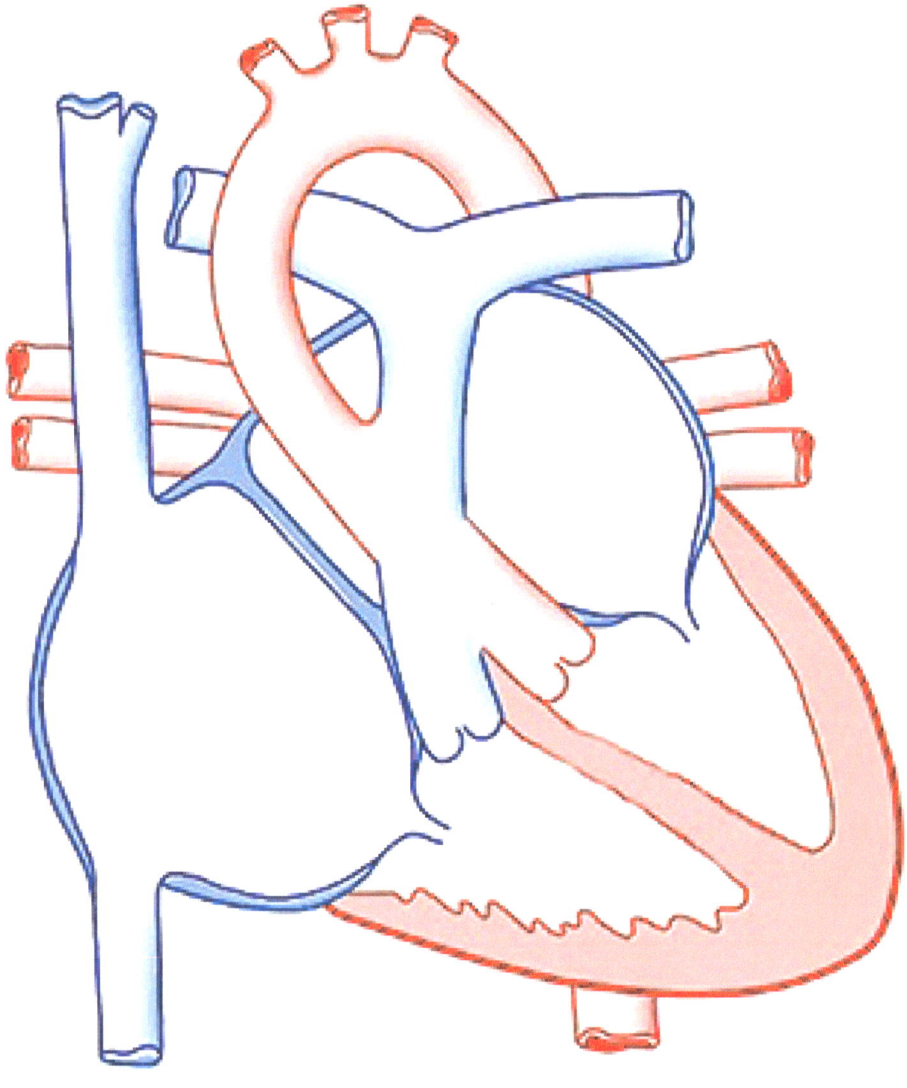

Figure 2: Congenital aortopulmonary window, Congenital aortopulmonary window.

*Corresponding author Oran B: Medicana International Hospital, Department of Pediatric Cardiology, İzmir, Turkey
E-mail:boran@medicana.com.tr and bulentoran@hotmail.com

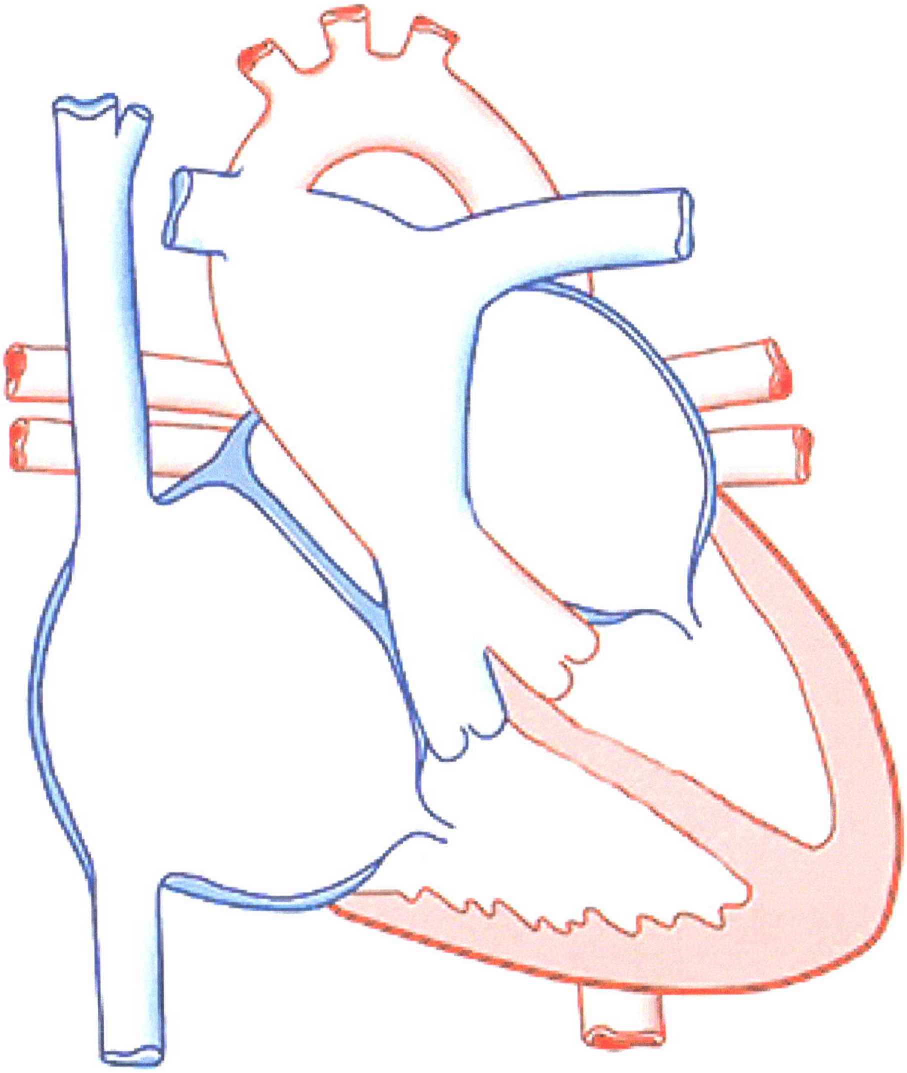

Figure 3: Congenital aortopulmonary window.

*Corresponding author Oran B: Medicana International Hospital, Department of Pediatric Cardiology, İzmir, Turkey
E-mail:boran@medicana.com.tr and bulentoran@hotmail.com

Truncus Arteriosus / Common Arterial Trunk

A common arterial trunk arises from the heart and gives rise to the aorta, coronary arteries, and pulmonary arteries. There is a semilunar "truncal" valve that has three or more leaflets and a VSD. It is impossible for these patients to survive into adulthood without surgery. This defect is associated with an interrupted aortic arch, coarctation of the aorta, coronary anomalies, and DiGeorge syndrome.

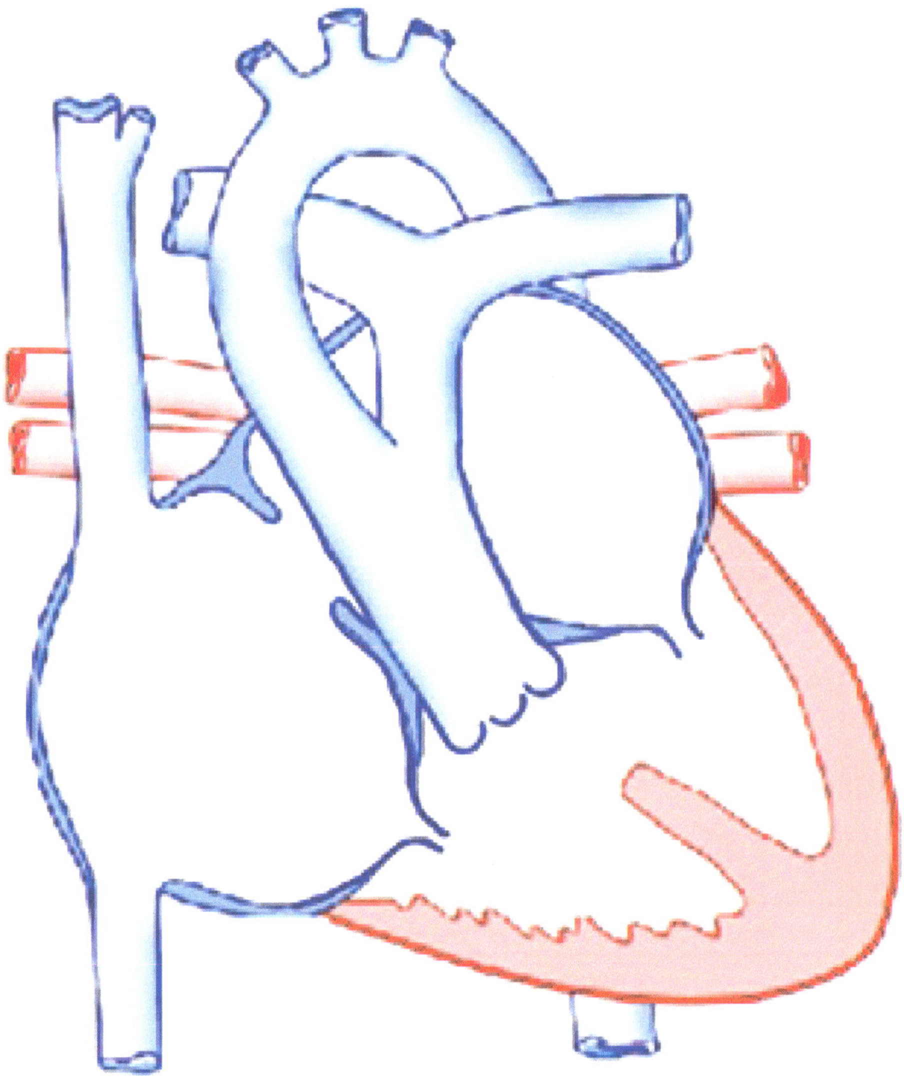

Figure 4: Truncus Arteriosus, type 1. Common arterial trunk with aortic dominance, main pulmonary artery arising from trunk.

*Corresponding author Oran B: Medicana International Hospital, Department of Pediatric Cardiology, İzmir, Turkey
E-mail:boran@medicana.com.tr and bulentoran@hotmail.com

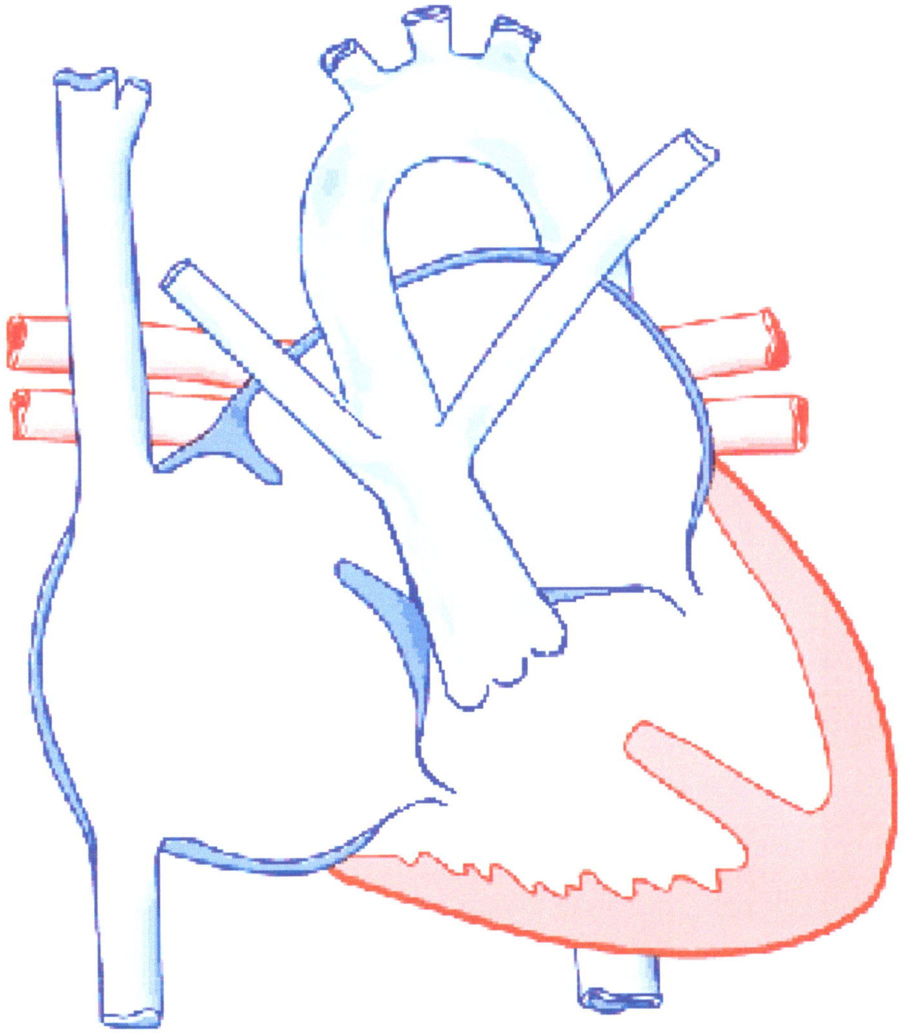

Figure 5: Truncus Arteriosus, type ll. Common arterial trunk with aortic dominance, and both pulmonary arteries arising from trunk. Right and left pulmonary artery from ascending aorta.

*Corresponding author Oran B: Medicana International Hospital, Department of Pediatric Cardiology, İzmir, Turkey
E-mail:boran@medicana.com.tr and bulentoran@hotmail.com

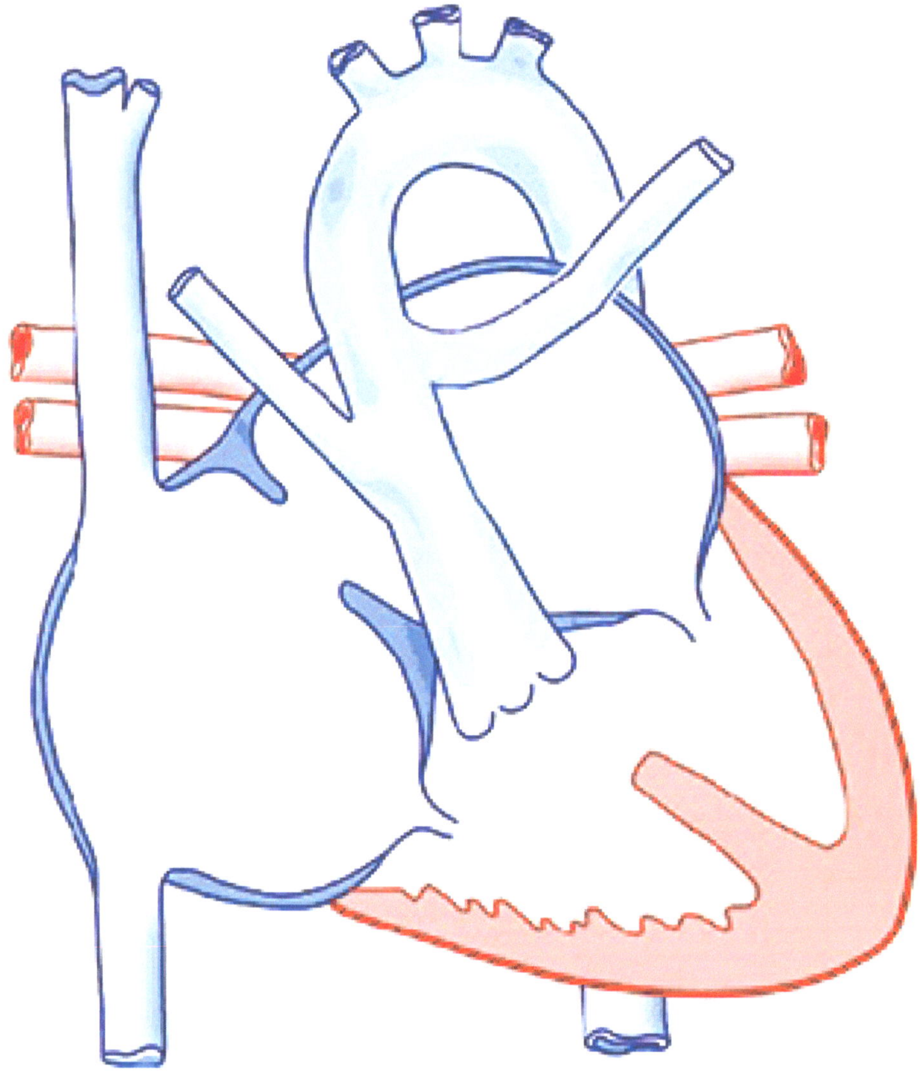

Figure 6: Truncus Arteriosus, type lll. Common arterial trunk, VSD. Common arterial trunk with aortic dominance, and both pulmonary arteries arising from trunk.

*Corresponding author Oran B: Medicana International Hospital, Department of Pediatric Cardiology, İzmir, Turkey
E-mail:boran@medicana.com.tr and bulentoran@hotmail.com

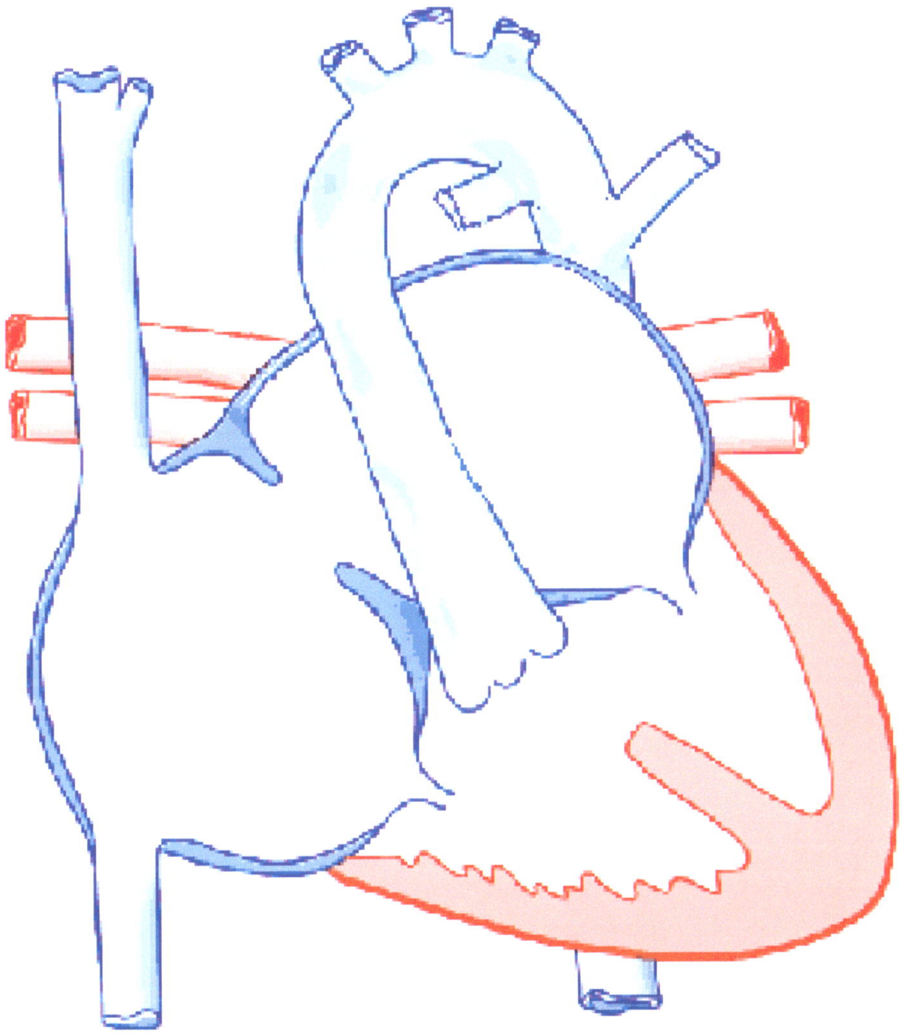

Figure 7: Truncus Arteriosus, type IV, VSD. Common arterial trunk with aortic dominance, and both pulmonary arteries arising from descending aorta and ventricular septal defect.

*Corresponding author Oran B: Medicana International Hospital, Department of Pediatric Cardiology, İzmir, Turkey
E-mail:boran@medicana.com.tr and bulentoran@hotmail.com

Coarctation of aorta

Coarctation of the aorta represents 7% of reported congenital heart defects and involves stenosis in the aortic arch. The anatomy varies from mild, localized obstruction to interruption or hypoplasia of the aortic arch. The stenosis is typically located at or beyond the aortic arch, occasionally at the site of the duct. Affected adults commonly exhibit an obstruction with segmental narrowing distal to the left subclavian artery. A bicuspid aortic valve is present in up to 80% of patients. Coarctation of the aorta is associated with VSDs, PDA, Turner syndrome, and brain aneurysm of the circle of Willis.

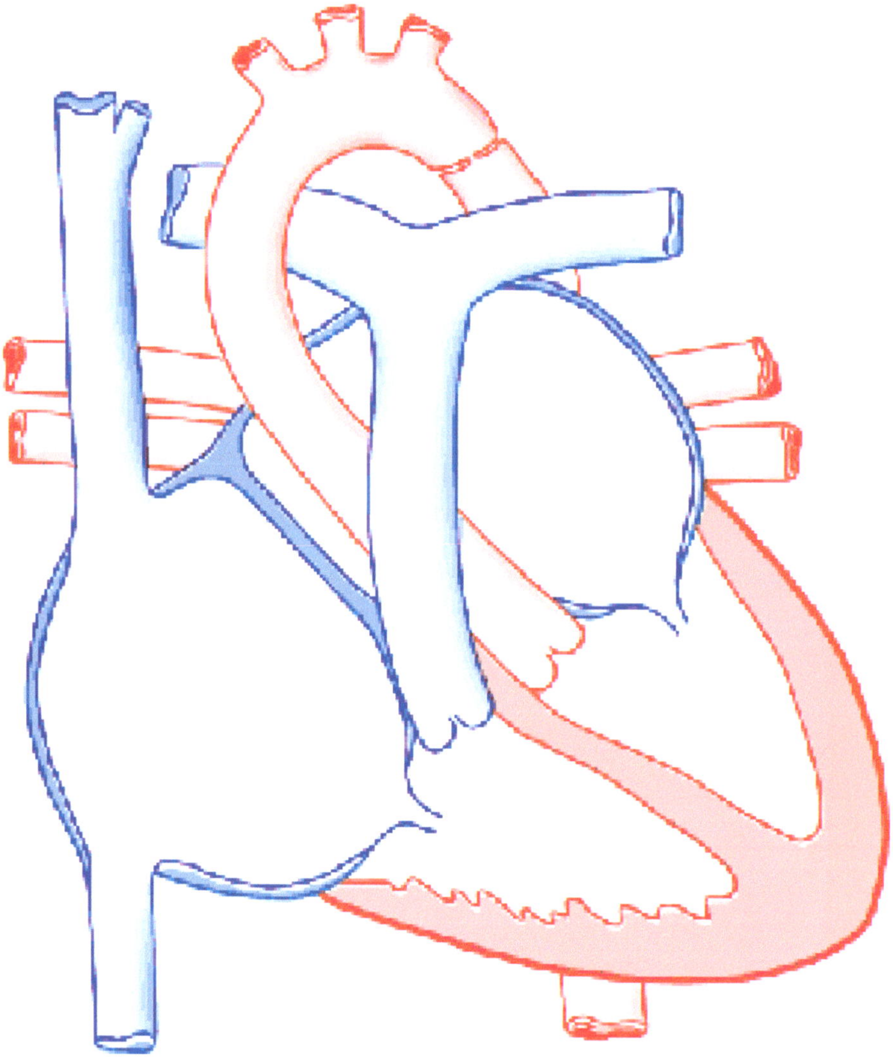

Figure 8: Aortic coarctation, Coarctation of aorta. Common arterial trunk with pulmonary dominance and aortic coarctation.

*Corresponding author Oran B: Medicana International Hospital, Department of Pediatric Cardiology, İzmir, Turkey
E-mail:boran@medicana.com.tr and bulentoran@hotmail.com

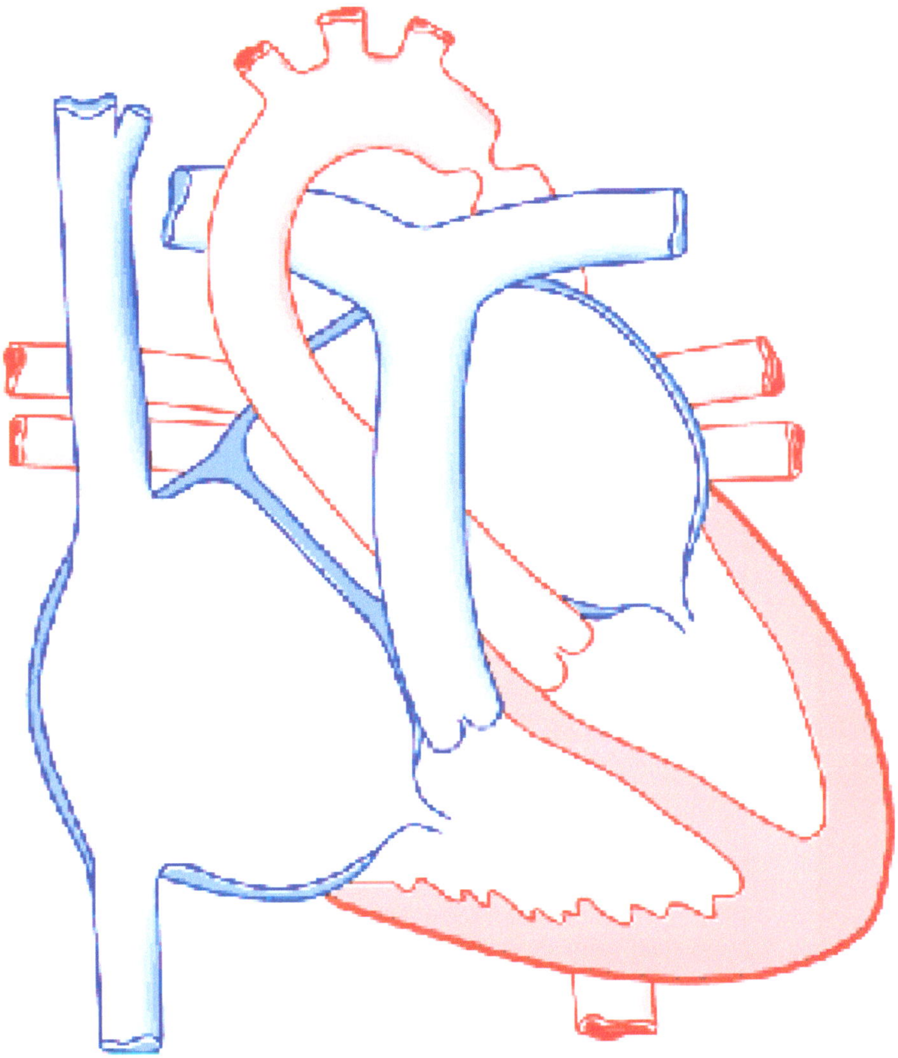

Figure 9: Aortic arch hypoplasia (tubular). Hypoplasia of the aortic arch. (Common arterial trunk with pulmonary dominance and aortic arch obstruction)

*Corresponding author Oran B: Medicana International Hospital, Department of Pediatric Cardiology, İzmir, Turkey
E-mail:boran@medicana.com.tr and bulentoran@hotmail.com

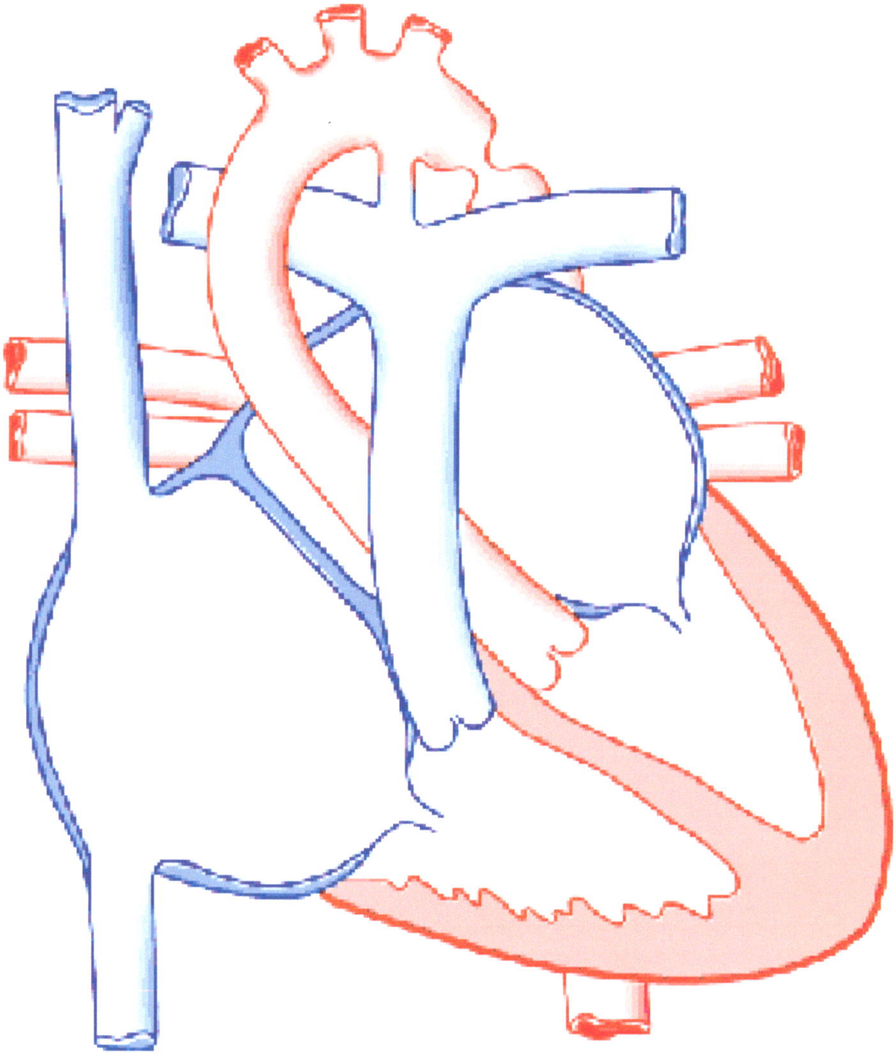

Figure 10: Aortic arch hypoplasia (tubular) and PDA. Hypoplasia of the aortic arch. (Common arterial trunk with pulmonary dominance and aortic arch obstruction) with patent arterial duct.

*Corresponding author Oran B: Medicana International Hospital, Department of Pediatric Cardiology, İzmir, Turkey
E-mail:boran@medicana.com.tr and bulentoran@hotmail.com

Interrupted Aortic Arch

The interrupted aortic arch is a serious duct-dependent anomaly for which the immediate removal of the stenosis is indicated at birth. End-to-end or end-to-side anastomosis of the aortic arch is performed, and any VSDs are closed. Aortic stenosis is eliminated. Some patients may require Ross-Kono surgery. All surgical interventions should occur during childhood; survival to adulthood is impossible without reconstruction of the aortic arch.

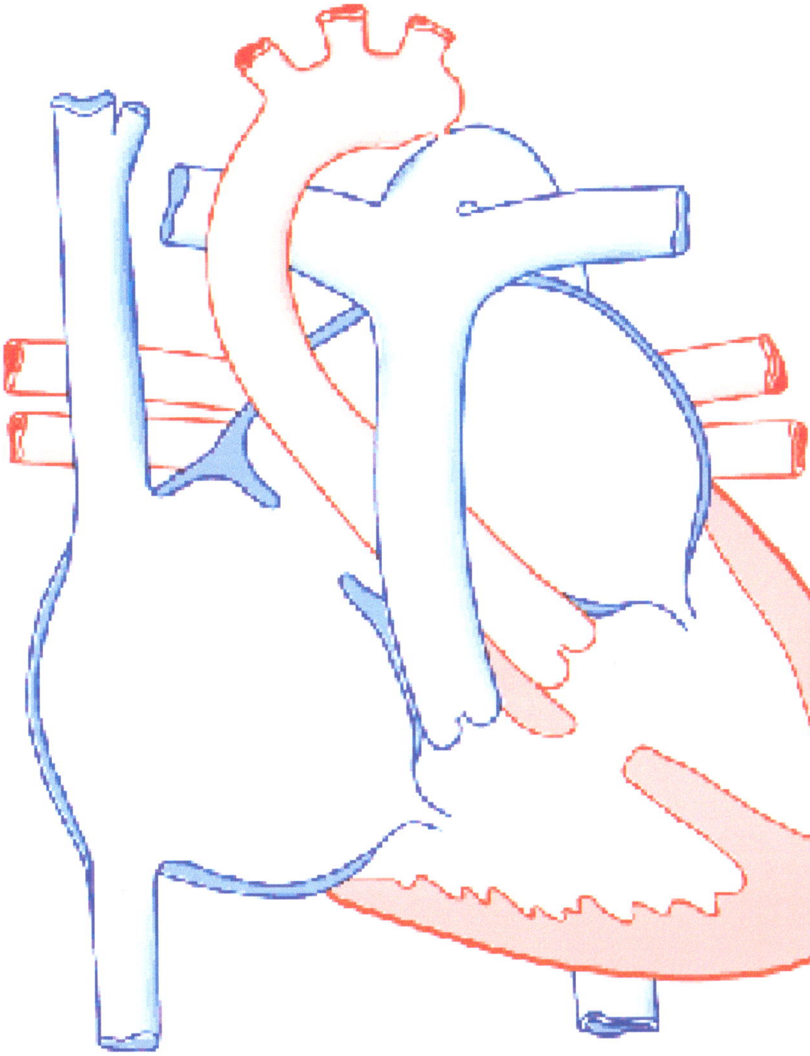

Figure 11: Interrupted aortic arch, type l.Interrupted aortic arch distal to subclavian artery, type A.

*Corresponding author Oran B: Medicana International Hospital, Department of Pediatric Cardiology, İzmir, Turkey
E-mail:boran@medicana.com.tr and bulentoran@hotmail.com

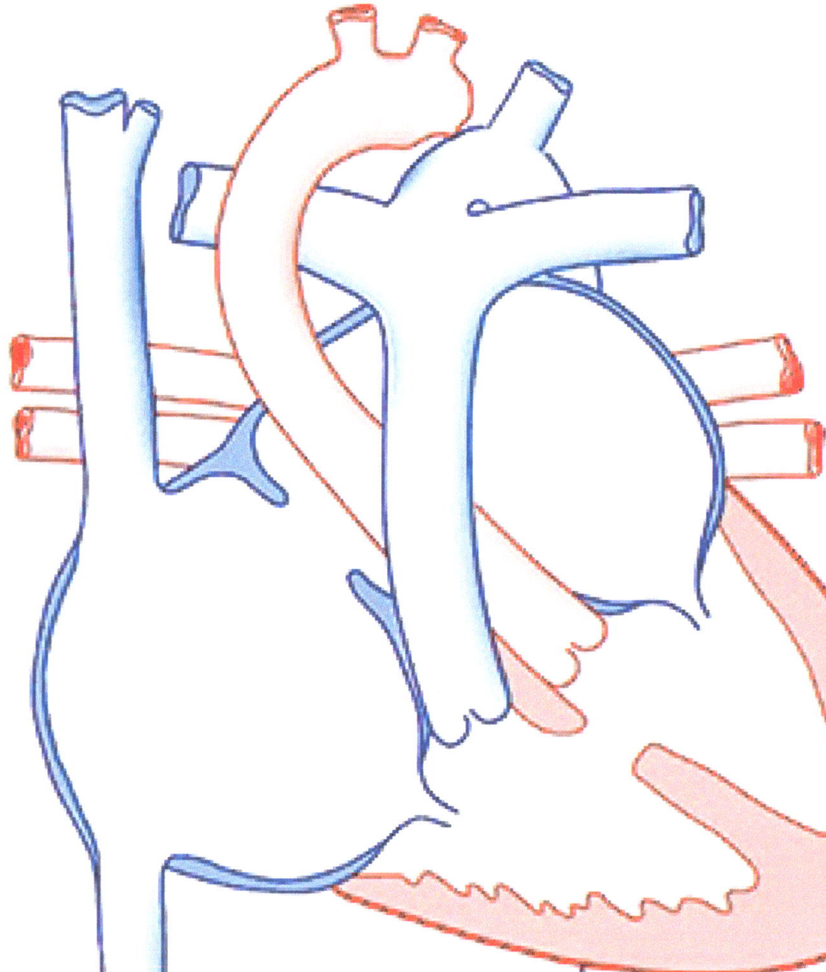

Figure 12: Interrupted aortic arch, type ll. ASD, and VSD. Interrupted aortic arch between subclavian and common carotid arteries, type B with ASD and VSD.

*Corresponding author Oran B: Medicana International Hospital, Department of Pediatric Cardiology, İzmir, Turkey
E-mail:boran@medicana.com.tr and bulentoran@hotmail.com

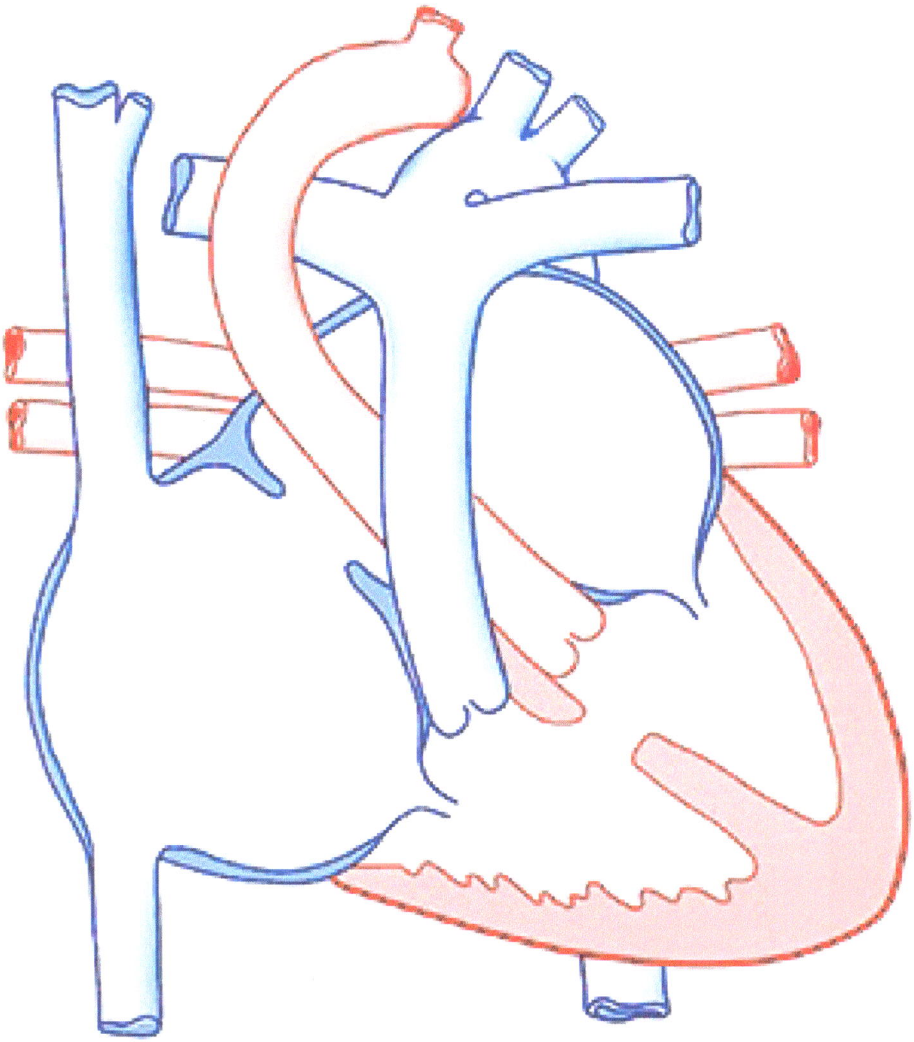

Figure 13: Interrupted aortic arch, type lll. ASD, and VSD. Interrupted aortic arch between carotid arteries, type C, ASD, and VSD.

*Corresponding author Oran B: Medicana International Hospital, Department of Pediatric Cardiology, İzmir, Turkey
E-mail:boran@medicana.com.tr and bulentoran@hotmail.com

Congenital Aortic Valvar Stenosis

Congenital aortic valvar stenosis is characterized by deformed aortic valves and a narrow valve annulus. Stenosis in children is most commonly associated with bicuspid valve development, in which only two dimorphic cusps develop. It is rare for these patients to survive into adulthood without Interventional procedures or surgery.

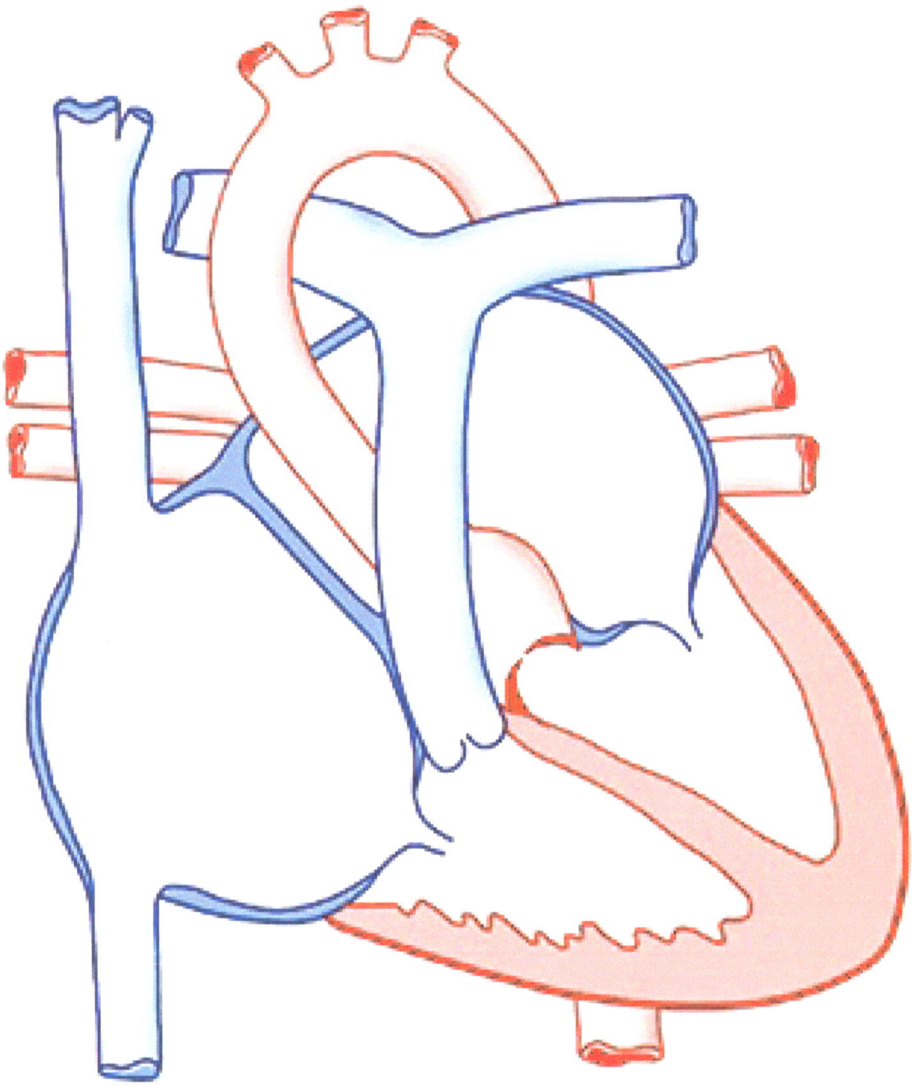

Figure 14: Aortic stenosis, valvar. Congenital aortic valvar stenosis.

*Corresponding author Oran B: Medicana International Hospital, Department of Pediatric Cardiology, İzmir, Turkey
E-mail:boran@medicana.com.tr and bulentoran@hotmail.com

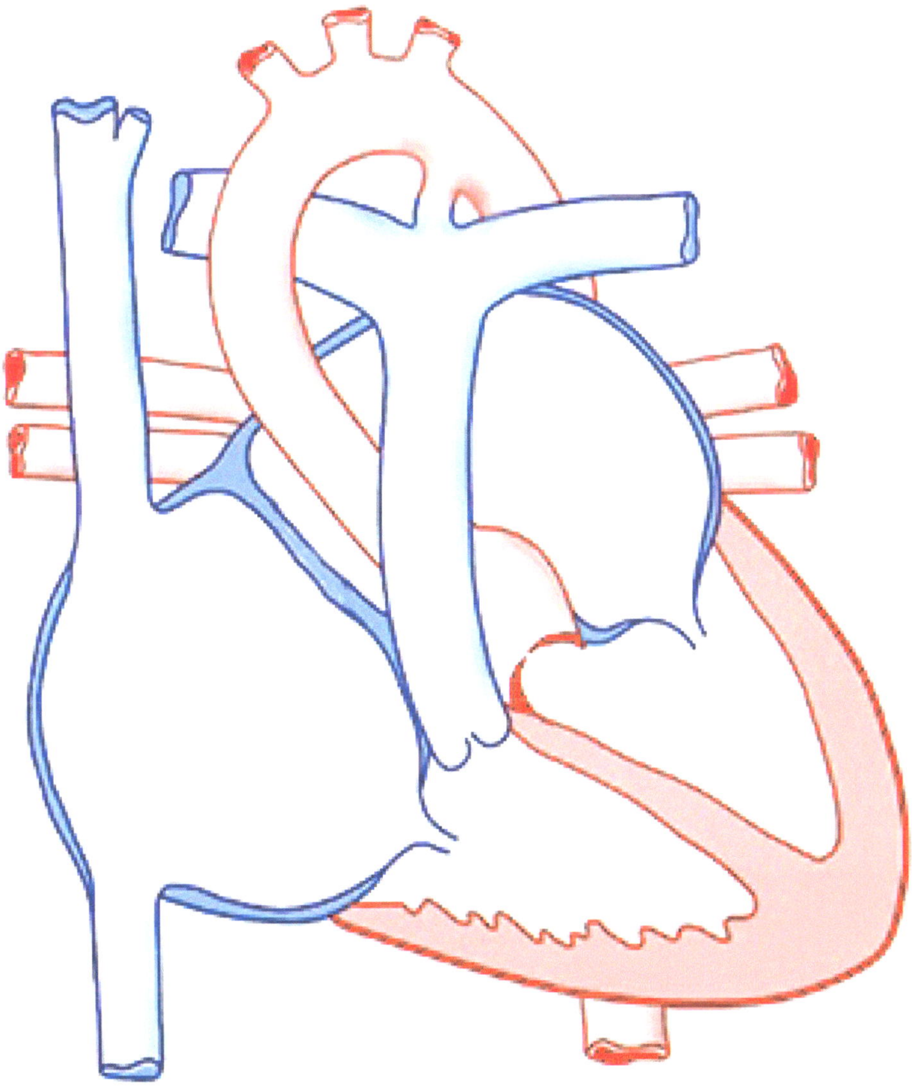

Figure 15: Aortic stenosis, valvar with PDA. Congenital aortic valvar stenosis with patent arterial duct.

*Corresponding author Oran B: Medicana International Hospital, Department of Pediatric Cardiology, İzmir, Turkey
E-mail:boran@medicana.com.tr and bulentoran@hotmail.com

Congenital Aortic Subvalvar Stenosis

In congenital aortic subvalvar stenosis, the shapes of the valves and annulus are normal, but there is a discrete subaortic membrane (ridge of 90%) or fibromuscular tunnel.

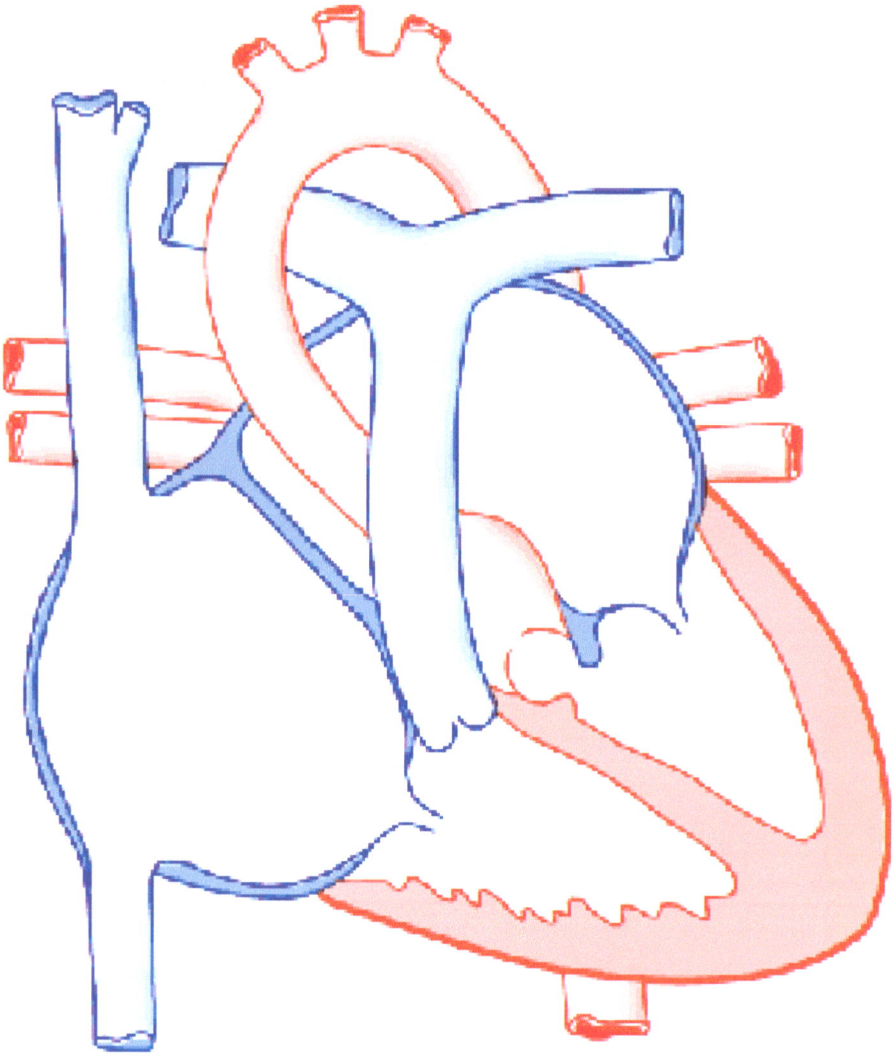

Figure 16: Aortic stenosis, subvalvar. Congenital subaortic stenosis.

*Corresponding author Oran B: Medicana International Hospital, Department of Pediatric Cardiology, İzmir, Turkey
E-mail:boran@medicana.com.tr and bulentoran@hotmail.com

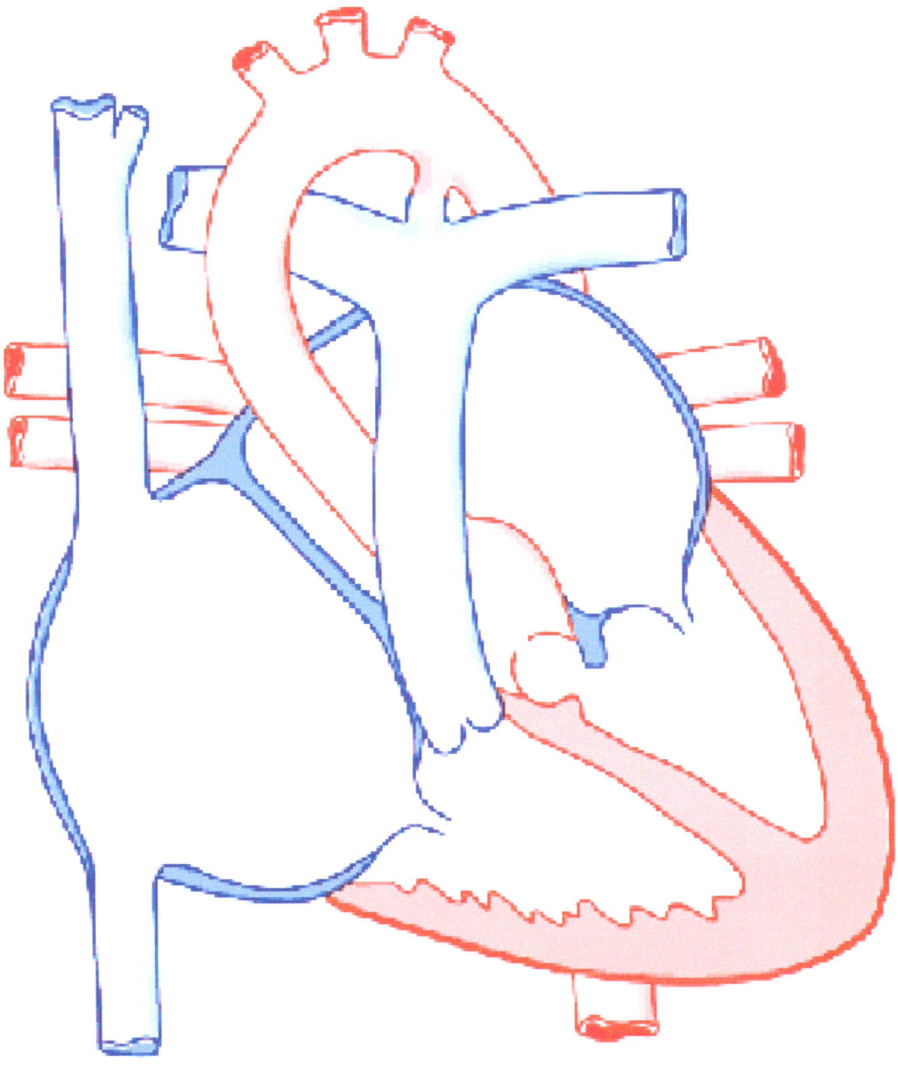

Figure 17: Aortic stenosis, subvalvar, PDA. Congenital subaortic stenosis with patent arterial duct.

*Corresponding author Oran B: Medicana International Hospital, Department of Pediatric Cardiology, İzmir, Turkey
E-mail:boran@medicana.com.tr and bulentoran@hotmail.com

Congenital Aortic Supravalvar Stenosis

Congenital aortic supravalvar stenosis typically involves focal or diffuse stenosis in the distal aspect of the synotubular junction. Rarely, stenosis covers the entire aortic arch. Fibromuscular thickening of coronary artery outflow has been reported in some affected patients. These thickenings prevent coronary circulation. Furthermore, because the coronary arteries are located on the proximal side of the aortic stenosis, they are exposed to high left ventricular pressure. Other anomalies and associated syndromes include aortic insufficiency, hypoplastic left heart syndrome, mitral valve anomalies, aortic arch anomalies, coarctation of the aorta, VSDs, AVSDs, Shone syndrome, sinus valsalva aneurysm (common in Marfan syndrome), and Williams syndrome.

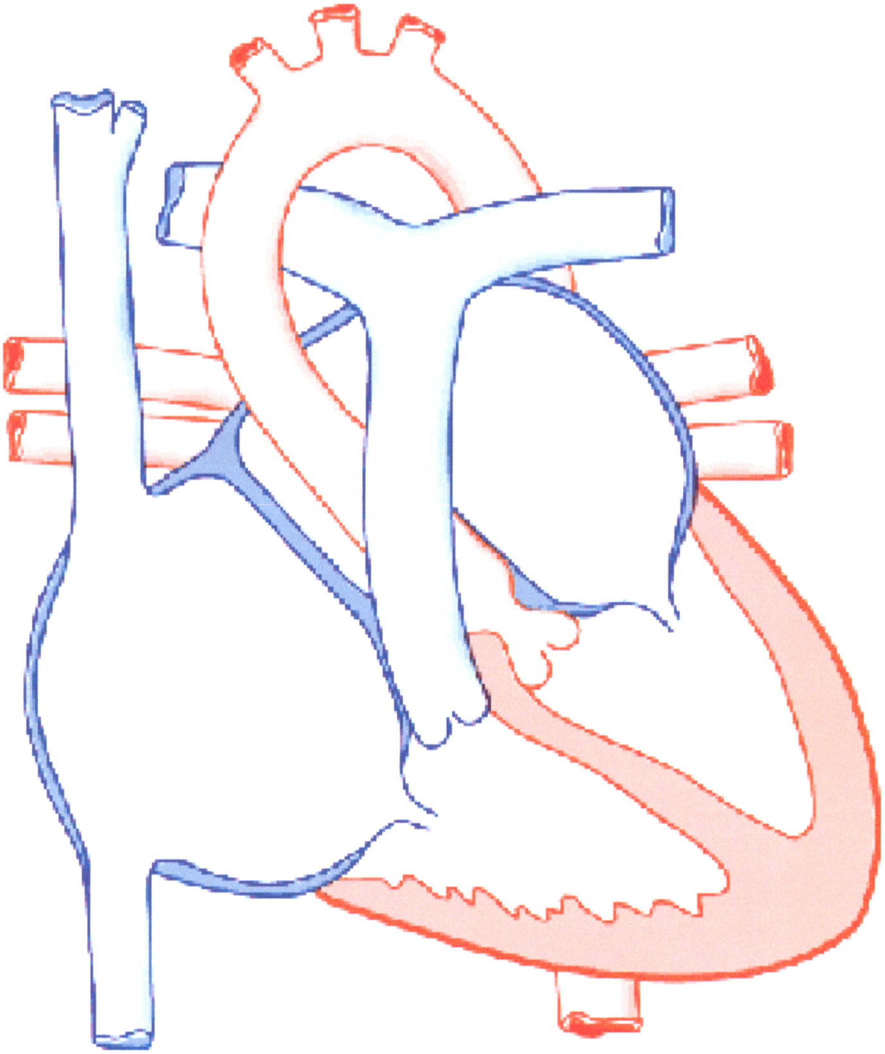

Figure 18: Aortic stenosis, supravalvar. Congenital aortic supravalvar stenosis. Congenital supravalvar aortic stenosis.

*Corresponding author Oran B: Medicana International Hospital, Department of Pediatric Cardiology, İzmir, Turkey
E-mail:boran@medicana.com.tr and bulentoran@hotmail.com

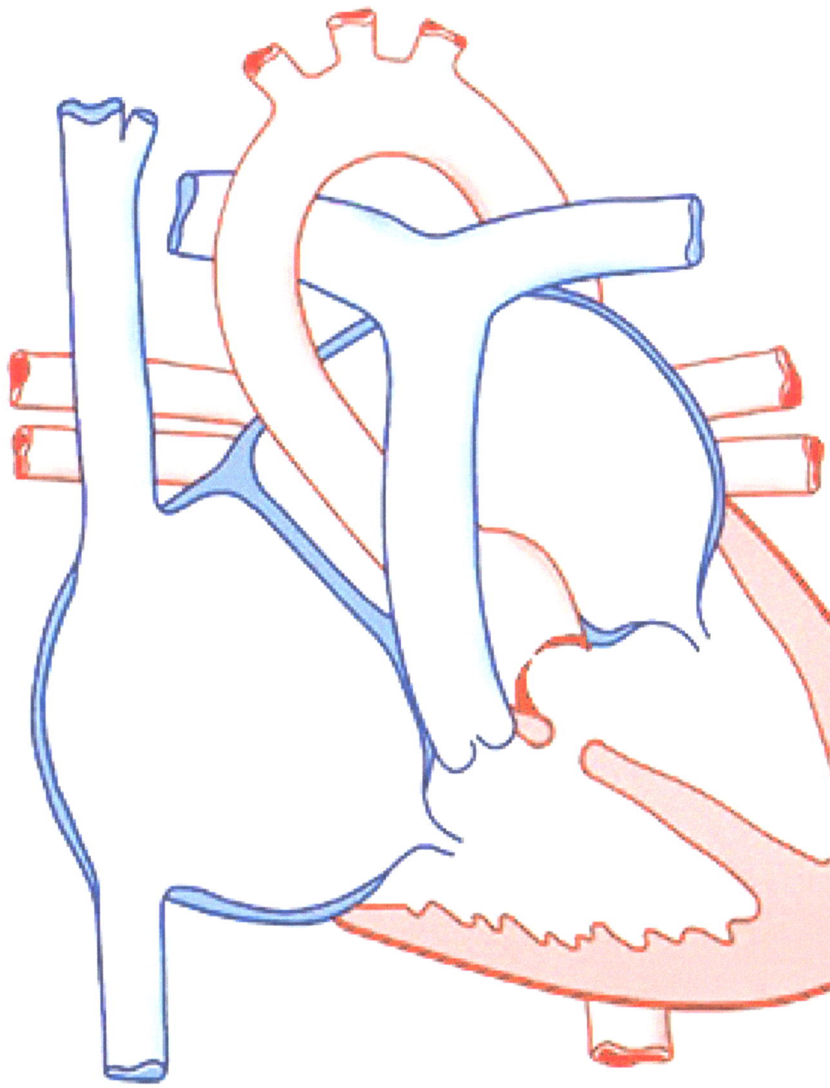

Figure 19: Aortic stenosis, supravalvar, VSD. Congenital aortic supravalvar stenosis. Congenital supravalvar aortic stenosis with ventricular septal defect.

*Corresponding author Oran B: Medicana International Hospital, Department of Pediatric Cardiology, İzmir, Turkey
E-mail:boran@medicana.com.tr and bulentoran@hotmail.com

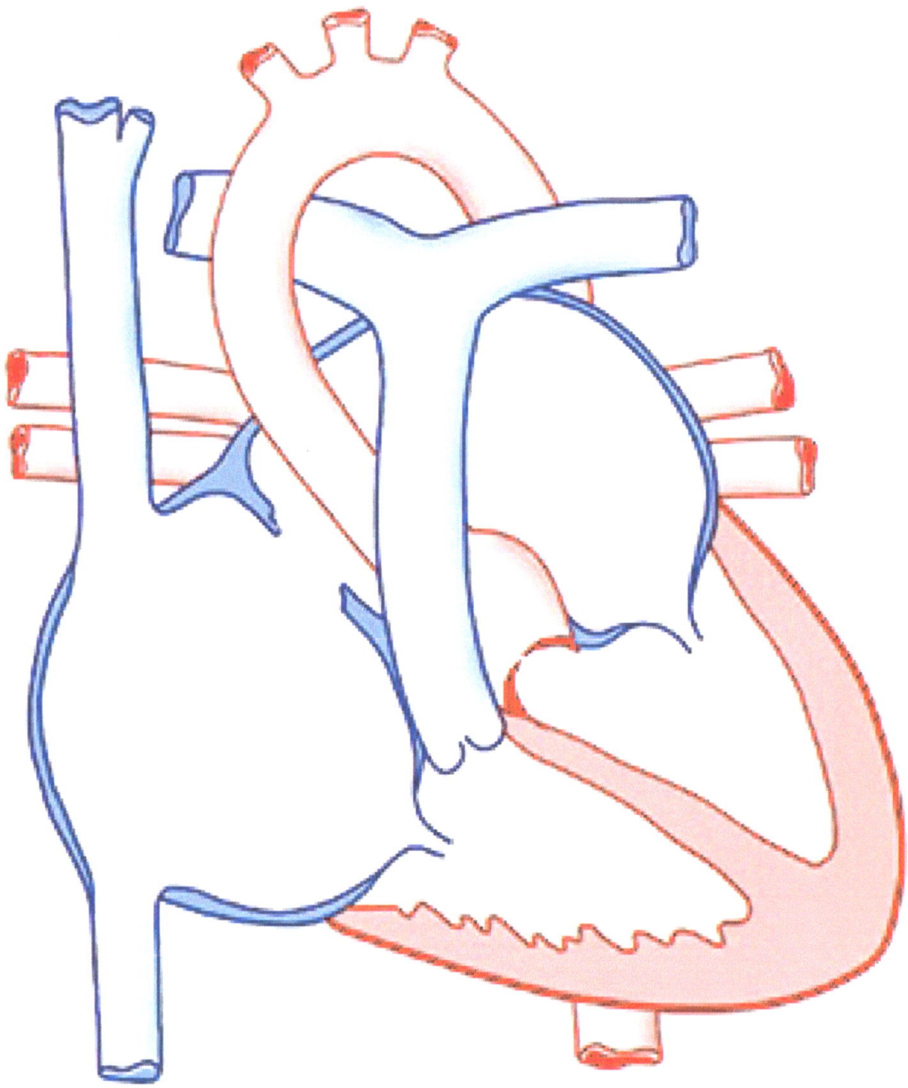

Figure 20: Aortic stenosis, supravalvar, ASD. Congenital aortic supravalvar stenosis. Congenital supravalvar aortic stenosis with atrial septal defect.

*Corresponding author Oran B: Medicana International Hospital, Department of Pediatric Cardiology, İzmir, Turkey
E-mail:boran@medicana.com.tr and bulentoran@hotmail.com

Subaortic Stenosis Due To Fibromuscular Shelf And Fibromuscular Tunnel

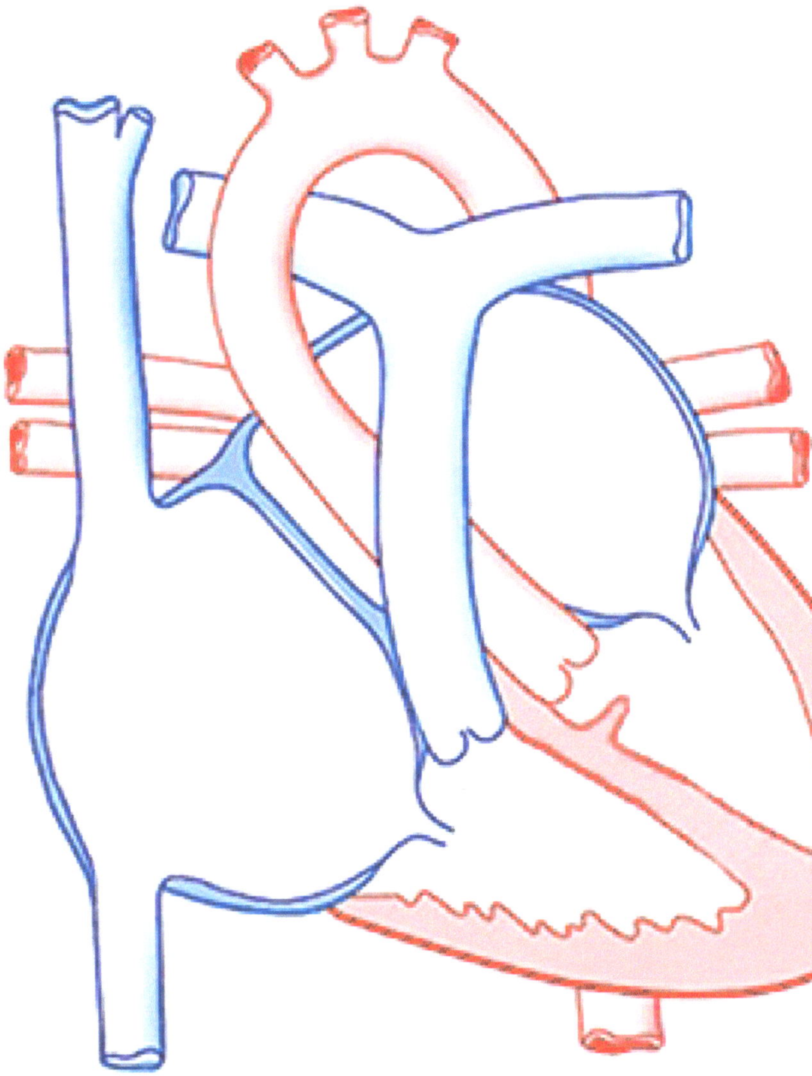

Figure 21: Subaortic stenosis due to fibromuscular shelf and fibromuscular tunnel

*Corresponding author Oran B: Medicana International Hospital, Department of Pediatric Cardiology, İzmir, Turkey
E-mail:boran@medicana.com.tr and bulentoran@hotmail.com

Congenital Aortic Valvar Atresia

Aortic atresia with an associated ventricular septal defect and adequate sized left ventricle is extremely rare and it is often associated with left ventricular hypoplasia. It is impossible for these patients to survive into adulthood without Interventional procedures or surgery.

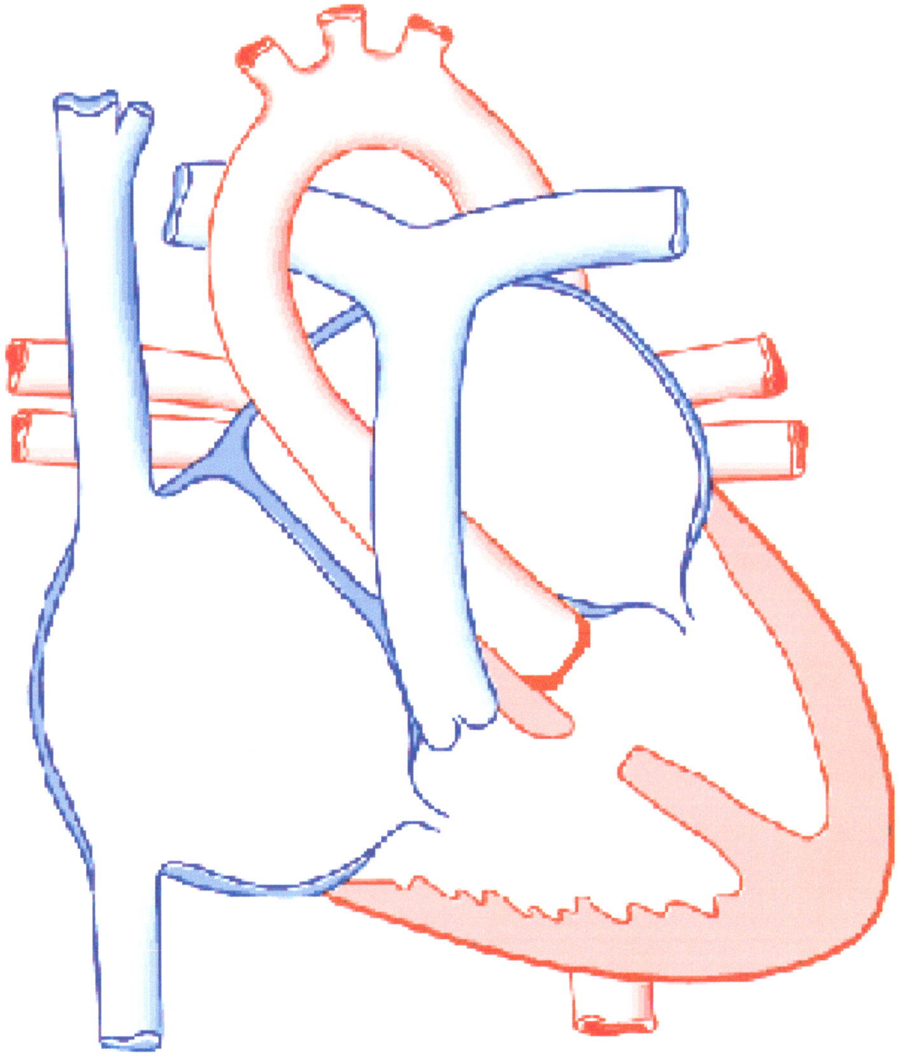

Figure 22: Congenital aortic valvar atresia. Aortic valve atresia.

*Corresponding author Oran B: Medicana International Hospital, Department of Pediatric Cardiology, İzmir, Turkey
E-mail:boran@medicana.com.tr and bulentoran@hotmail.com

Systemic-to-pulmonary collateral arteries

Small or nonexistent pulmonary arteries are associated with partial or complete blood flow that originates from aortopulmonary collateral vessels; Major Aorto Pulmonary Collateral Arteries (MAPCA).

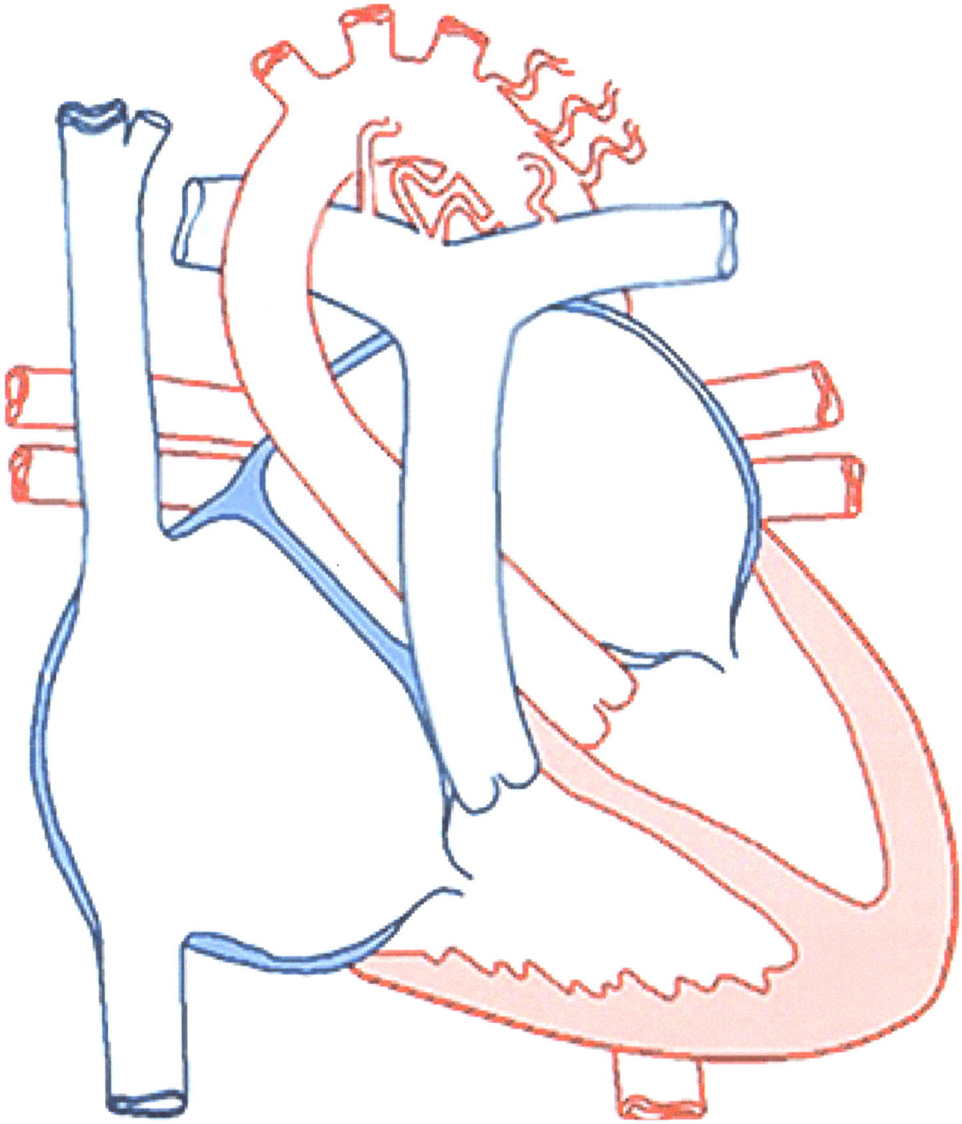

Figure 23: Systemic to pulmonary collateral arteries (Major Aorto Pulmoner Collateral Arteries - MAPCA). Systemic pulmonary collaterals. Systemic-to-pulmonary collateral arteries.

*Corresponding author Oran B: Medicana International Hospital, Department of Pediatric Cardiology, İzmir, Turkey
E-mail:boran@medicana.com.tr and bulentoran@hotmail.com

Aortoventricular Tunnels

Left and right aortoventricular tunnels are congenital extracardiac channels with progressive ventricular dilatation.

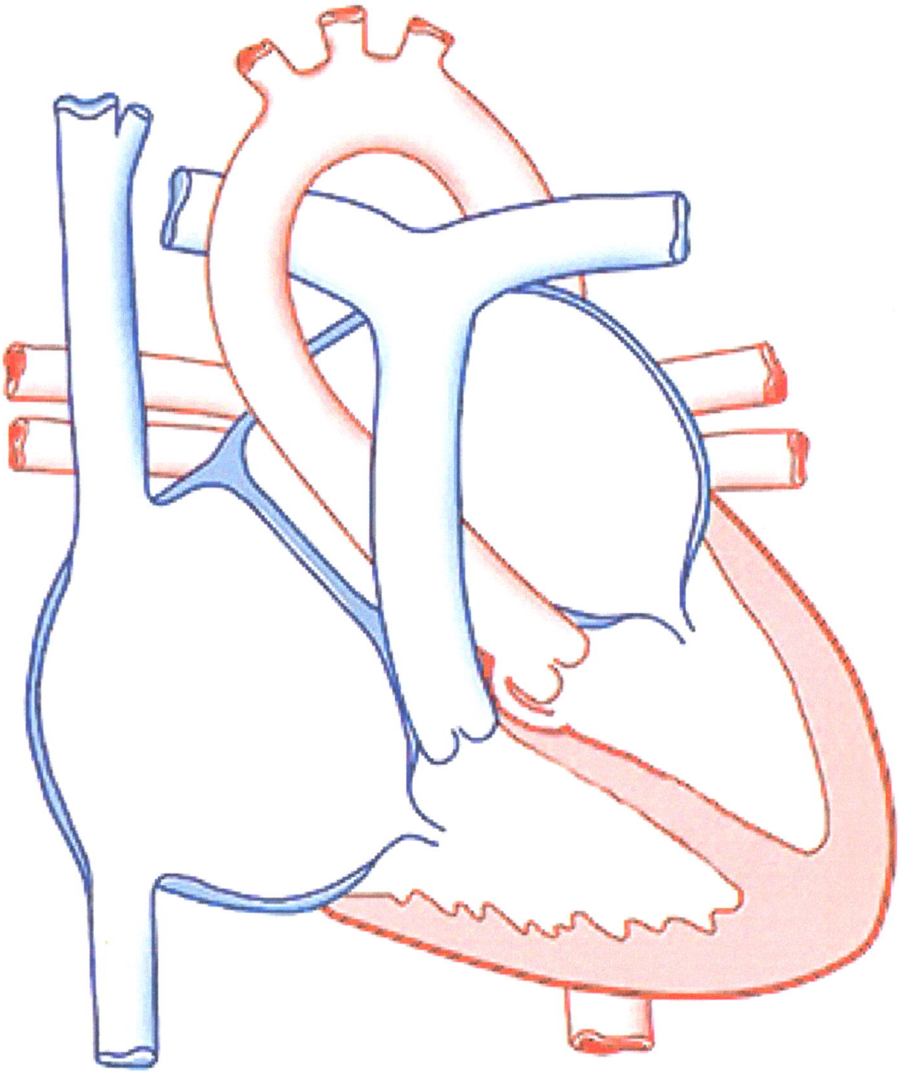

Figure 24: Aorto-left ventricular tunnel, Left ventricle to aorta tunnel.

*Corresponding author Oran B: Medicana International Hospital, Department of Pediatric Cardiology, İzmir, Turkey
E-mail:boran@medicana.com.tr and bulentoran@hotmail.com

Aorto-Right Ventricular Tunnel

An aorto-right ventricular tunnel is a rare congenital, extracardiac channel that connects the ascending aorta above the sinutubular junction to the right ventricle cavity.

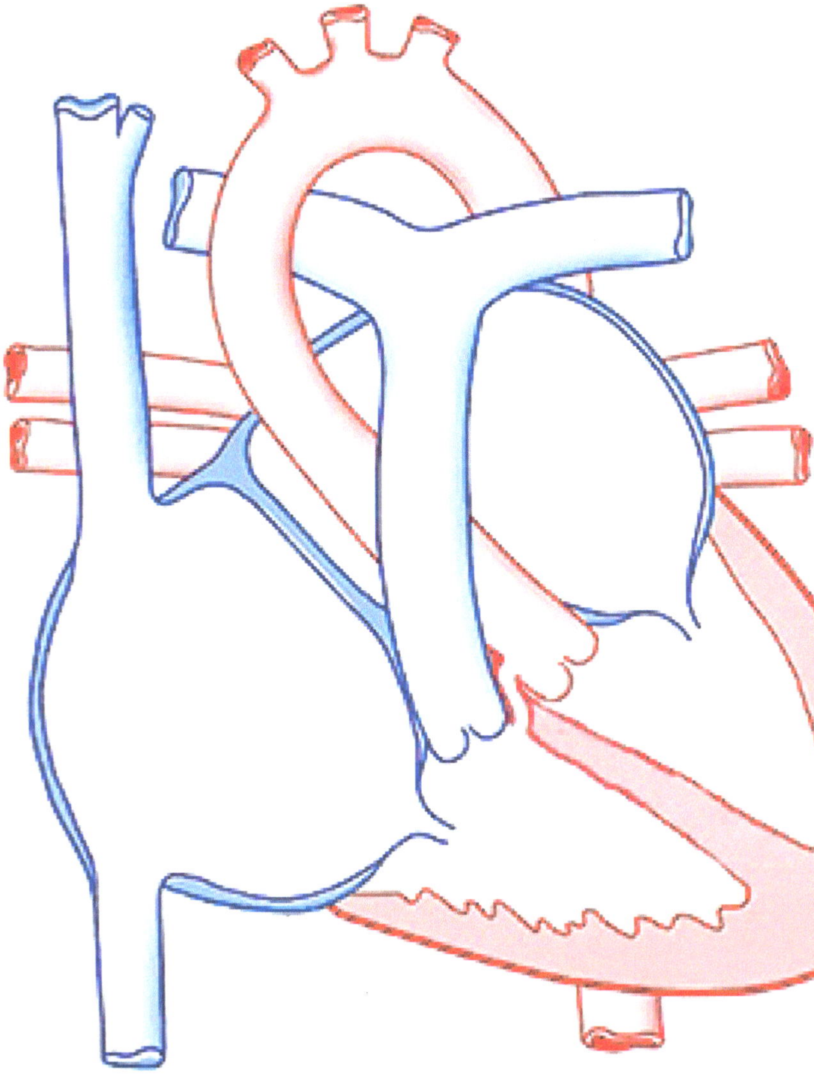

Figure 25: Aorto-right ventricular tunnel, Right ventricle to aorta tunnel.

*Corresponding author Oran B: Medicana International Hospital, Department of Pediatric Cardiology, İzmir, Turkey
E-mail:boran@medicana.com.tr and bulentoran@hotmail.com

Right Aortic Arch

Right aortic arch occurs as an isolated anomaly or in combination with congenital heart disease. It is especially common in patients with tetralogy of Fallot and truncus arteriosus. The aortic arch is observed as a mirror image of the normal left arch aorta.

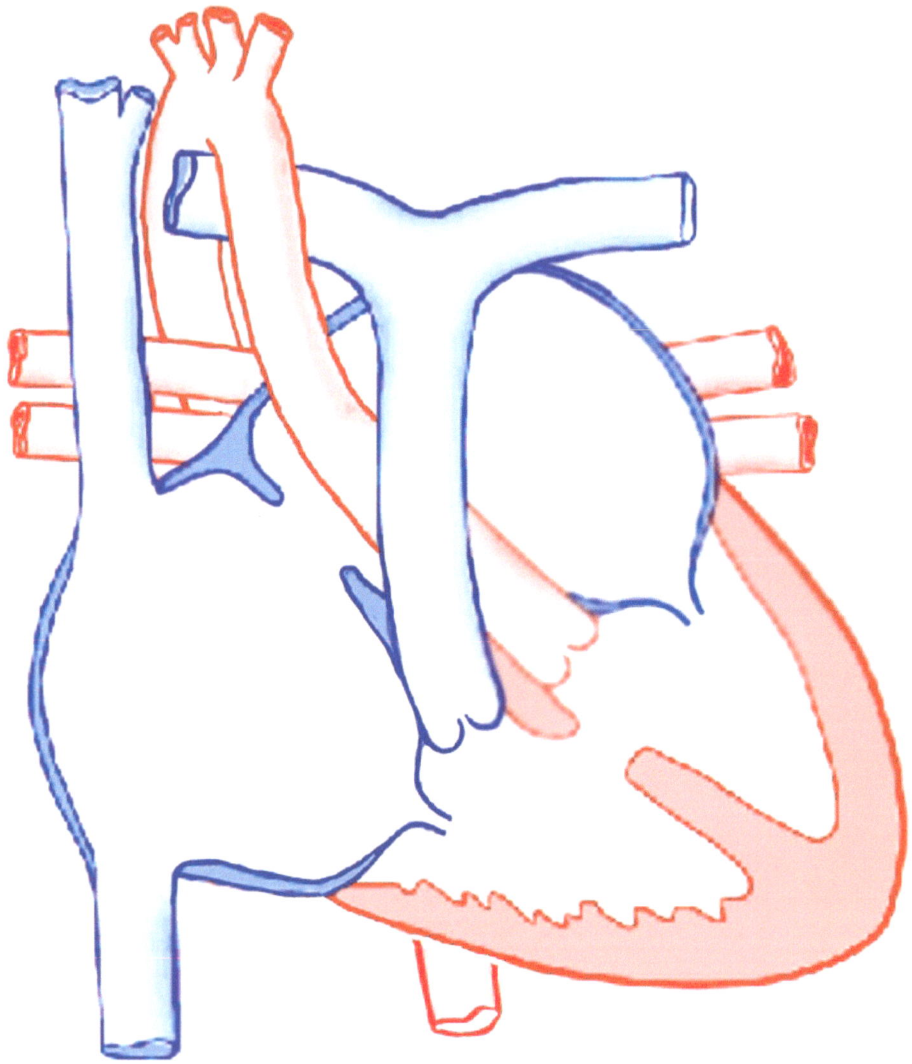

Figure 26: Right aortic arch.

*Corresponding author Oran B: Medicana International Hospital, Department of Pediatric Cardiology, İzmir, Turkey
E-mail:boran@medicana.com.tr and bulentoran@hotmail.com

Hemitruncus arteriosus

Hemitruncus arteriosus refers to the anomalous origin of one pulmonary artery from arcus aorta. It is rare for these patients to survive into adulthood without Interventional procedures or surgery.

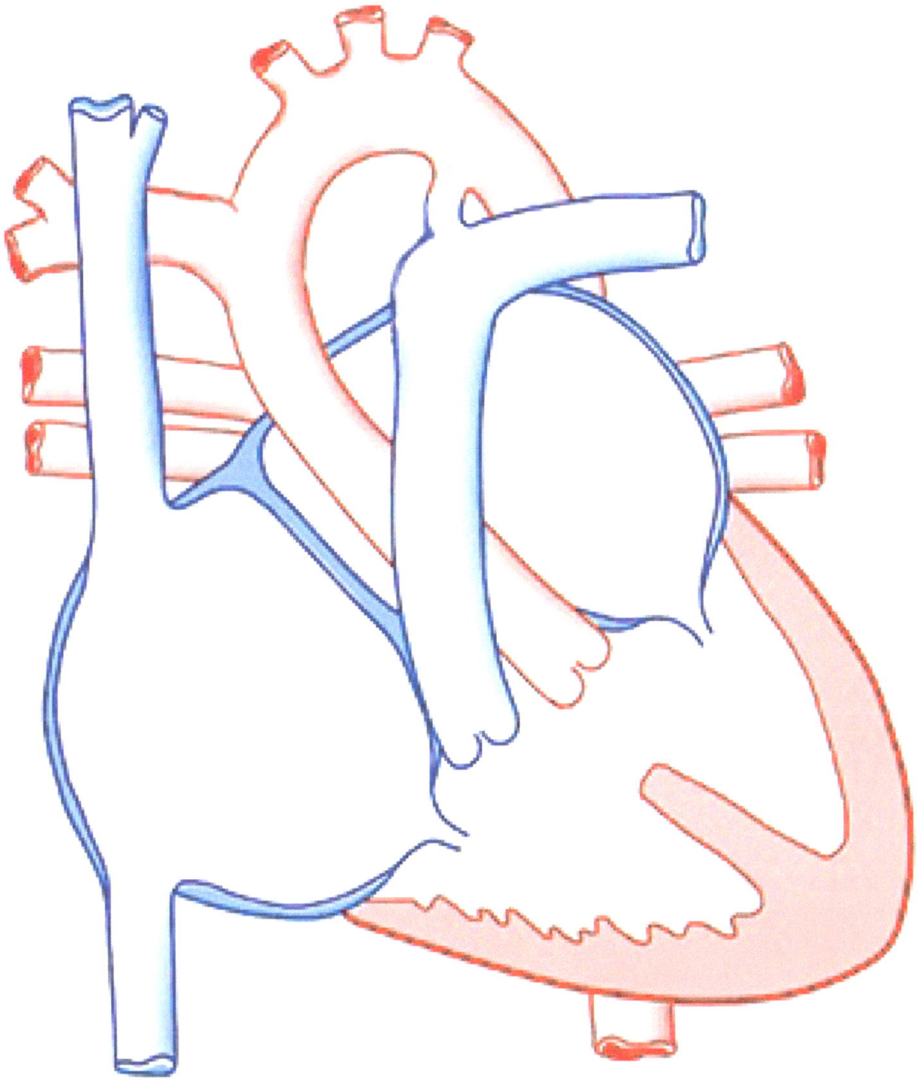

Figure 27: One of the two pulmonary artery origin from ascending aorta (hemitruncus), VSD. Hemitruncus. Common arterial trunk with aortic dominance and absent or atretic right pulmonary artery with ventricular septal defect.

*Corresponding author Oran B: Medicana International Hospital, Department of Pediatric Cardiology, İzmir, Turkey
E-mail:boran@medicana.com.tr and bulentoran@hotmail.com

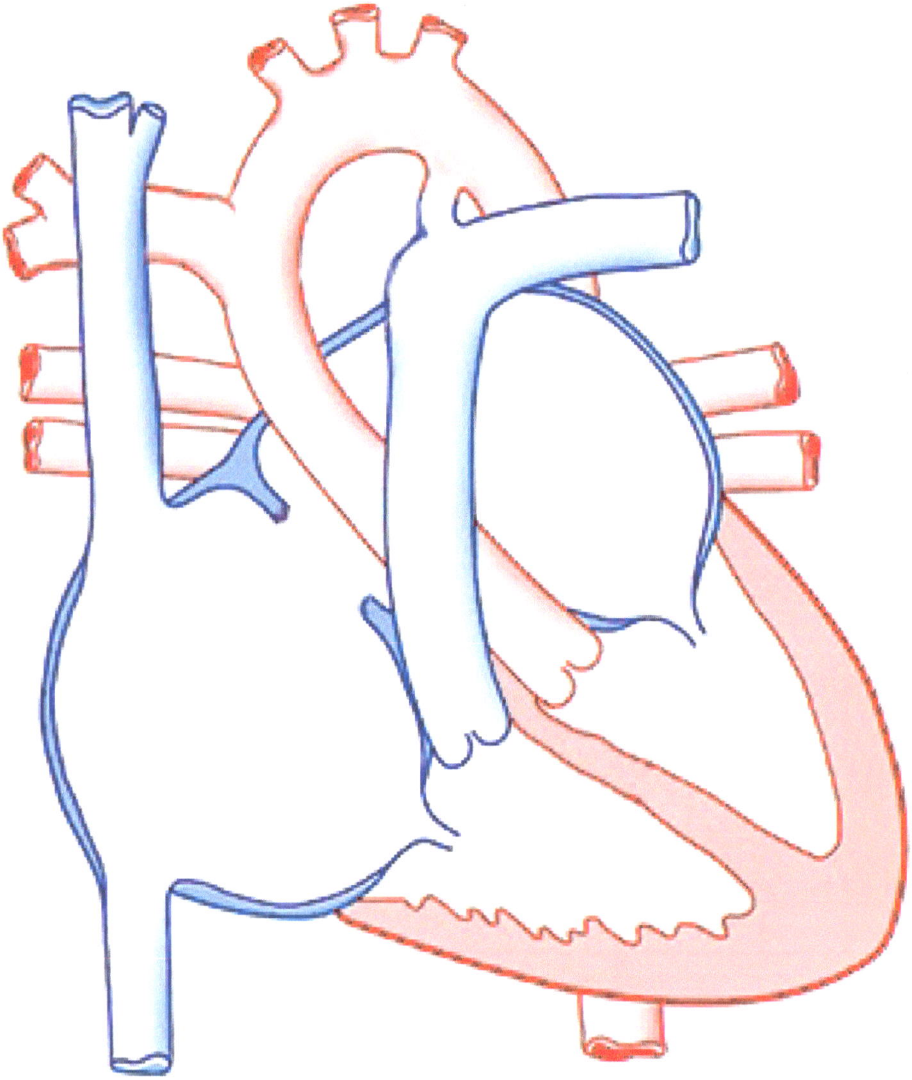

Figure 28: One of the two pulmonary artery origin from ascending aorta (hemitruncus), ASD. Hemitruncus. Common arterial trunk with aortic dominance and absent or atretic right pulmonary artery with atrial septal defect.

*Corresponding author Oran B: Medicana International Hospital, Department of Pediatric Cardiology, İzmir, Turkey
E-mail:boran@medicana.com.tr and bulentoran@hotmail.com

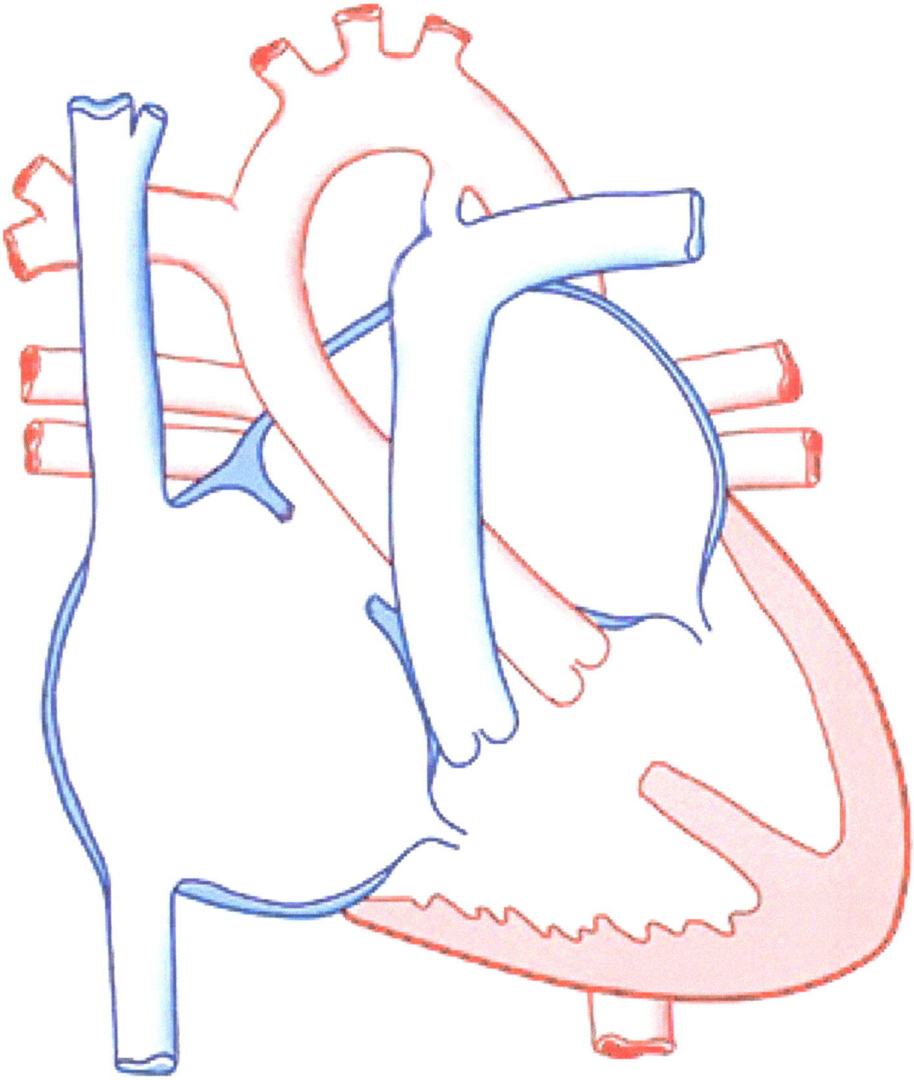

Figure 29: One of the two pulmonary artery origin from ascending aorta (hemitruncus), ASD, VSD, and PDA. Hemitruncus. Common arterial trunk with aortic dominance and absent or atretic right pulmonary artery with atrial septal defect. ventricular septal defect.

*Corresponding author Oran B: Medicana International Hospital, Department of Pediatric Cardiology, İzmir, Turkey
E-mail:boran@medicana.com.tr and bulentoran@hotmail.com

Patent Ductus Arteriosus

Patent ductus arteriosus (PDA) is a hole in the vessel connecting the pulmonary artery to the aorta. This structure is vital during fetal heart development. The size and shape of the PDA varies greatly. From a clinical perspective, PDA is graded as (1) silent: tiny defect without audible heart murmurs; (2) small: no hemodynamic significance, normal left atrial and left ventricular sizes without pulmonary hypertension; (3) moderate: enlargement of the left atrium and left ventricle, with some degree of pulmonary hypertension; or (4) large: typically observed in adults with Eisenmenger physiology and signs of pulmonary hypertension. This malformation is associated with coarctation of the aorta, VSDs, and vascular ring anomalies.

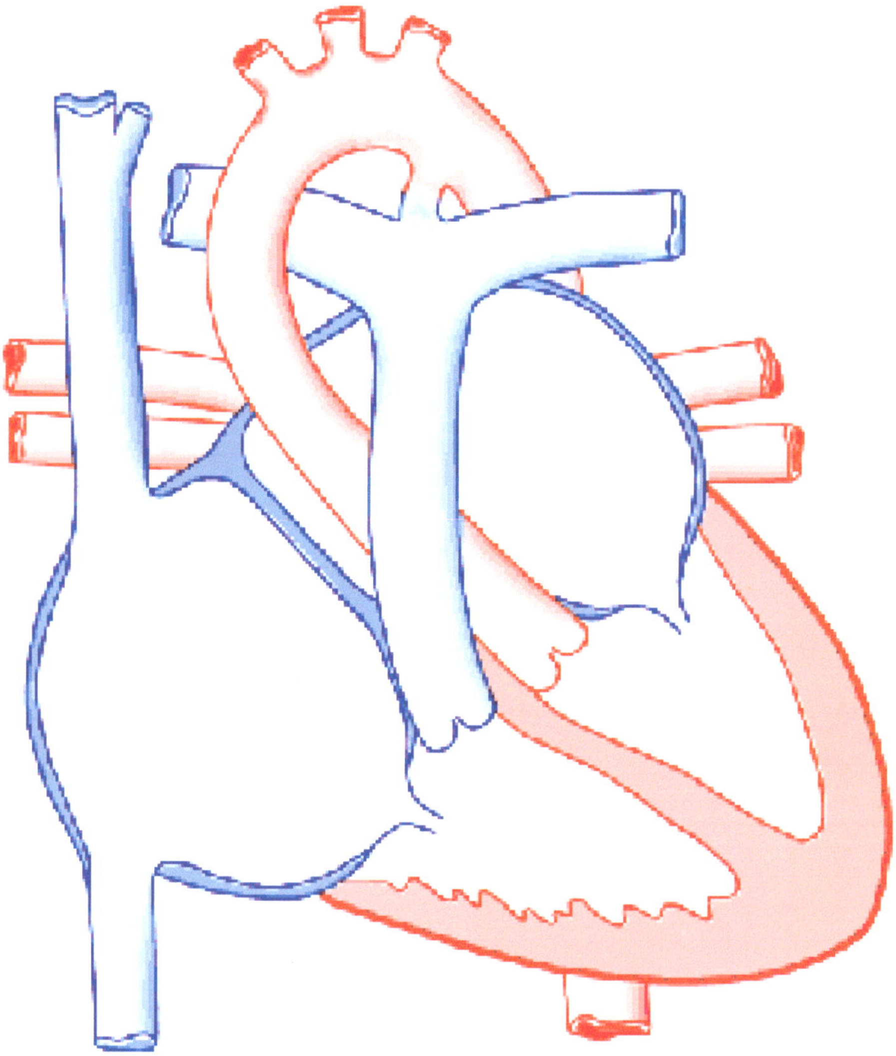

Figure 30: Patent ductus arteriosus. Patent arterial duct (PDA).

*Corresponding author Oran B: Medicana International Hospital, Department of Pediatric Cardiology, İzmir, Turkey
E-mail:boran@medicana.com.tr and bulentoran@hotmail.com

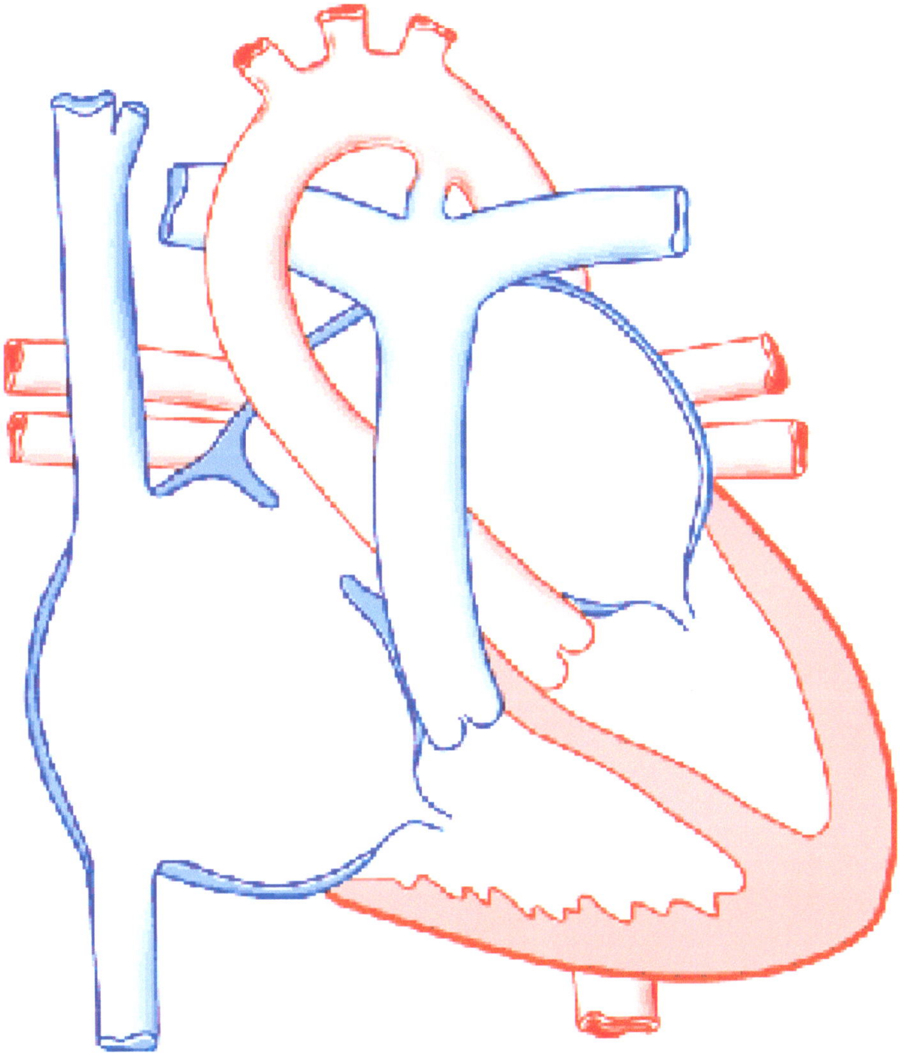

Figure 31: Patent ductus arteriosus with secundum atrial septal defect. Patent arterial duct (PDA) with atrial septal defect, secundum.

*Corresponding author Oran B: Medicana International Hospital, Department of Pediatric Cardiology, İzmir, Turkey
E-mail:boran@medicana.com.tr and bulentoran@hotmail.com

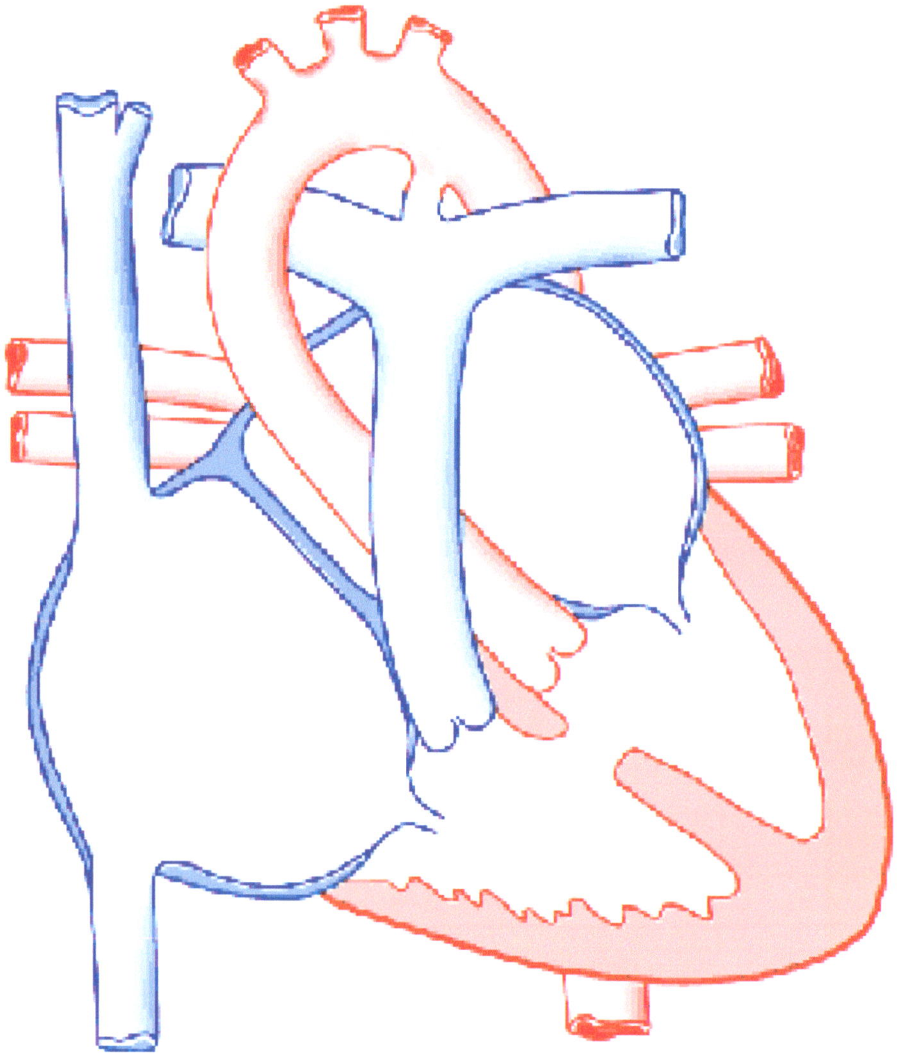

Figure 32: Patent ductus arteriosus with ventricular septal defect. Patent arterial duct (PDA) with ventricular septal defect.

*Corresponding author Oran B: Medicana International Hospital, Department of Pediatric Cardiology, İzmir, Turkey
E-mail:boran@medicana.com.tr and bulentoran@hotmail.com

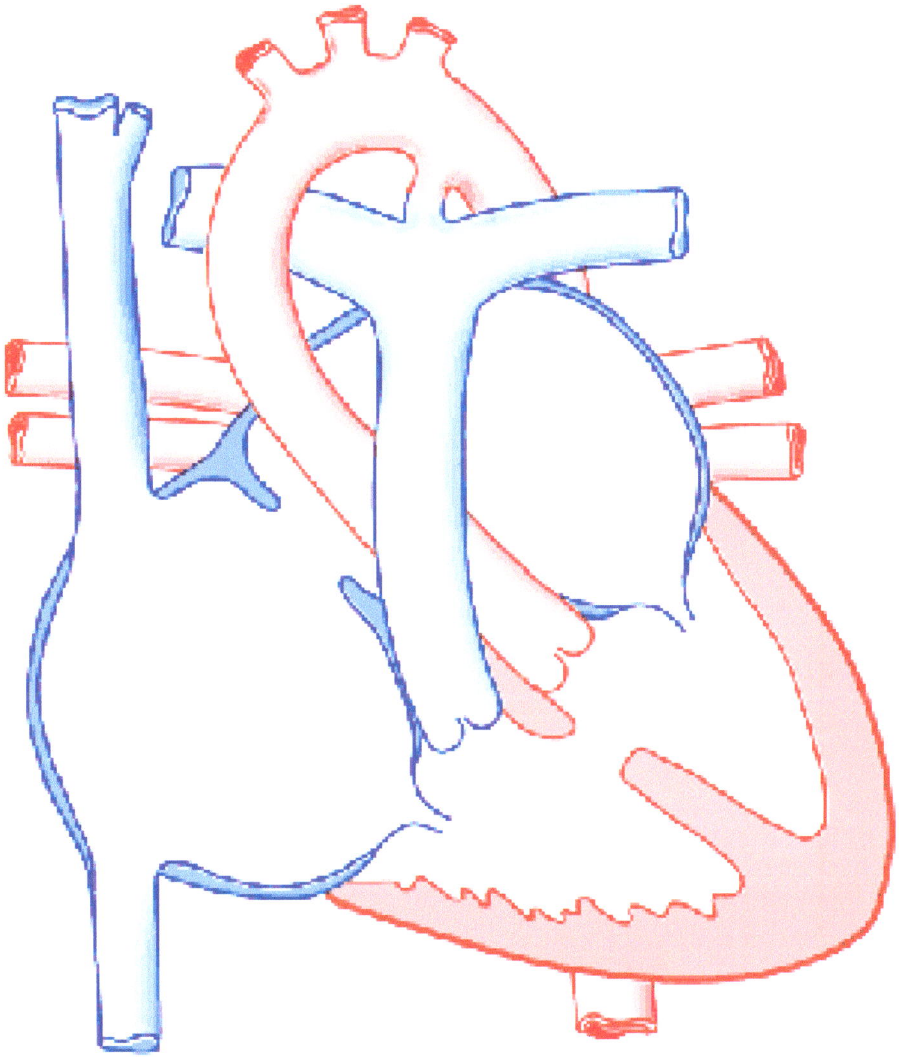

Figure 33: Patent ductus arteriosus, atrial septal defect, and ventricular septal defect. Patent arterial duct (PDA).

*Corresponding author Oran B: Medicana International Hospital, Department of Pediatric Cardiology, İzmir, Turkey
E-mail:boran@medicana.com.tr and bulentoran@hotmail.com

*Corresponding author Oran B: Medicana International Hospital, Department of Pediatric Cardiology, İzmir, Turkey
E-mail:boran@medicana.com.tr and bulentoran@hotmail.com

CHAPTER 3

Pulmonary Artery Anomalies

Oran B.

Medicana International Hospital, Department of Pediatric Cardiology, İzmir, Turkey

*Corresponding author Oran B: Medicana International Hospital, Department of Pediatric Cardiology, İzmir, Turkey
E-mail:boran@medicana.com.tr and bulentoran@hotmail.com

Pulmonary Valve Stenosis

There are various levels of right ventricular outflow tract obstruction: pulmonary valve stenosis, supravalvar pulmonary stenosis, infundibular stenosis, pulmonary artery stenosis (main pulmonary artery and/or peripheral branches) and double-chambered right ventricle. Pulmonary artery stenosis is a rare condition, characterized by dysplastic pulmonary valves with thickened and immobile leaflets. It most often affects the main pulmonary artery and/or peripheral branches. Valvar stenosis affects leaflet commissures, ranging from minimal adhesion to severe deformity or atresia. In each systole, the pulmonary valves adopt a dome shape; they are thick and myxomatous. Valvar stenosis causes expansion of the main pulmonary artery diameter due to jet flow (post-stenotic dilatation). Additional anomalies and associated syndromes include pulmonary artery branch stenosis, VSD, tetralogy of Fallot, Noonan syndrome, Williams syndrome, and Alagilli syndrome.

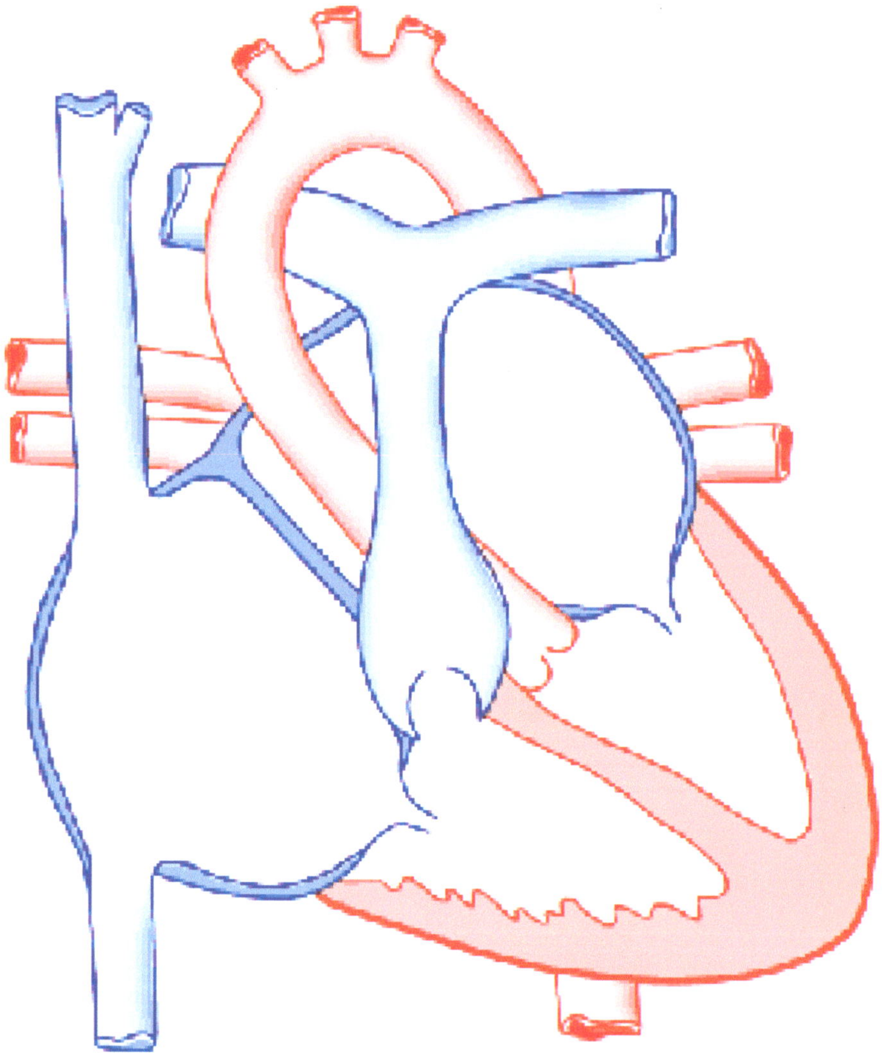

Figure 1: Pulmonary valve stenosis. Congenital pulmonary valvar stenosis.

*Corresponding author Oran B: Medicana International Hospital, Department of Pediatric Cardiology, İzmir, Turkey
E-mail:boran@medicana.com.tr and bulentoran@hotmail.com

Subvalvar Pulmonary Stenosis

Also known as infundibular stenosis, subvalvar pulmonary stenosis is associated with valvar stenosis. Infundibular hypertrophy of the right ventricular outflow tract causes pulmonary obstruction.

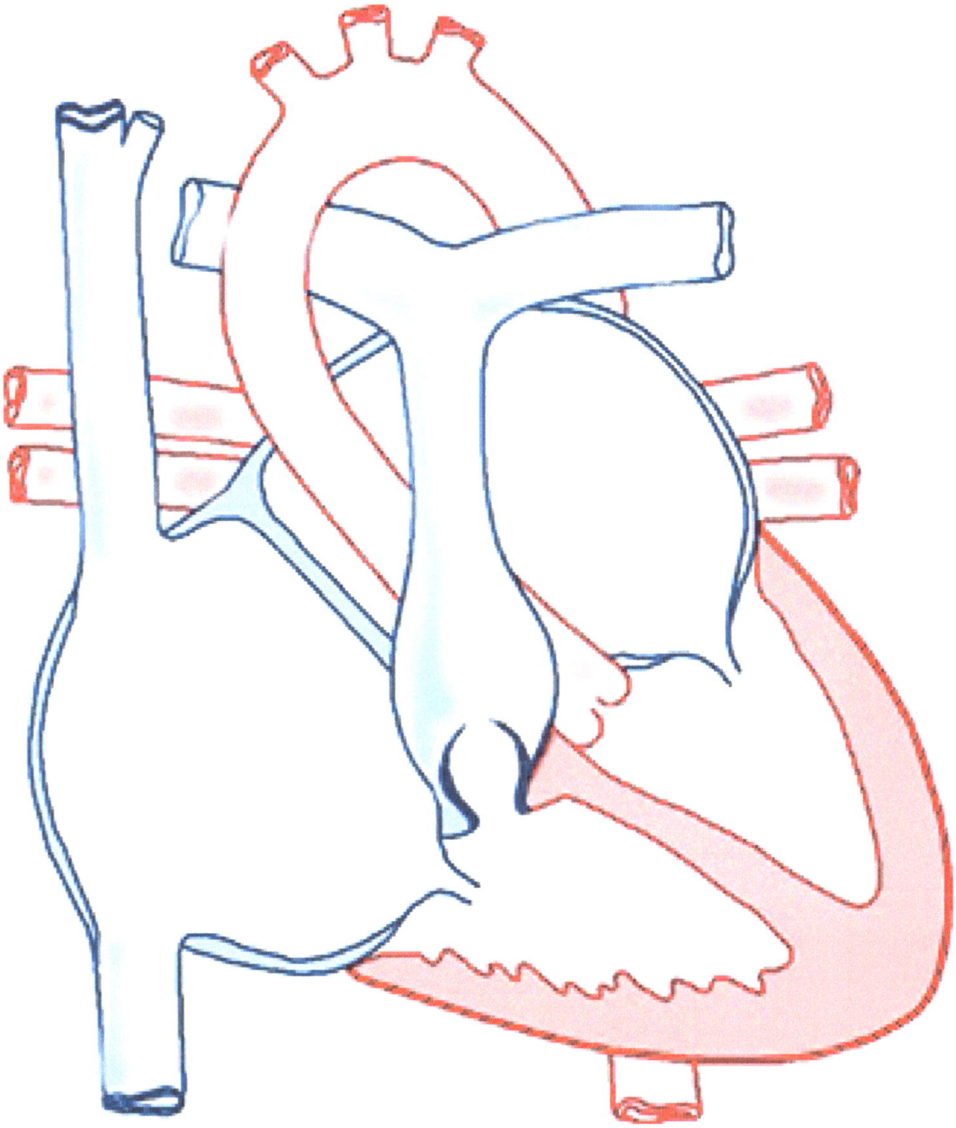

Figure 2: Subvalvar or infundibular pulmonary stenosis. Congenital subpulmonary stenosis.

*Corresponding author Oran B: Medicana International Hospital, Department of Pediatric Cardiology, İzmir, Turkey
E-mail:boran@medicana.com.tr and bulentoran@hotmail.com

Supravalvar Pulmonary Stenosis

Supravalar pulmonary stenosis is characterized by a hypoplastic main pulmonary artery annulus with right and left pulmonary artery branch stenosis. It is frequently reported in patients with rubella and Williams Syndrome. Iatrogenic stenosis may also develop after surgery.

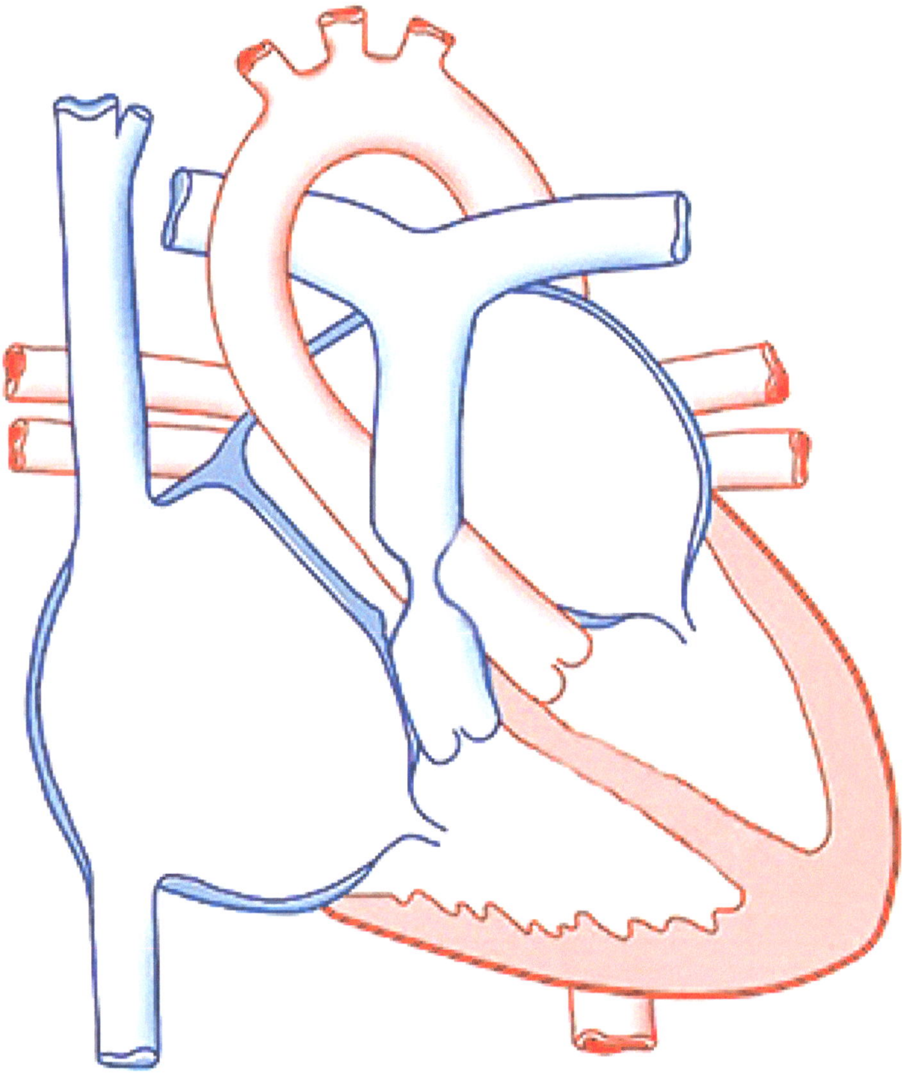

Figure 3: Supravalvar pulmonary stenosis. Congenital supravalvar pulmonary stenosis.

*Corresponding author Oran B: Medicana International Hospital, Department of Pediatric Cardiology, İzmir, Turkey
E-mail:boran@medicana.com.tr and bulentoran@hotmail.com

Main pulmonary Artery Stenosis

Pulmonary artery stenosis is a narrowing of the pulmonary artery that impairs oxygenation of the blood by obstructing flow to the lungs.

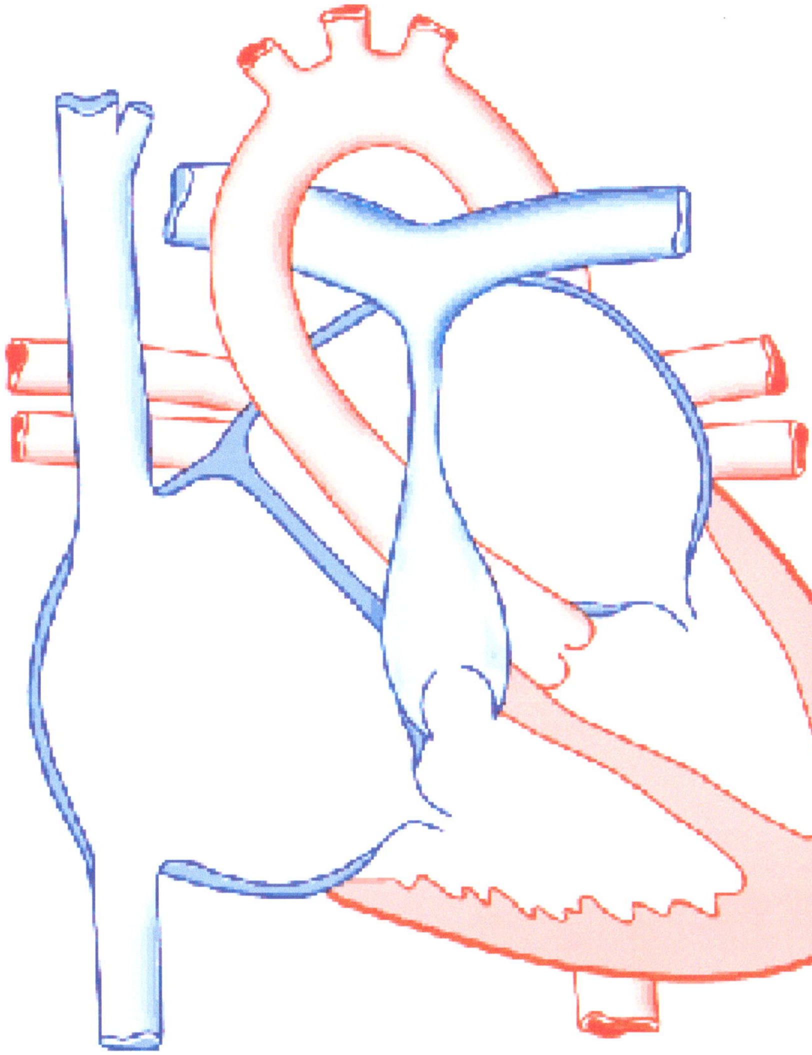

Figure 4: Main pulmonary artery stenosis. Pulmonary 'annular' hypoplasia.

*Corresponding author Oran B: Medicana International Hospital, Department of Pediatric Cardiology, İzmir, Turkey
E-mail:boran@medicana.com.tr and bulentoran@hotmail.com

Peripheral Pulmonary Artery Stenosis, Hilar, Bifurcation Level

Narrowing of pulmonary arteries may occur in the main pulmonary artery and/or in the left or right pulmonary artery branches. The resulting reduction in oxygen leads to cardiovascular deficiency.

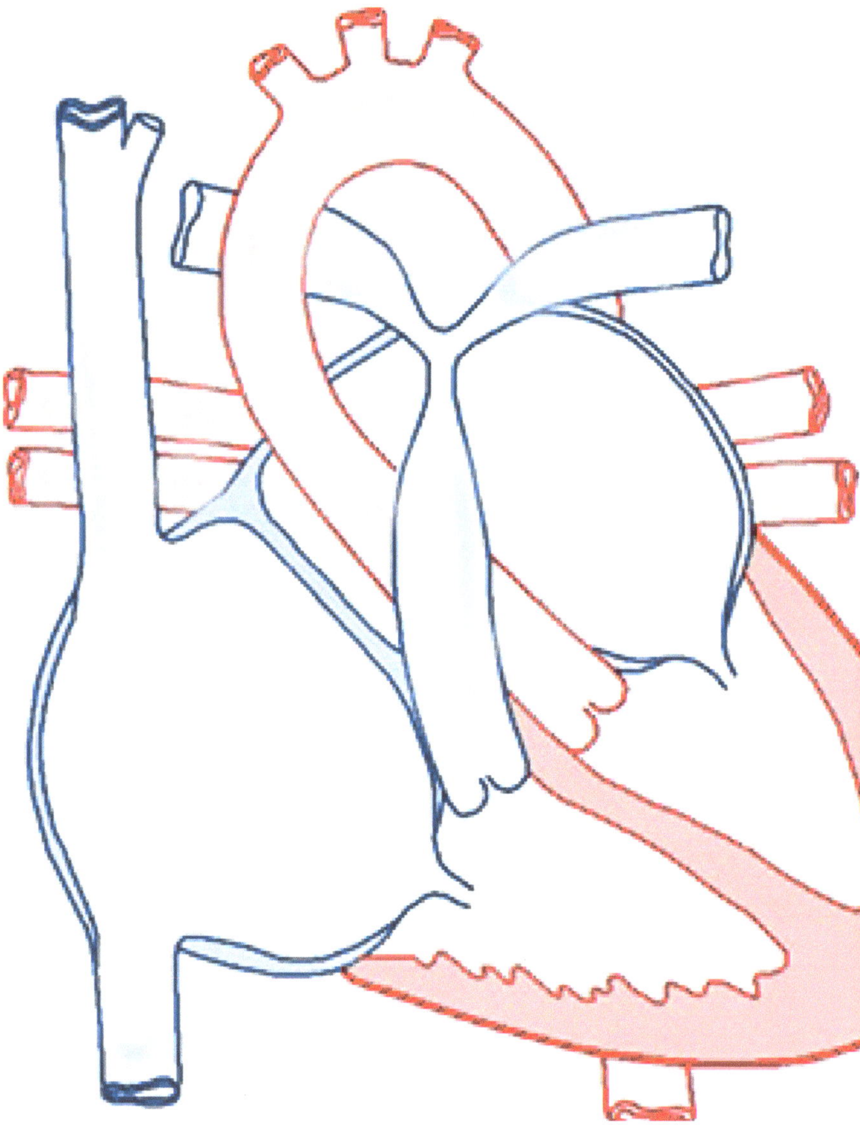

Figure 5: Peripheral pulmonary artery stenosis, hilar, bifurcation level. Congenital central pulmonary arterial stenosis or hypoplasia proximal to hilar bifurcation.

*Corresponding author Oran B: Medicana International Hospital, Department of Pediatric Cardiology, İzmir, Turkey
E-mail:boran@medicana.com.tr and bulentoran@hotmail.com

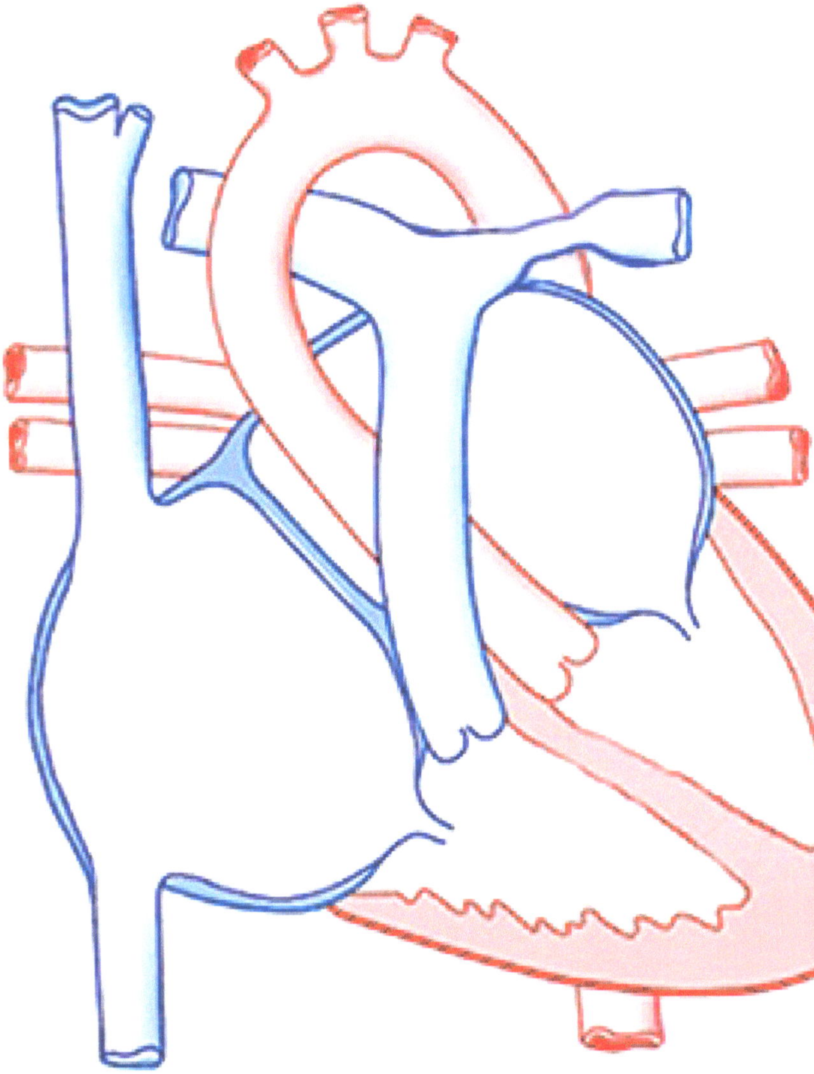

Figure 6: Congenital left pulmonary arterial stenosis.

*Corresponding author Oran B: Medicana International Hospital, Department of Pediatric Cardiology, İzmir, Turkey
E-mail:boran@medicana.com.tr and bulentoran@hotmail.com

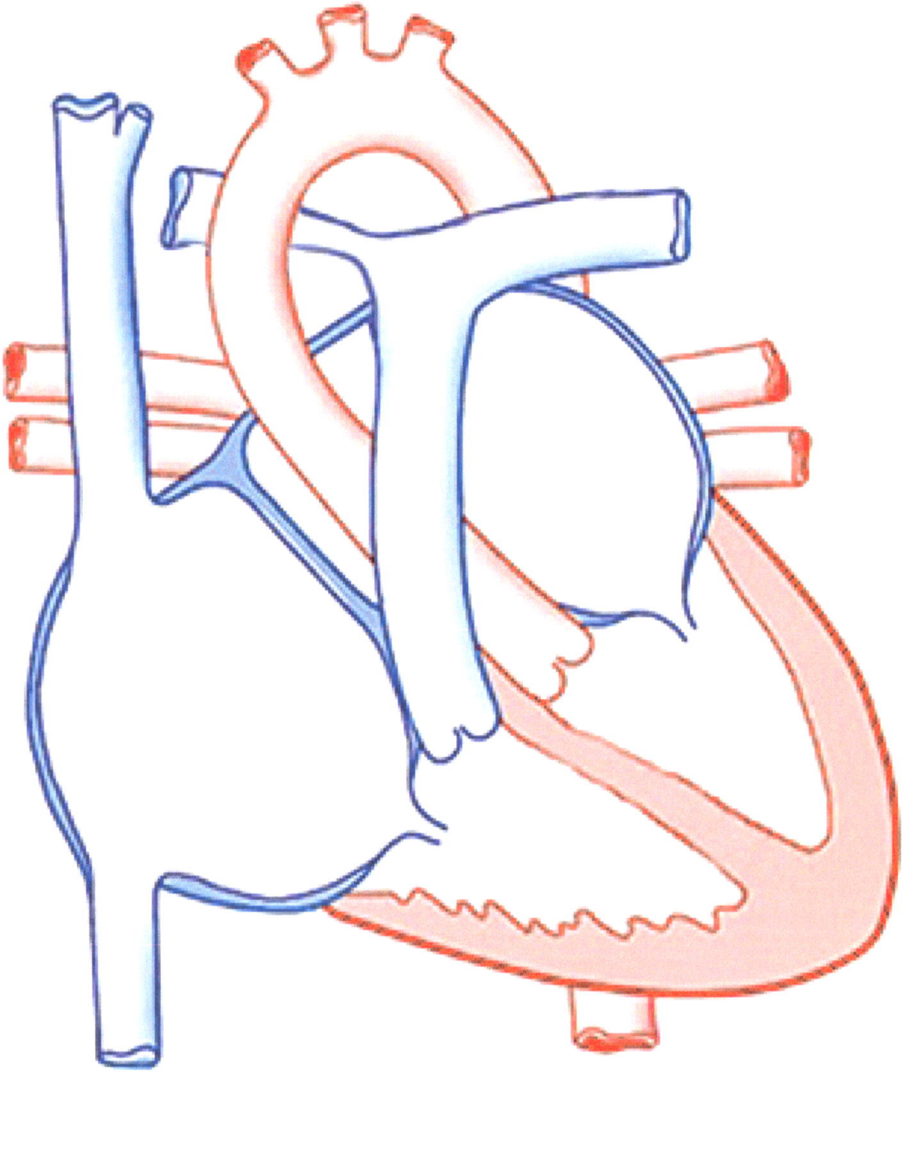

Figure 7: Congenital right pulmonary arterial stenosis.

*Corresponding author Oran B: Medicana International Hospital, Department of Pediatric Cardiology, İzmir, Turkey
E-mail:boran@medicana.com.tr and bulentoran@hotmail.com

Fallot Tetralogy

Tetralogy of Fallot is the most commonly diagnosed and surgically operated cyanotic congenital heart disease in adult patients. There are four main abnormalities: **overriding** (dextroposition) of the aorta, typically non-restrictive VSD, pulmonary and/or infundibular stenosis (with or without branch pulmonary artery stenosis), and right ventricular hypertrophy. This disease has various morphologies, ranging from minimal pulmonary stenosis to pulmonary atresia and from minimal aortic override to a double outlet right ventricle. Pentalogy of Fallot is diagnosed when ASD is present. Tetralogy of Fallot is associated with truncus arteriosus, pulmonary atresia, complete AVSD, abnormal pulmonary venous return, right aortic arch, interrupted aortic arch, and left persistent superior vena cava anomalies. It is commonly encountered in patients with 21q11 deletion, trisomy 21, Alagilli syndrome, pentalogy of Cantrell, or Goldenhar syndrome.

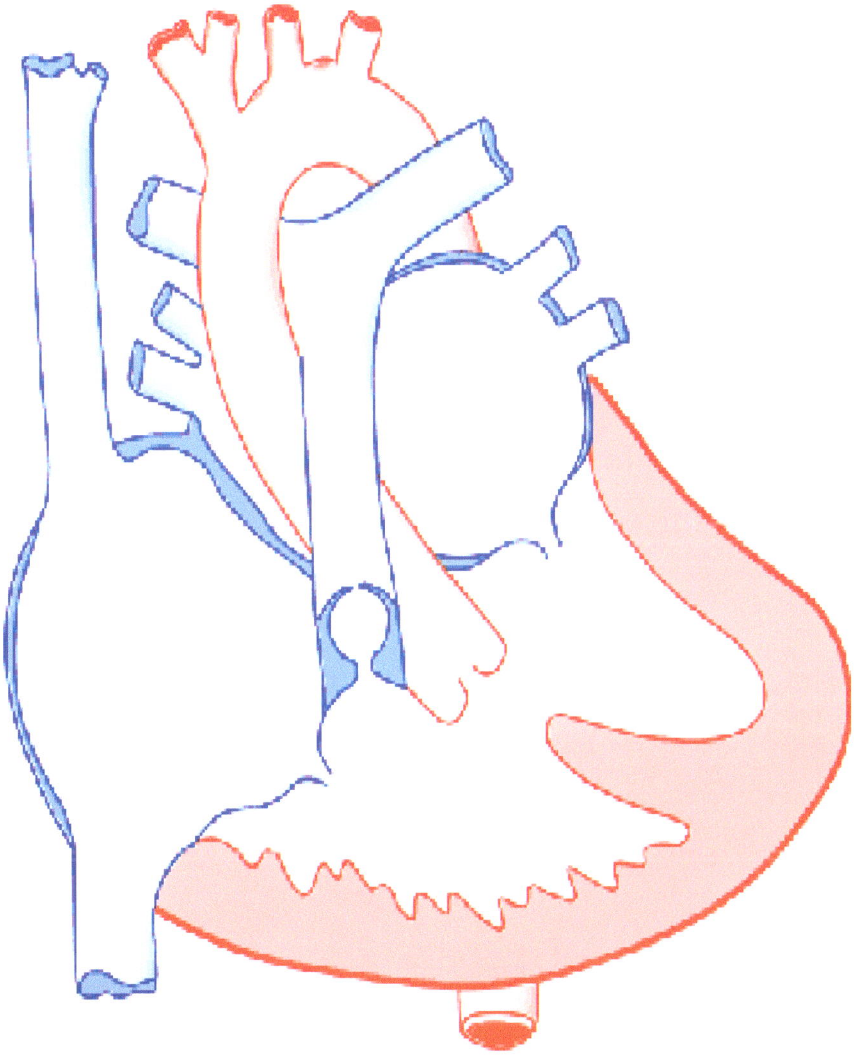

Figure 8: Fallot Tetralogy. Tetralogy of Fallot.

*Corresponding author Oran B: Medicana International Hospital, Department of Pediatric Cardiology, İzmir, Turkey
E-mail:boran@medicana.com.tr and bulentoran@hotmail.com

Tetralogy of Fallot with Pulmonary Atresia

This more severe form of tetralogy of Fallot is characterized by a VSD, overriding aorta, right ventricular hypertrophy, and complete pulmonary obstruction. The pulmonary valve is absent and aortopulmonary circulation is provided by numerous multiple systemic to pulmonary arterial collaterals (MAPCAs).

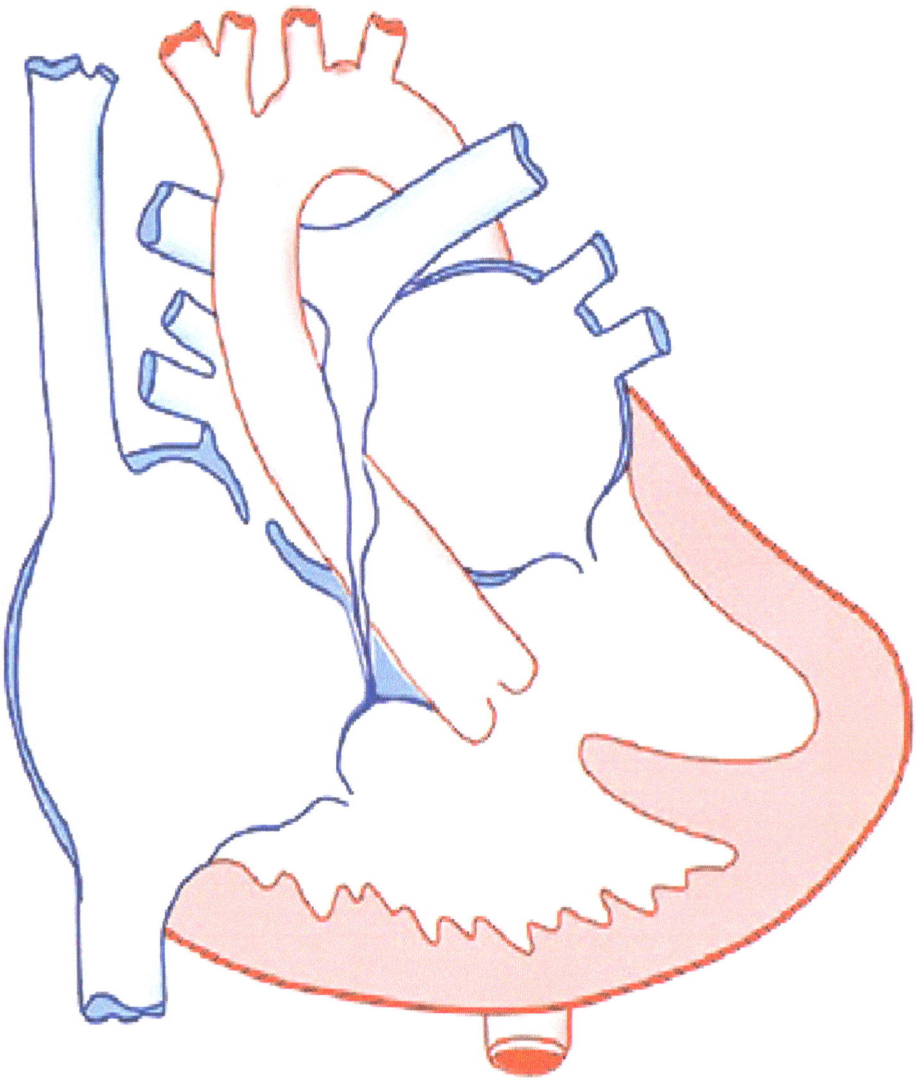

Figure 9: Tetralogy of Fallot with pulmonary atresia**.** Tetralogy of Fallot with pulmonary atresia.

*Corresponding author Oran B: Medicana International Hospital, Department of Pediatric Cardiology, İzmir, Turkey
E-mail:boran@medicana.com.tr and bulentoran@hotmail.com

Tetralogy of Fallot with Absence of Pulmonary Valve

Tetralogy of Fallot with absent pulmonary valve represents a rare variant of congenital heart disease. The anatomic features consist of a rudimentary pulmonary valve (stenotic and regurgitant valve), dilated pulmonary arteries, and a large VSD. This disease occurs in 2.5% of patients diagnosed with tetralogy of Fallot. Of these, 75% have the 22q11 deletion.

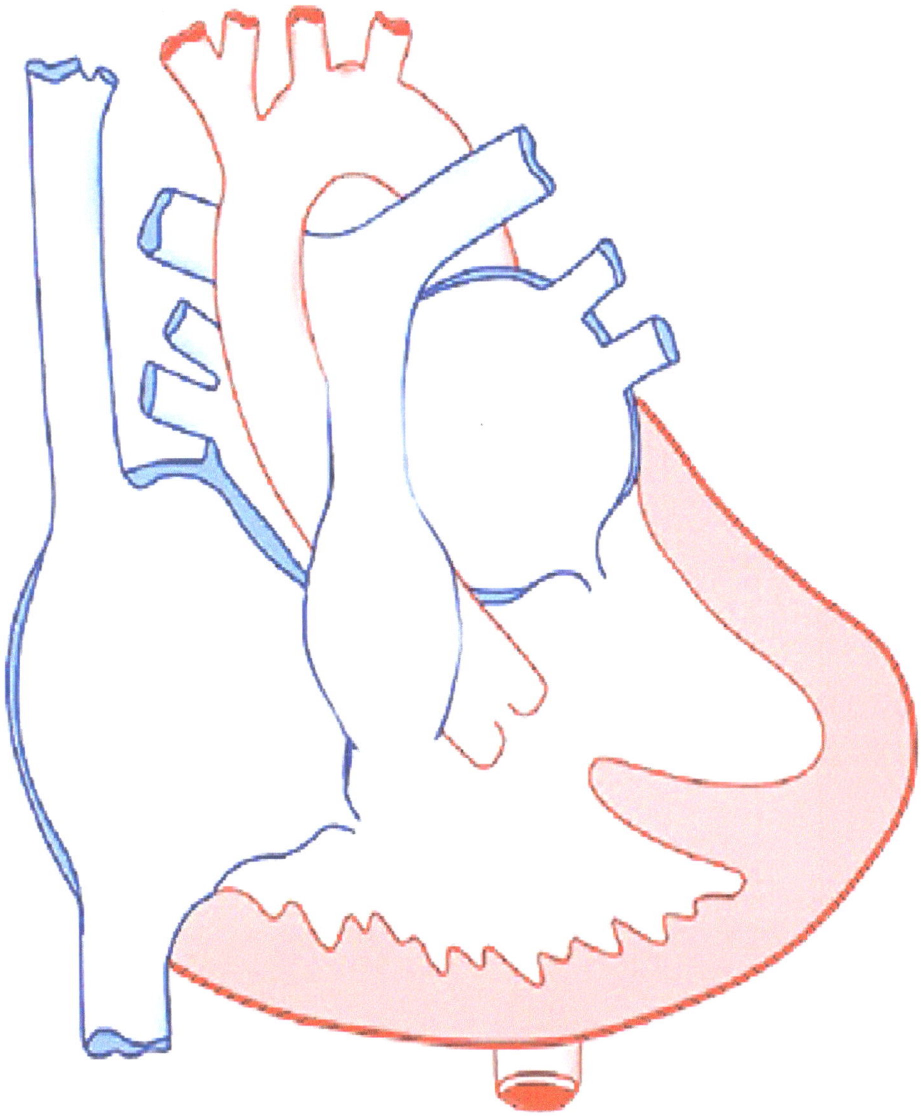

Figure 10: Tetralogy of Fallot with absence of pulmonary valve. Tetralogy of Fallot with absent pulmonary valve syndrome.

*Corresponding author Oran B: Medicana International Hospital, Department of Pediatric Cardiology, İzmir, Turkey
E-mail:boran@medicana.com.tr and bulentoran@hotmail.com

Pulmonary Atresia with Intact Ventricular Septum, PDA

Pulmonary atresia with intact ventricular septum is a rare congenital cardiac lesion characterized by heterogeneous right ventricular development, an imperforate pulmonary valve, and possible extensive ventriculocoronary connections. This severe heart valve lesion requires surgical intervention for survival to adulthood.

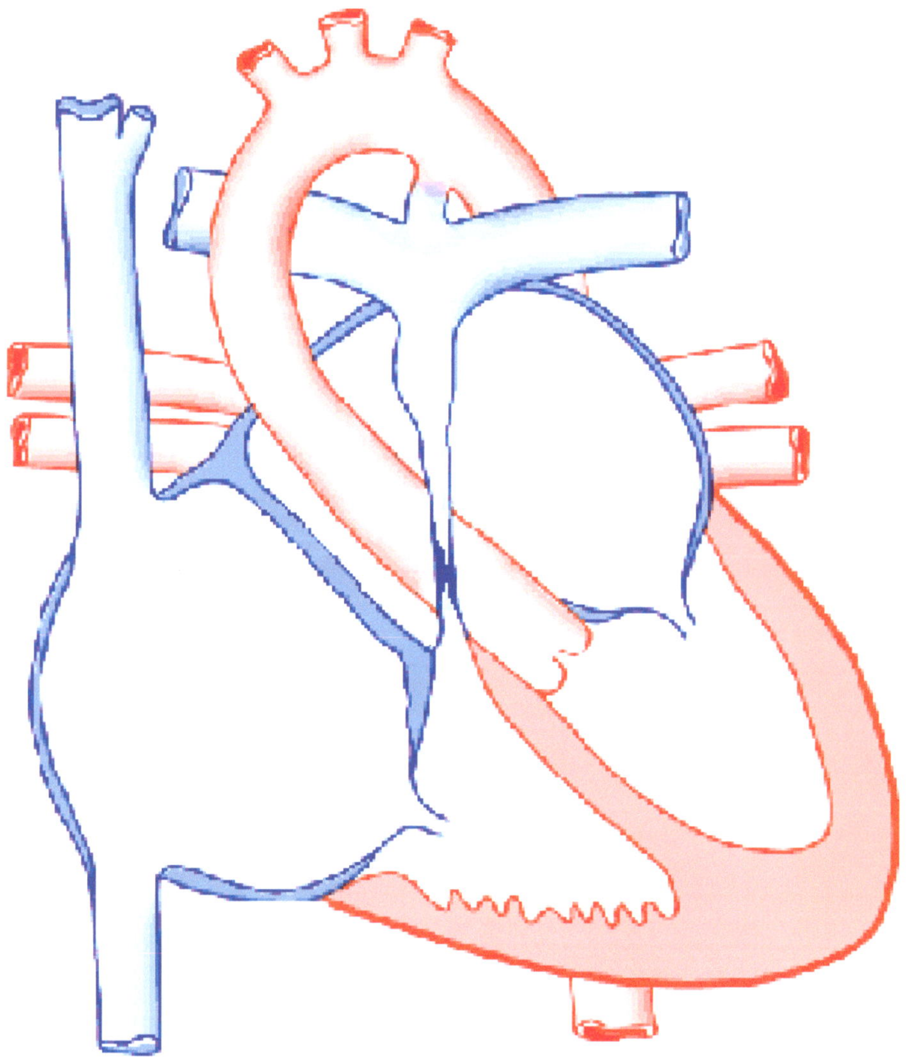

Figure 11: Pulmonary atresia with intact ventricular septum, PDA. Congenital pulmonary atresia with intact ventricular septum and patent arterial duct.

*Corresponding author Oran B: Medicana International Hospital, Department of Pediatric Cardiology, İzmir, Turkey
E-mail:boran@medicana.com.tr and bulentoran@hotmail.com

Pulmonary Atresia, Intact Ventricular Septum, Secundum ASD, PDA

Pulmonary atresia, intact ventricular septum is a severe heart valve defect. Due to the presence of secundum ASDs and PDA, a partial left-right shunt is placed in these patients.

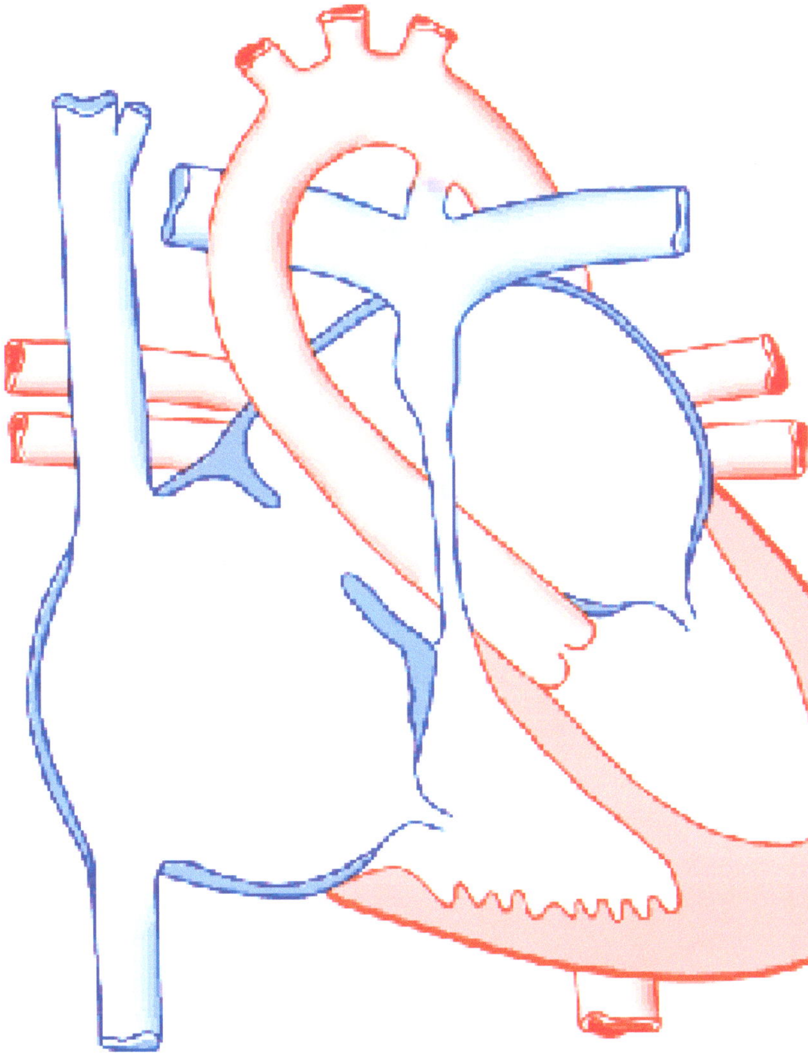

Figure 12: Pulmonary atresia with intact ventricular septum, secundum ASD, PDA. Congenital pulmonary atresia with intact ventricular septum and atrial septal defects within oval fossa, patent arterial duct.

*Corresponding author Oran B: Medicana International Hospital, Department of Pediatric Cardiology, İzmir, Turkey
E-mail:boran@medicana.com.tr and bulentoran@hotmail.com

Pulmonary Atresia, VSD, Fallot type-Secundum ASD

Unlike tetralogy of Fallot, which is characterized by pulmonary stenosis, this defect is characterized by a "malaligned" VSD with pulmonary valve atresia. There are three patterns of pulmonary vascular flow: confluent pulmonary arteries, a PDA, and systemic circulation. Features include multiple systemic to pulmonary arterial collaterals (MAPCAs) that arise from the descending aorta, a right aortic arch, and an ASD.

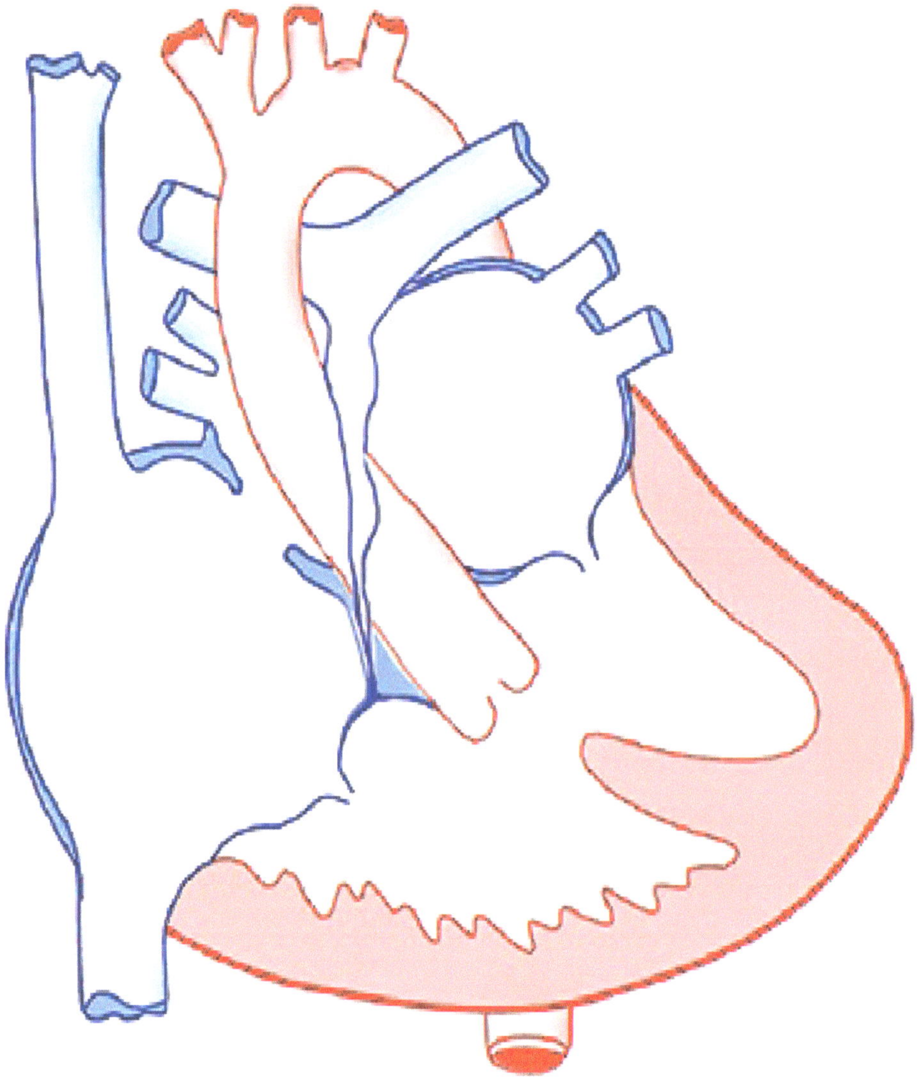

Figure 13: Pulmonary atresia, VSD, Fallot type-secundum ASD. Congenital pulmonary atresia, tetralogy of Fallot type, ventricular septal defect, atrial septal defects within oval fossa.

*Corresponding author Oran B: Medicana International Hospital, Department of Pediatric Cardiology, İzmir, Turkey
E-mail:boran@medicana.com.tr and bulentoran@hotmail.com

Pulmonary Atresia with ASD. VSD, PDA

In pulmonary atresia with a "malaligned" VSD, pulmonary circulation is provided by a PDA. It is rare for these patients to survive into adulthood without interventional procedures or surgery.

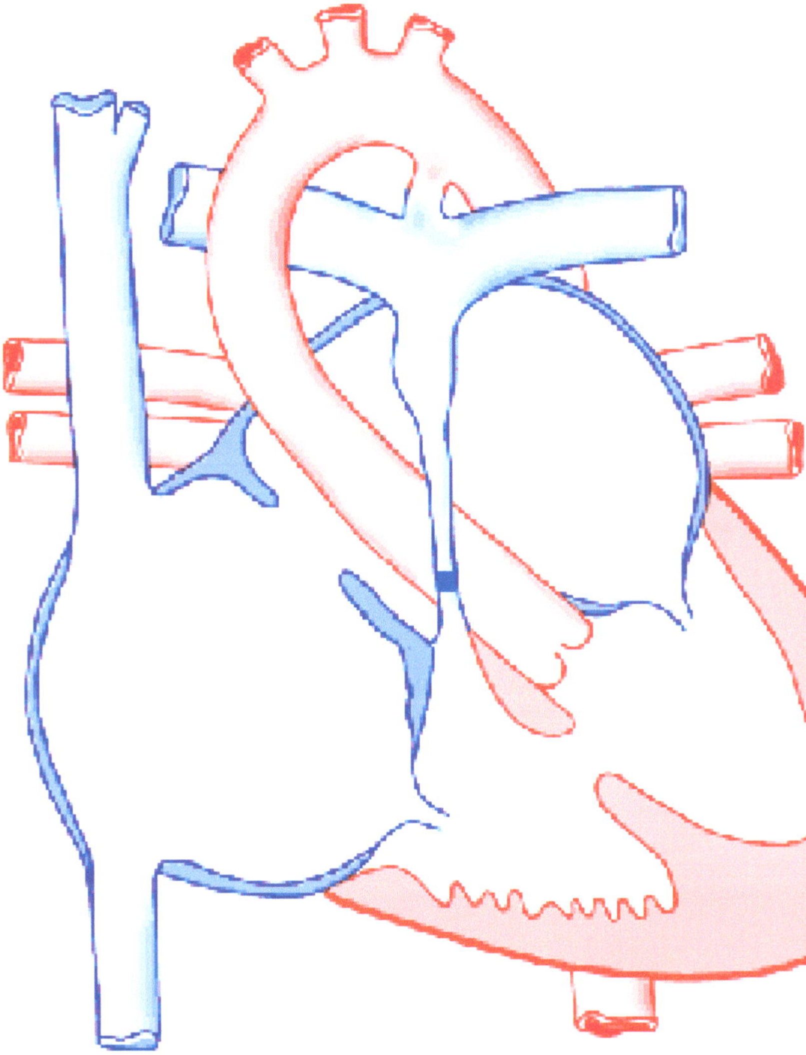

Figure 14: Pulmonary atresia ASD, VSD, PDA. Congenital pulmonary atresia, ventricular septal defect, atrial septal defects within oval fossa, and patent arterial duct.

*Corresponding author Oran B: Medicana International Hospital, Department of Pediatric Cardiology, İzmir, Turkey
E-mail:boran@medicana.com.tr and bulentoran@hotmail.com

Pulmonary Atresia, Secundum ASD

In this form of pulmonary atresia, pulmonary circulation is provided by a secundum ASD and a PDA. It is rare for these patients to survive into adulthood without interventional procedures or surgery.

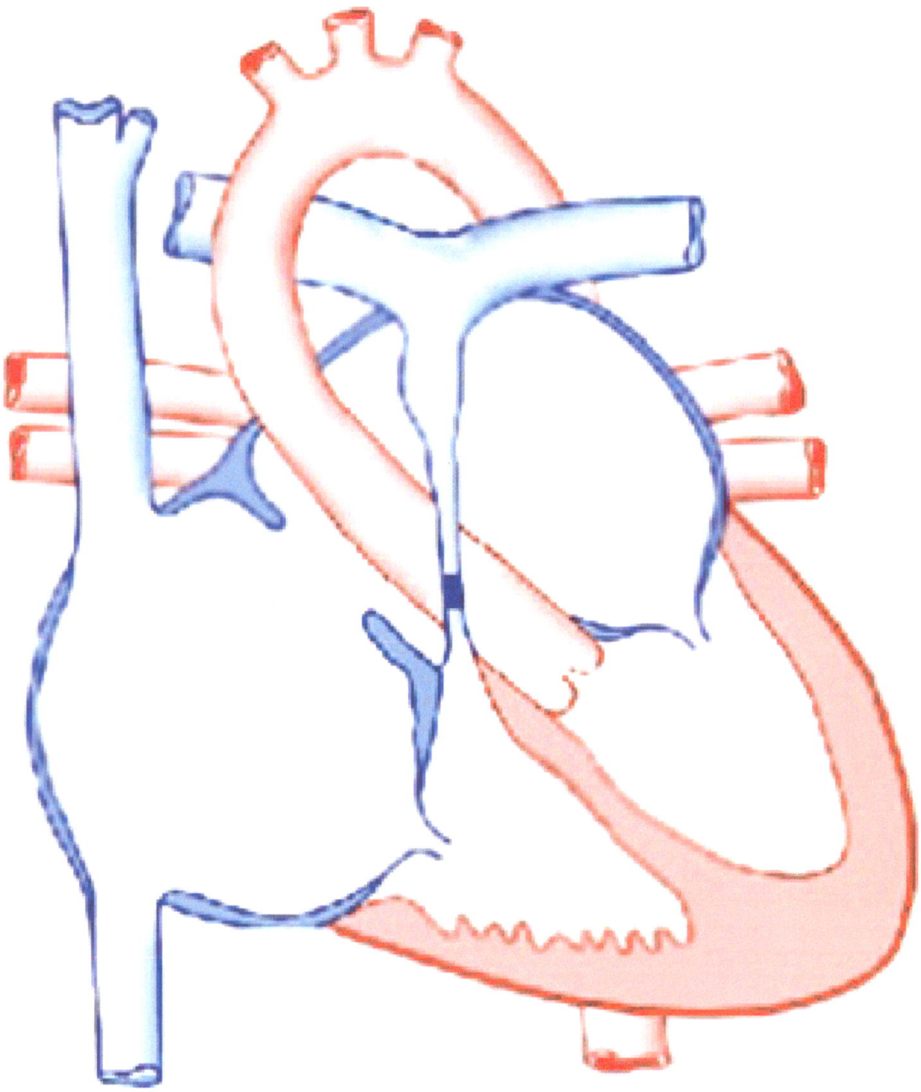

Figure 15: Pulmonary atresia, intact ventricular septum, secundum ASD. Congenital pulmonary atresia with intact ventricular septum and atrial septal defects within oval fossa.

*Corresponding author Oran B: Medicana International Hospital, Department of Pediatric Cardiology, İzmir, Turkey
E-mail:boran@medicana.com.tr and bulentoran@hotmail.com

Pulmonary Atresia, 'MAPCA'

In this form of pulmonary atresia, MAPCAs typically arise from the descending aorta. It is rare for these patients to survive into adulthood without interventional procedures or surgery.

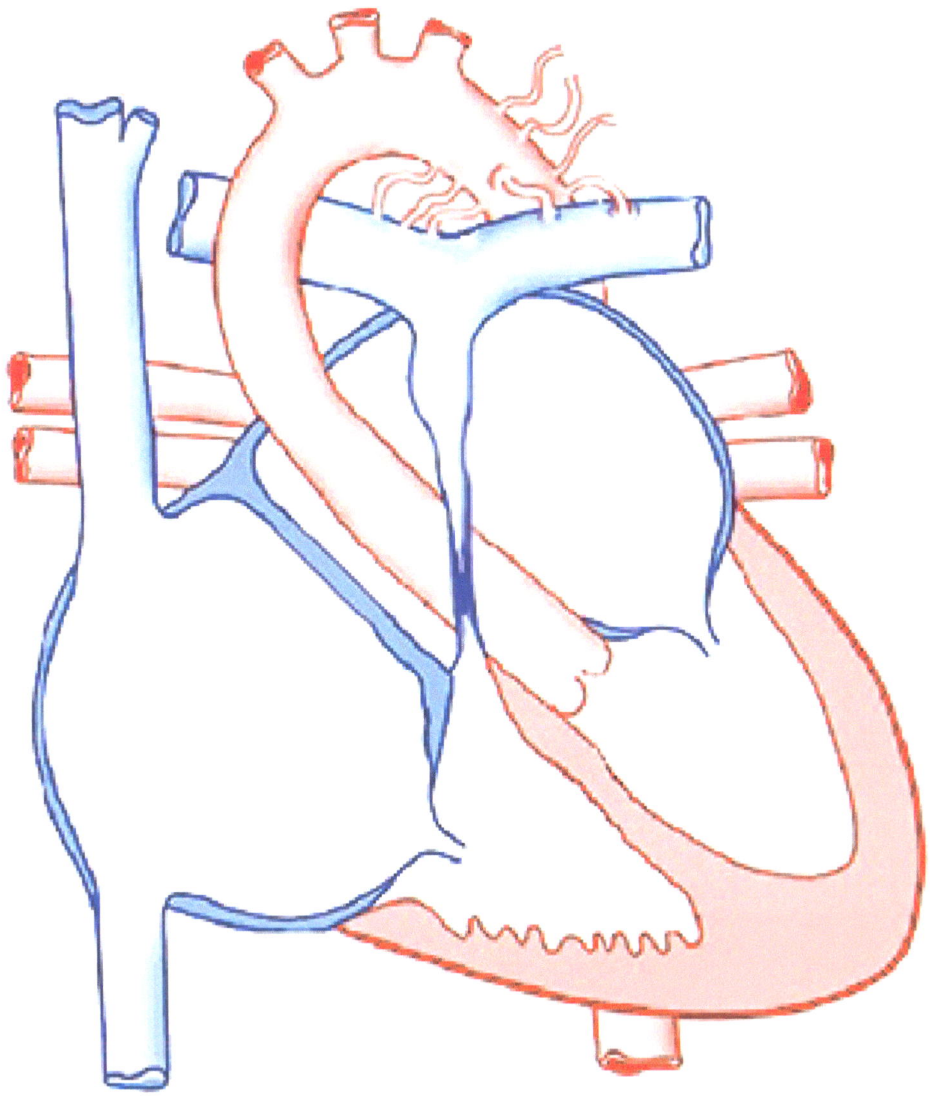

Figure 16: Pulmonary atresia, 'MAPCA'. Congenital pulmonary atresia with sistemic to pulmoner collaterals.

*Corresponding author Oran B: Medicana International Hospital, Department of Pediatric Cardiology, İzmir, Turkey
E-mail:boran@medicana.com.tr and bulentoran@hotmail.com

*Corresponding author Oran B: Medicana International Hospital, Department of Pediatric Cardiology, İzmir, Turkey
E-mail:boran@medicana.com.tr and bulentoran@hotmail.com

CHAPTER 4

Pulmonary Venous Anomalies

Oran B.

Medicana International Hospital, Department of Pediatric Cardiology, İzmir, Turkey

*Corresponding author Oran B: Medicana International Hospital, Department of Pediatric Cardiology, İzmir, Turkey
E-mail:boran@medicana.com.tr and bulentoran@hotmail.com

Total Abnormal Pulmonary Venous Return supracardiac

Total anomalous pulmonary venous return is a rare congenital malformation. All four pulmonary veins drain to the right heart chambers, instead of the left heart chambers. Pulmonary veins either drain directly into the right atrium or through a common vein into one of the systemic veins. Various forms have been documented: supracardiac, cardiac, infracardiac, mixed, and obstructed. It is impossible for these patients to survive into adulthood without Interventional procedures or surgery. Additional anomalies include ASDs, PDA, right atrial isomerism, and complex cyanotic congenital heart disease. The supracardiac form of abnormal pulmonary venous return is characterized by an abnormal pulmonary venous connection and discharge to the superior vena cava via the left vertical vein, the innominate vein, or the azygos vein.

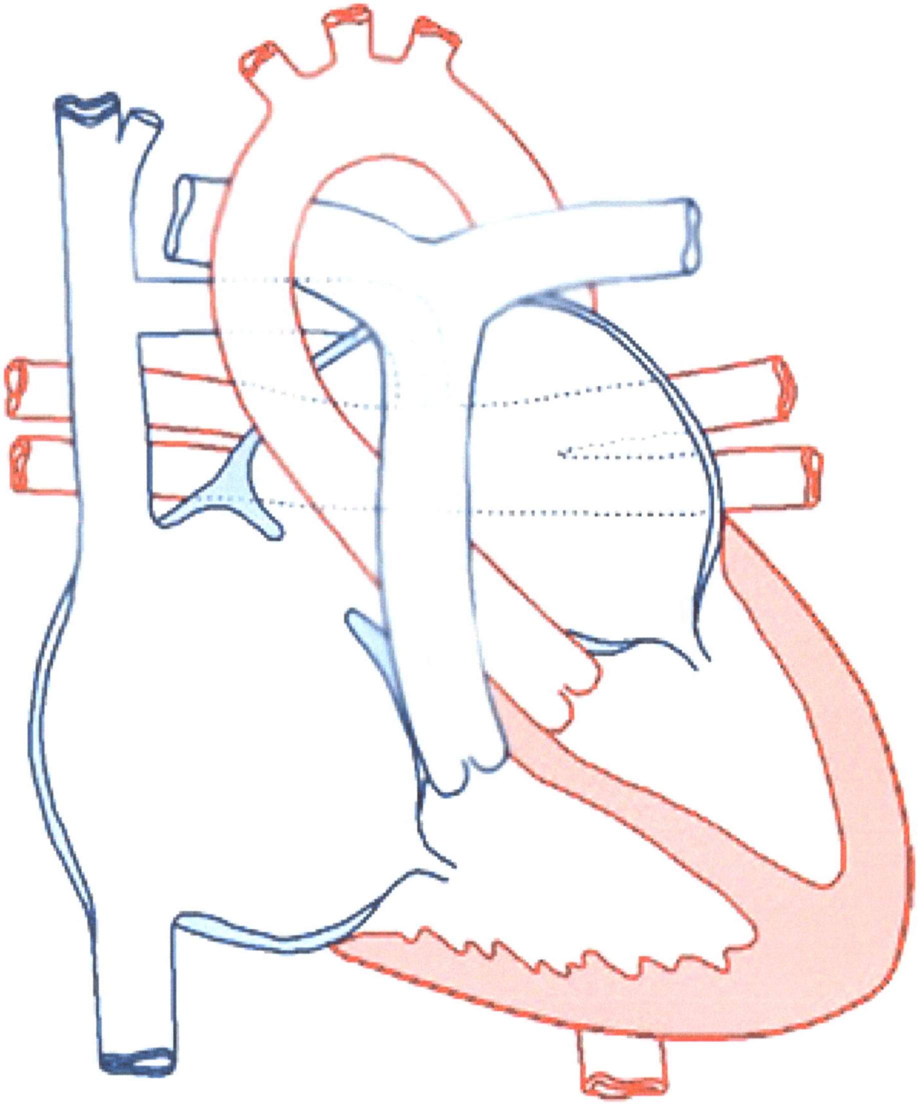

Figure 1: Total abnormal pulmonary venous return, supracardiac. Total anomalous pulmonary venous connection of the supracardiac type.

*Corresponding author Oran B: Medicana International Hospital, Department of Pediatric Cardiology, İzmir, Turkey
E-mail:boran@medicana.com.tr and bulentoran@hotmail.com

Total Abnormal Pulmonary Venous Return, Cardiac

The cardiac form of abnormal pulmonary venous connection is characterized by discharge into the right atrium via the left persistent superior vena cava and coronary sinus.

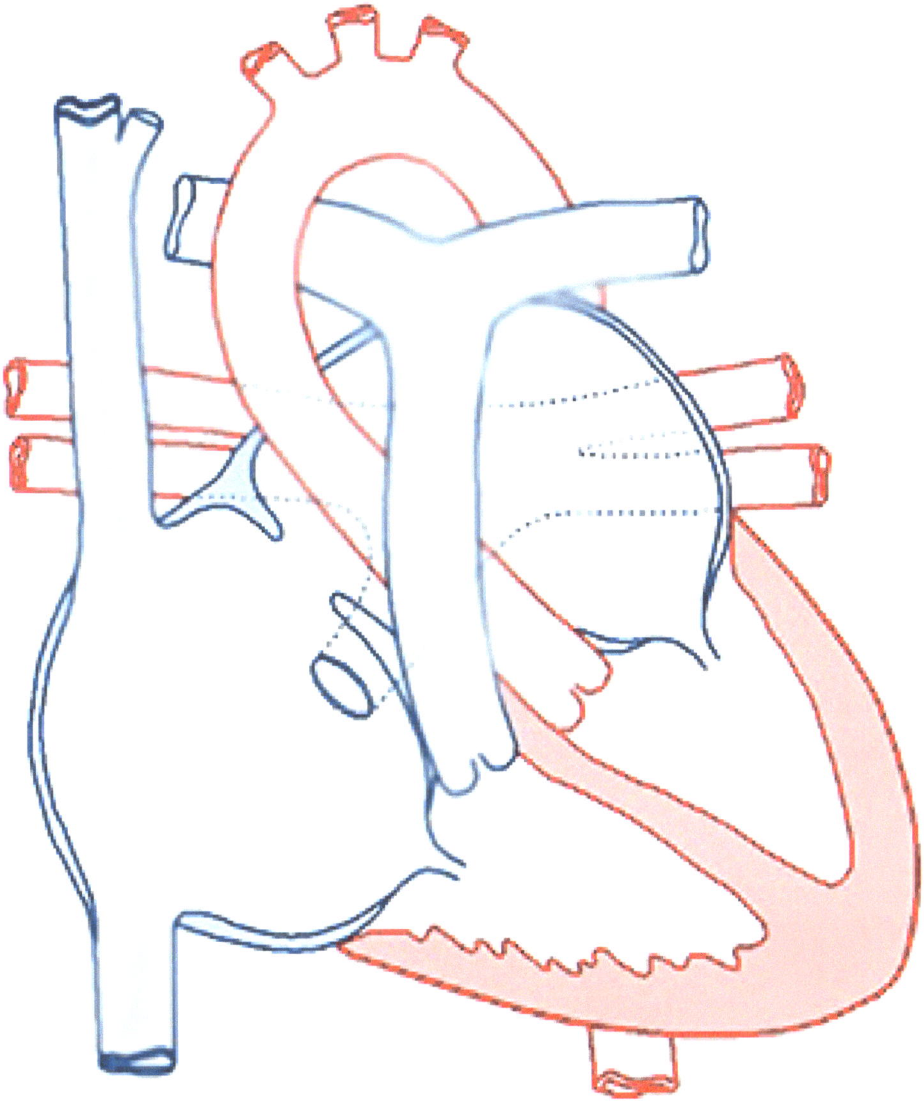

Figure 2: Total abnormal pulmonary venous return, cardiac. Total anomalous pulmonary venous connection of the cardiac type.

*Corresponding author Oran B: Medicana International Hospital, Department of Pediatric Cardiology, İzmir, Turkey
E-mail:boran@medicana.com.tr and bulentoran@hotmail.com

Total Abnormal Pulmonary Venous Return, Infracardiac

The infracardiac form of abnormal pulmonary venous connection is characterized by drainage through the intraabdominal veins below the diaphragm, the portal vein, or the inferior vena cava.

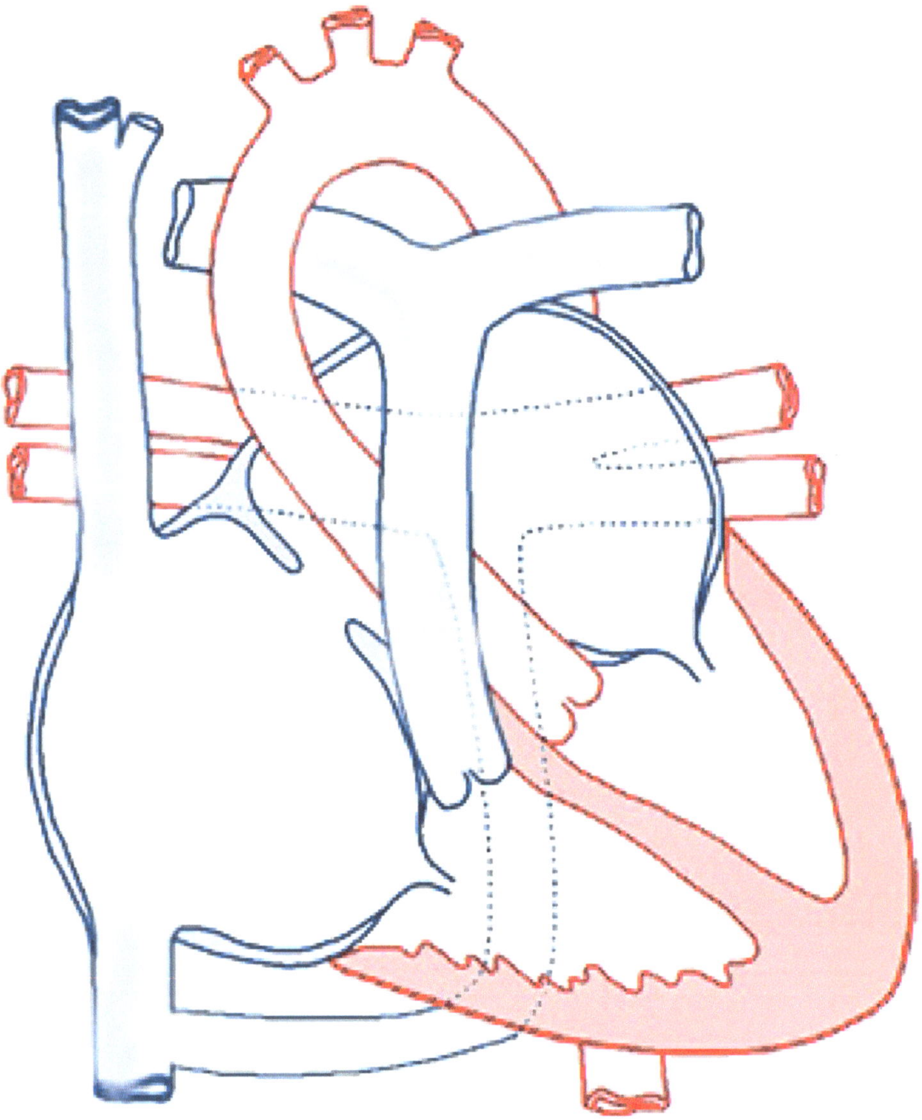

Figure 3: Total abnormal pulmonary venous return, infracardiac. Total anomalous pulmonary venous connection of the infracardiac type.

*Corresponding author Oran B: Medicana International Hospital, Department of Pediatric Cardiology, İzmir, Turkey
E-mail:boran@medicana.com.tr and bulentoran@hotmail.com

Partial Abnormal Pulmonary Venous Return Anomalies

Right pulmonary veins open to the right atrium, superior vena cava, or inferior vena cava, rather than to the left atrium. Although there are many variations, the most common is the opening of the right upper and middle pulmonary veins to the superior vena cava (90%). Another anomaly is the opening of the left upper pulmonary vein to the innominate vein. Sinus venosus type ASDs (10-15%) are often reported.

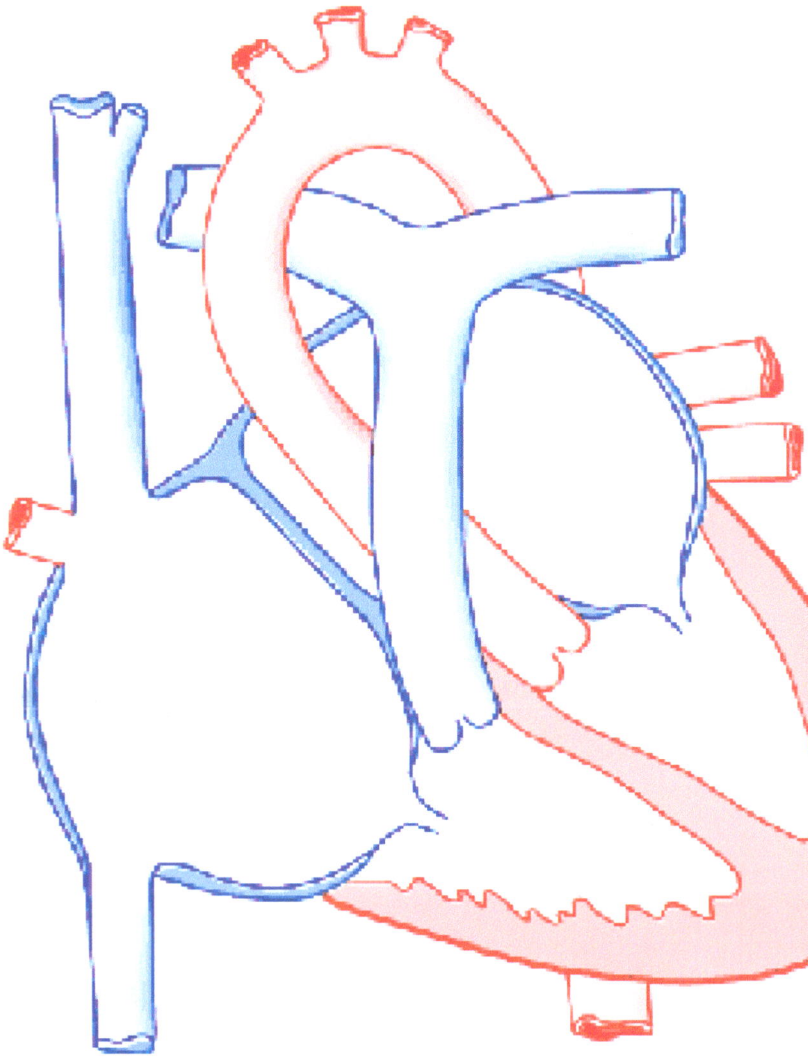

Figure 4: Partial abnormal pulmonary venous return anomalies. Partial anomalous pulmonary venous connection.

*Corresponding author Oran B: Medicana International Hospital, Department of Pediatric Cardiology, İzmir, Turkey
E-mail:boran@medicana.com.tr and bulentoran@hotmail.com

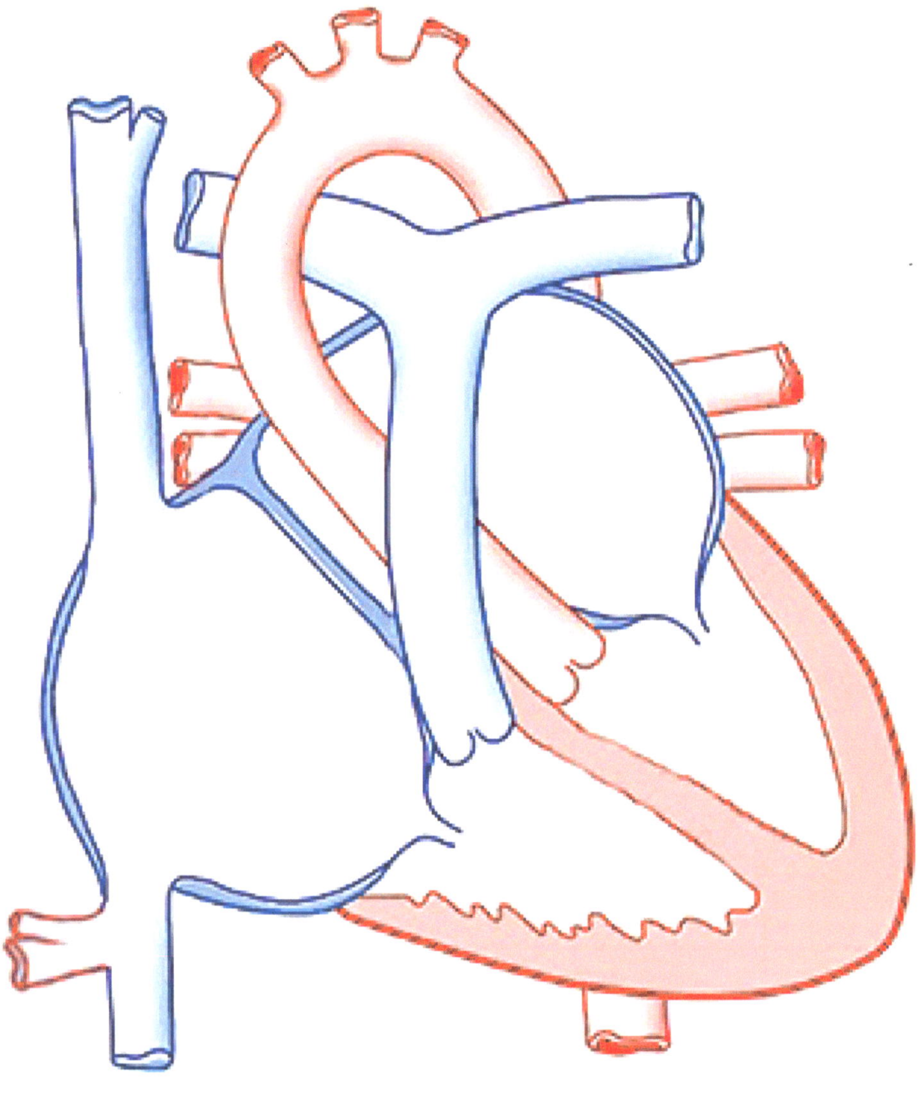

Figure 5: Partial abnormal pulmonary venous return anomalies. Partial anomalous pulmonary venous connection.

*Corresponding author Oran B: Medicana International Hospital, Department of Pediatric Cardiology, İzmir, Turkey
E-mail:boran@medicana.com.tr and bulentoran@hotmail.com

Scimitar Syndrome

Scimitar syndrome is a rare familial syndrome. The right lung is typically involved, but left lung involvement has been reported in rare cases. The lung on the affected side is usually hypoplastic. The lower-middle lobes of the affected lung receive their blood from the descending aorta, rather than from the pulmonary artery. Pulmonary veins drain to the inferior vena cava under the diaphragm, instead of the left atrium. Scimitar syndrome is associated with ASDs, VSDs, PDA, coarctation of the aorta, and tetralogy of Fallot.

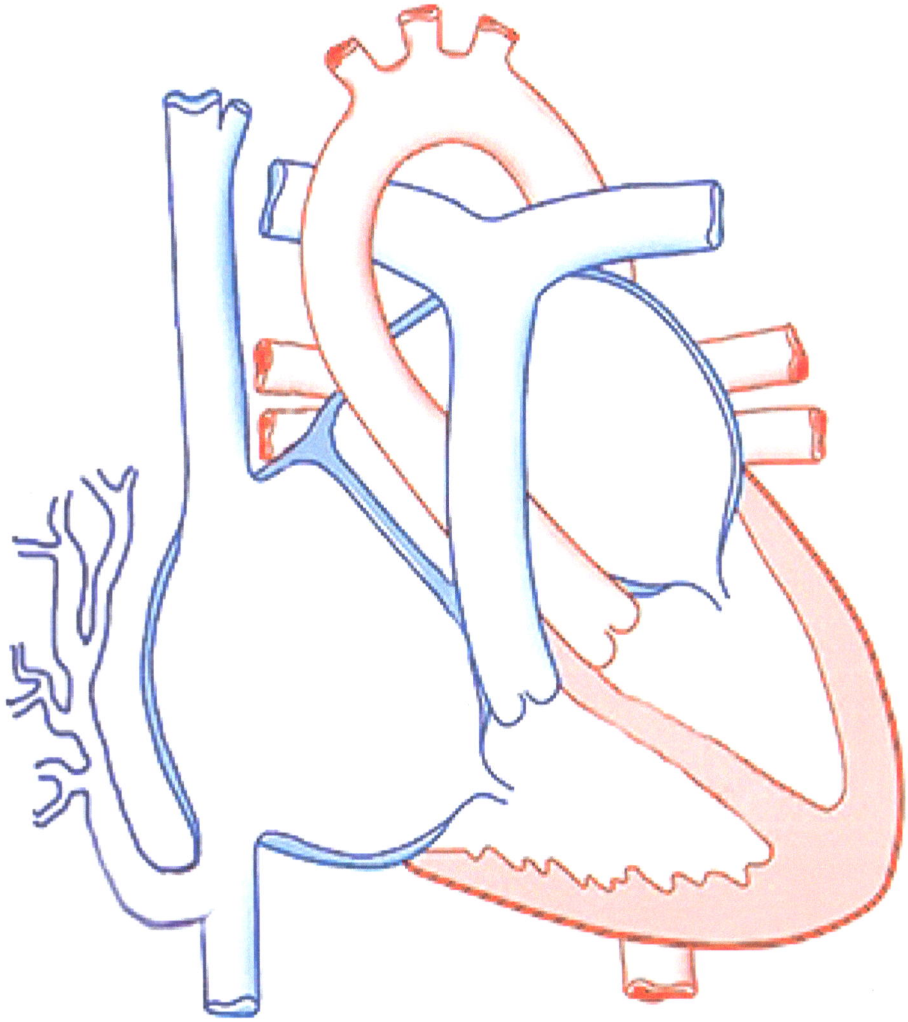

Figure 6: Scimitar syndrome. Partial anomalous pulmonary venous connection of Scimitar type.

*Corresponding author Oran B: Medicana International Hospital, Department of Pediatric Cardiology, İzmir, Turkey
E-mail:boran@medicana.com.tr and bulentoran@hotmail.com

Cor Triatriatum

In cor triatriatum, the left atrium is divided into a proximal chamber and a distal chamber by a fibromuscular membrane, thus causing the appearance of three atria. Pulmonary veins open to the proximal chamber of the left atrium; the left atrial appendage and mitral valve are located in the distal chamber. The membrane includes orifices with different diameters. There is often a connection between the right atrium and the distal chamber. Cor triatriatum is associated with secundum ASDs (50%), partial or total abnormal pulmonary venous return anomaly, PDA, and left persistent superior vena cava and pulmonary vein stenosis.

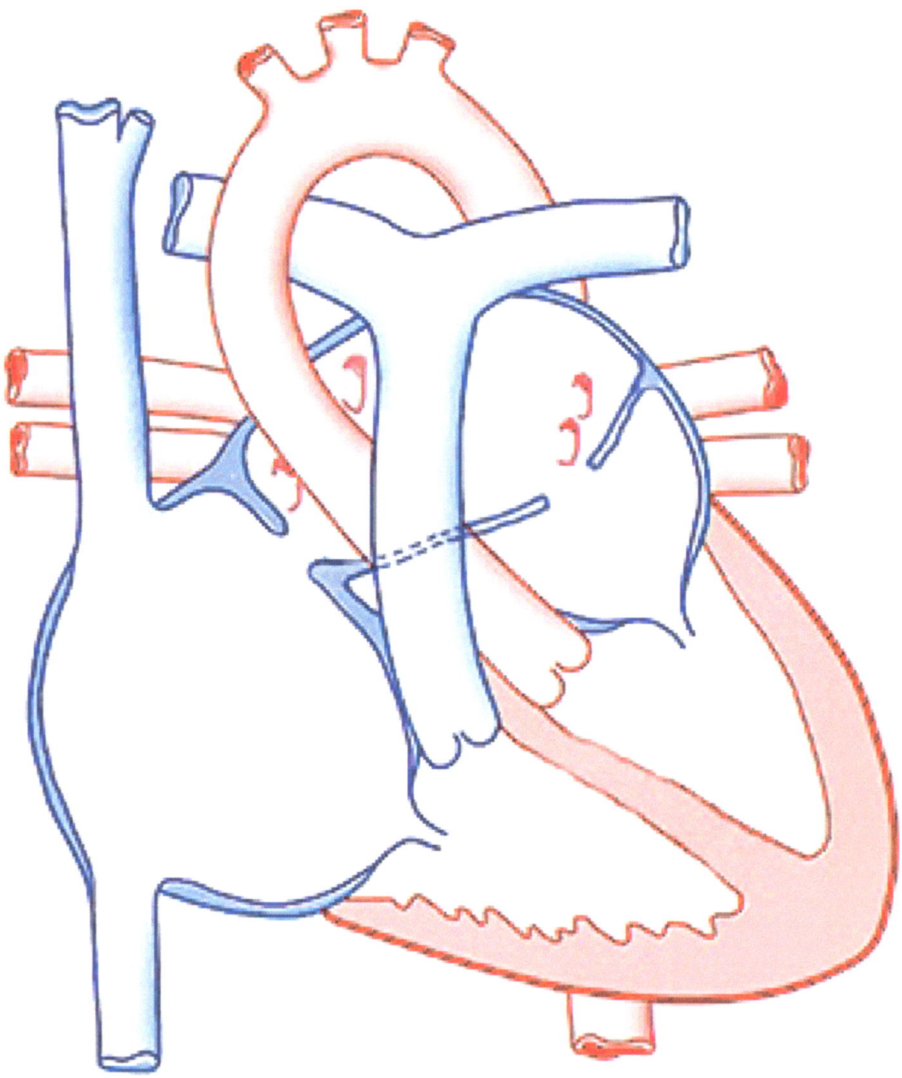

Figure 7: Cor triatriatum. Divided left atrium

*Corresponding author Oran B: Medicana International Hospital, Department of Pediatric Cardiology, İzmir, Turkey
E-mail:boran@medicana.com.tr and bulentoran@hotmail.com

Supravalvar Mitral Ring

The supravalvar mitral ring is characterized by an abnormal ridge of connective tissue on the atrial side of the mitral valve, which obstructs the mitral valve inflow.

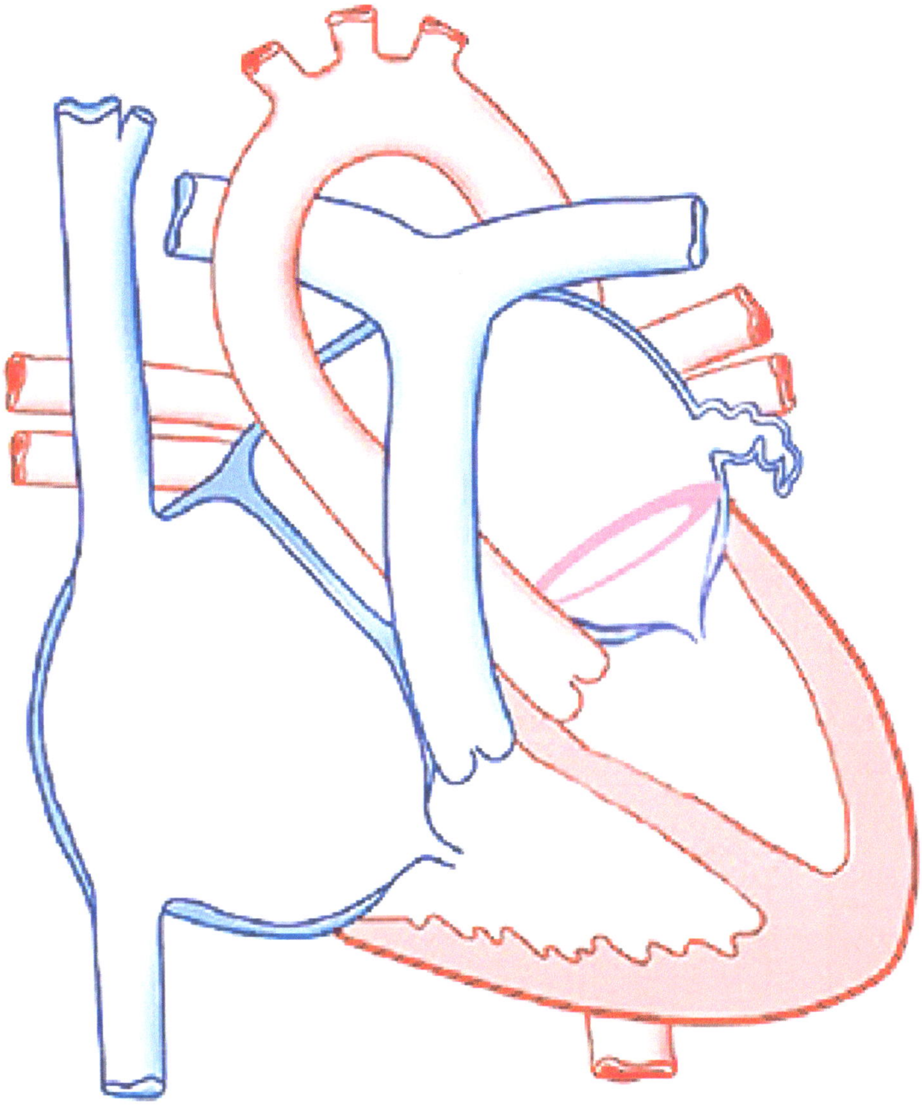

Figure 8: Supravalvar mitral ring.

*Corresponding author Oran B: Medicana International Hospital, Department of Pediatric Cardiology, İzmir, Turkey
E-mail:boran@medicana.com.tr and bulentoran@hotmail.com

Parachute Mitral Valve

A parachute mitral valve occurs when the mitral valve chordae insert into a single papillary muscle. This condition may contribute to mitral stenosis.

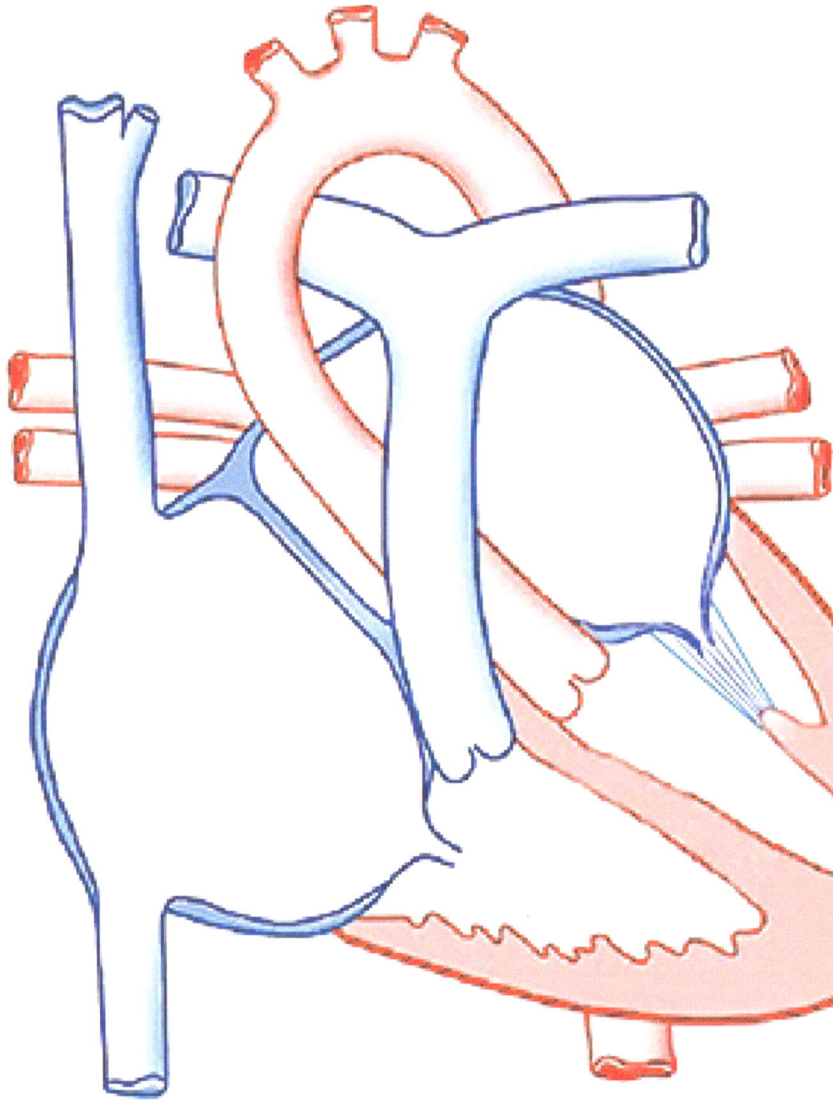

Figure 9: Parachute mitral valve. Parachute malformation of mitral valve.

*Corresponding author Oran B: Medicana International Hospital, Department of Pediatric Cardiology, İzmir, Turkey
E-mail:boran@medicana.com.tr and bulentoran@hotmail.com

CHAPTER 5
Systemic Venous Anomalies

Oran B.

Medicana International Hospital, Department of Pediatric Cardiology, İzmir, Turkey

*Corresponding author Oran B: Medicana International Hospital, Department of Pediatric Cardiology, İzmir, Turkey
E-mail:boran@medicana.com.tr and bulentoran@hotmail.com

Vena Cava Superior Anomalies

Persistent left superior vena cava drainage is the most common congenital anomaly of the systemic venous system. This condition lacks hemodynamic features; it is often recognized during transvenous pacemaker implantation and/or cardiac surgery. The superior vena cava typically opens to the right atrium via the coronary sinus. Tetralogy of Fallot is commonly reported as an associated anomaly.

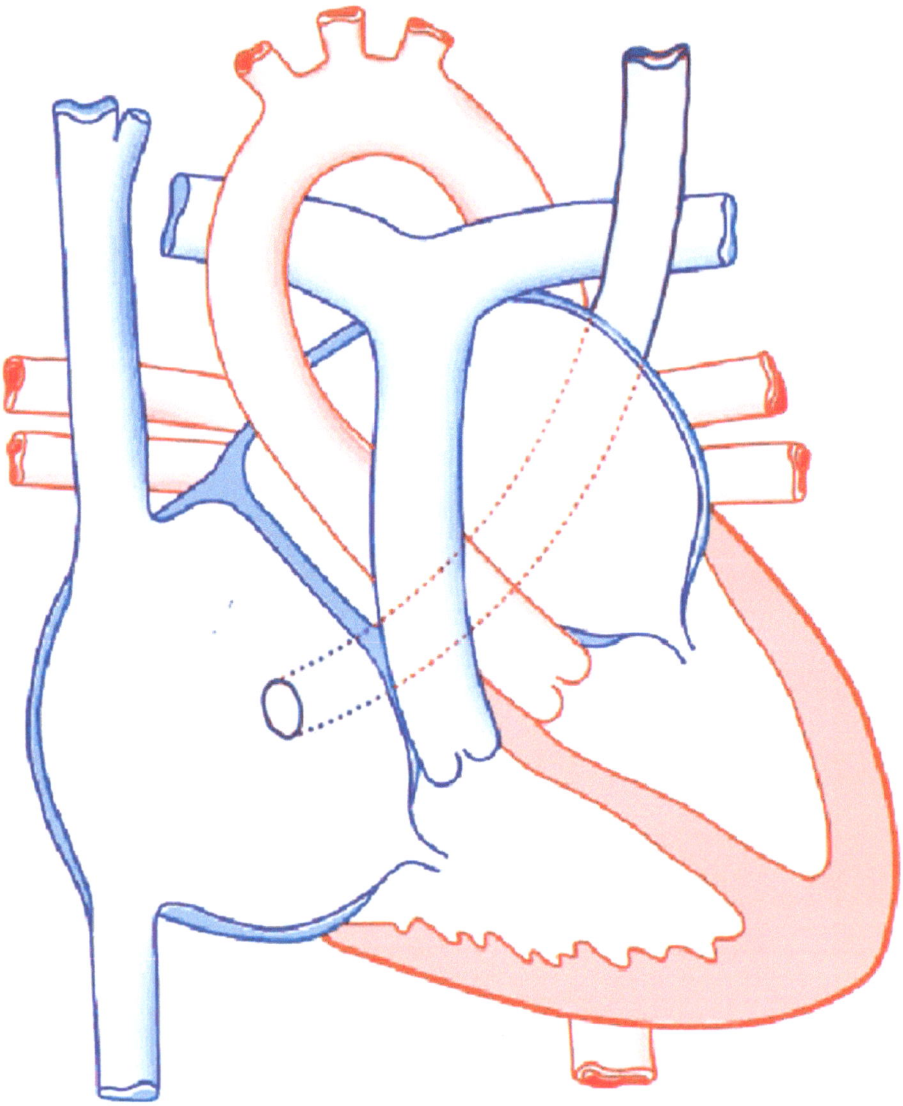

Figure 1: Left SVC persisting to coronary sinus. Left superior caval vein to coronary sinus.

*Corresponding author Oran B: Medicana International Hospital, Department of Pediatric Cardiology, İzmir, Turkey
E-mail:boran@medicana.com.tr and bulentoran@hotmail.com

Persistent Left Superior Vena Cava Draining Into the Left Atrium

Persistent drainage of the left superior vena cava into the left atrium is uncommon and causes minimal left-to-right shunting with mild cyanosis. The defect lies between the posterior wall of the left atrium and the coronary sinus (roofless coronary sinus).

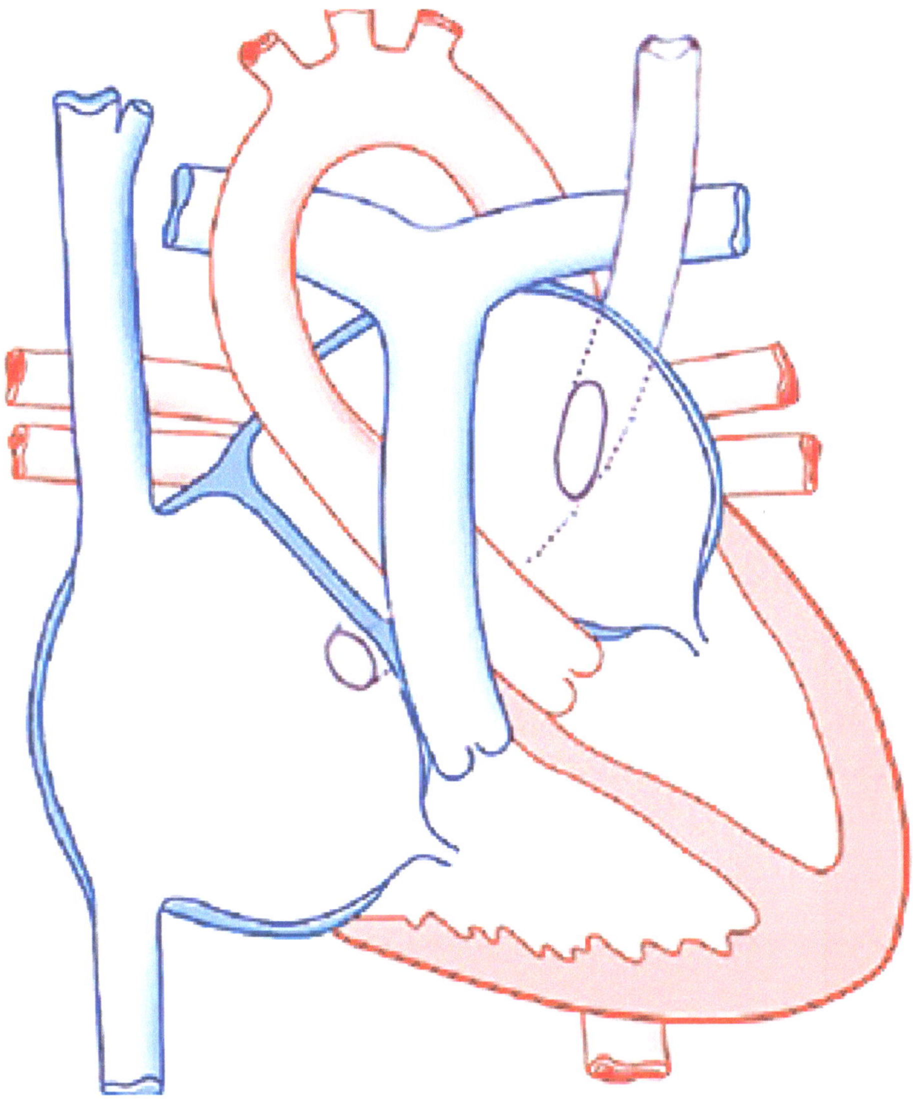

Figure 2: Left superior vena cava persisting to left atrium. Left superior caval vein to left-sided atrium, Unroofed coronary sinus.

*Corresponding author Oran B: Medicana International Hospital, Department of Pediatric Cardiology, İzmir, Turkey
E-mail:boran@medicana.com.tr and bulentoran@hotmail.com

Persistent Left Superior Vena Cava with Absent Right Superior Vena Cava

Persistent left superior vena cava with absent right superior vena cava (isolated left superior vena cava) is a very rare venous malformation. It is typically asymptomatic, but can impede central venous access, pacemaker implantation, and heart surgery.

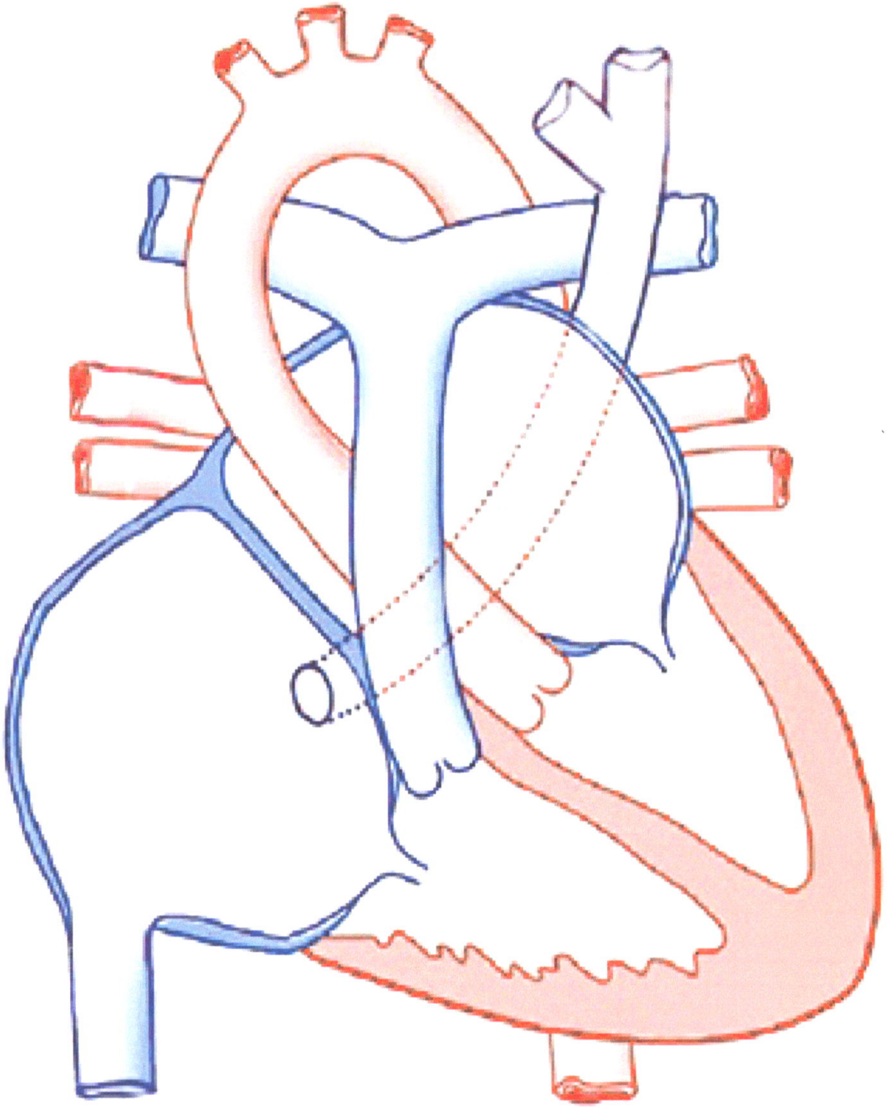

Figure 3: Persistent left superior vena cava with absent right superior vena cava. Absent right superior caval vein.

*Corresponding author Oran B: Medicana International Hospital, Department of Pediatric Cardiology, İzmir, Turkey
E-mail:boran@medicana.com.tr and bulentoran@hotmail.com

Inferior Vena Cava Anomalies

Inferior vena cava anomalies include azygos and hemiazygos continuation. The infrahepatic portion of the inferior vena cava is absent and the inferior vena cava is interrupted. In addition, the hepatic veins drain directly into the right atrium. The lower systemic venous return is mediated by the azygos or hemiazygos veins, which are enlarged. Among additional anomalies, left atrial isomerism is frequently reported.

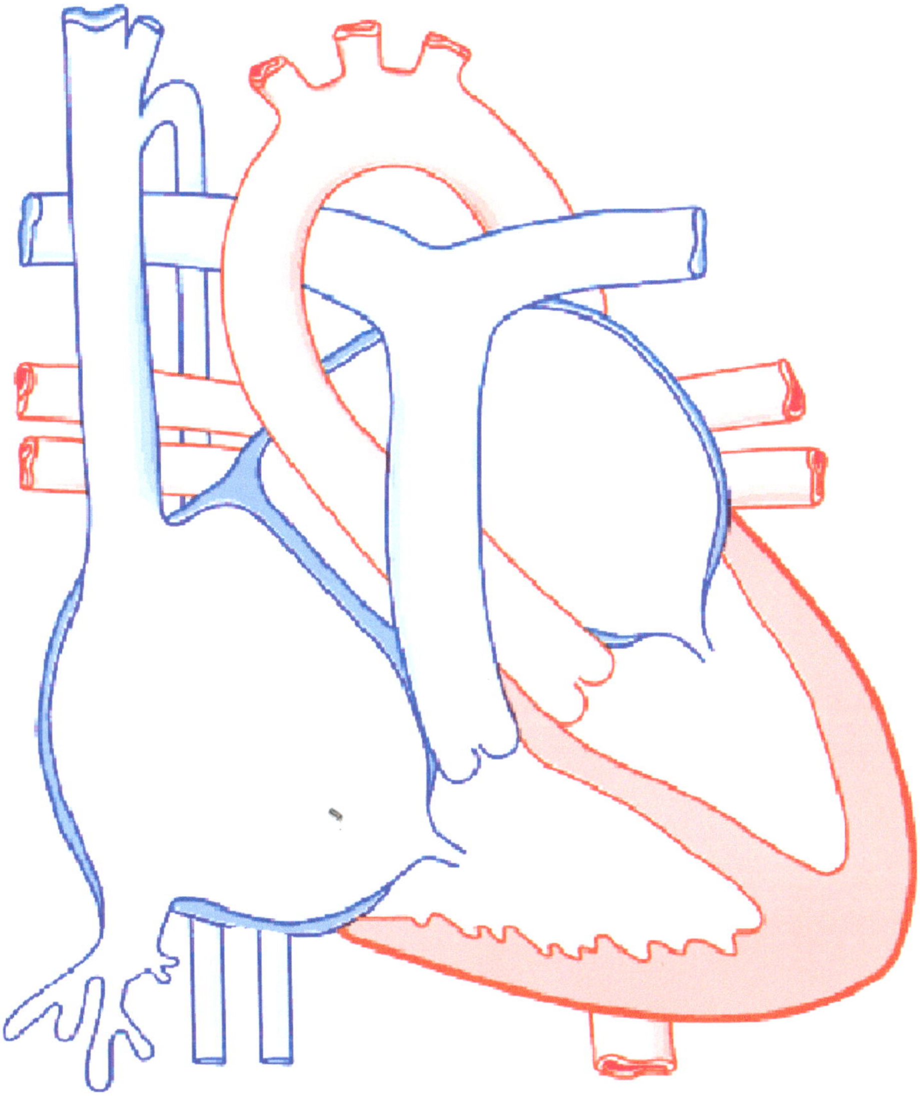

Figure 4: Vena azygos and hemi-azygos continuity of inferior vena cava. Interrupted inferior caval vein with absent suprarenal segment and azygos continuation.

*Corresponding author Oran B: Medicana International Hospital, Department of Pediatric Cardiology, İzmir, Turkey
E-mail:boran@medicana.com.tr and bulentoran@hotmail.com

*Corresponding author Oran B: Medicana International Hospital, Department of Pediatric Cardiology, İzmir, Turkey
E-mail:boran@medicana.com.tr and bulentoran@hotmail.com

CHAPTER 6

Right and Left Ventricular Anomalies

Oran B.

Medicana International Hospital, Department of Pediatric Cardiology, İzmir, Turkey

*Corresponding author Oran B: Medicana International Hospital, Department of Pediatric Cardiology, İzmir, Turkey
E-mail:boran@medicana.com.tr and bulentoran@hotmail.com

Ebstein Anomaly

The Ebstein anomaly is a rare condition in which the posterior and septal valves of the tricuspid valve are displaced into the right ventricle; this condition is characterized by tricuspid stiffness. The inlet portion of the right ventricle is connected to the right atrium and termed the "atrialized right ventricle." The anterior leaflet of the tricuspid valve is enlarged and appears sail-like; this promotes pulmonary stenosis due to shortened chordae. The right atrium is also considerably enlarged. ASDs, PDA, pulmonary stenosis or pulmonary atresia, Wolff-Parkinson-White syndrome, bicuspid aortic valve, aortic stenosis, coarctation of the aorta, and tetralogy of Fallot are malformations associated with Ebstein anomalies.

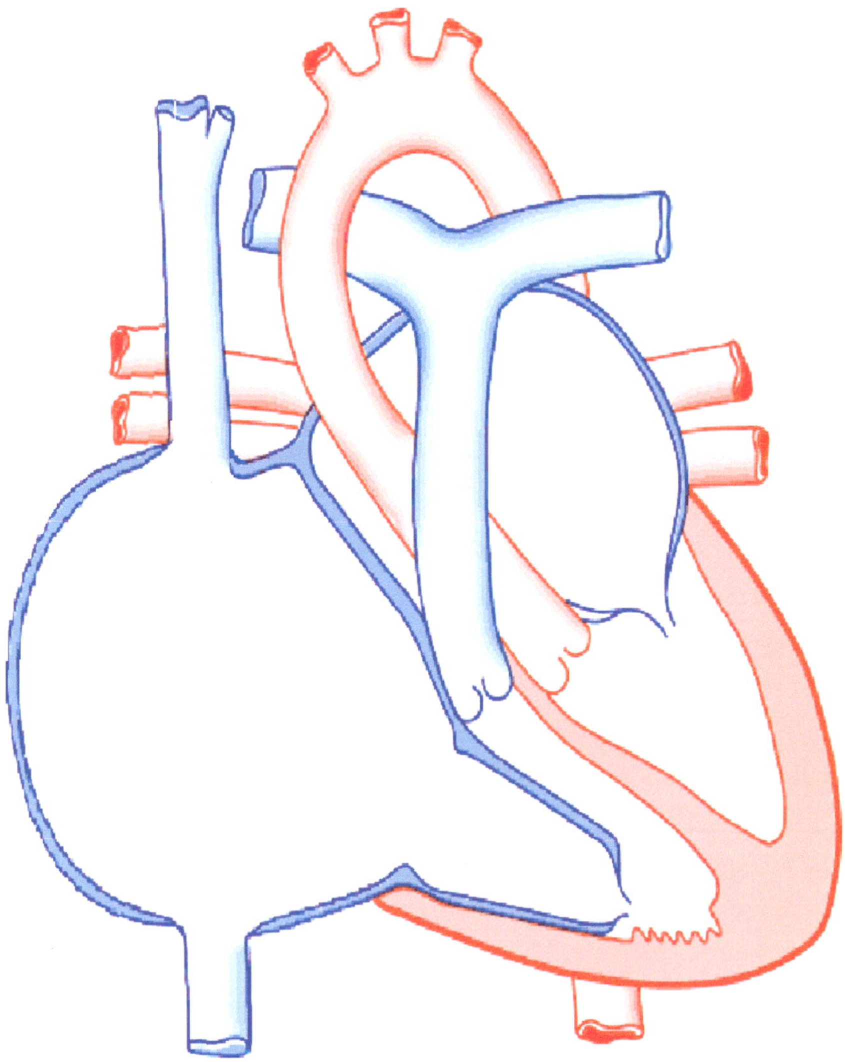

Figure 1: Ebstein anomaly (Ebstein's malformation of tricuspid valve). Ebstein malformation of tricuspid valve and congenital giant right atrium.

*Corresponding author Oran B: Medicana International Hospital, Department of Pediatric Cardiology, İzmir, Turkey
E-mail:boran@medicana.com.tr and bulentoran@hotmail.com

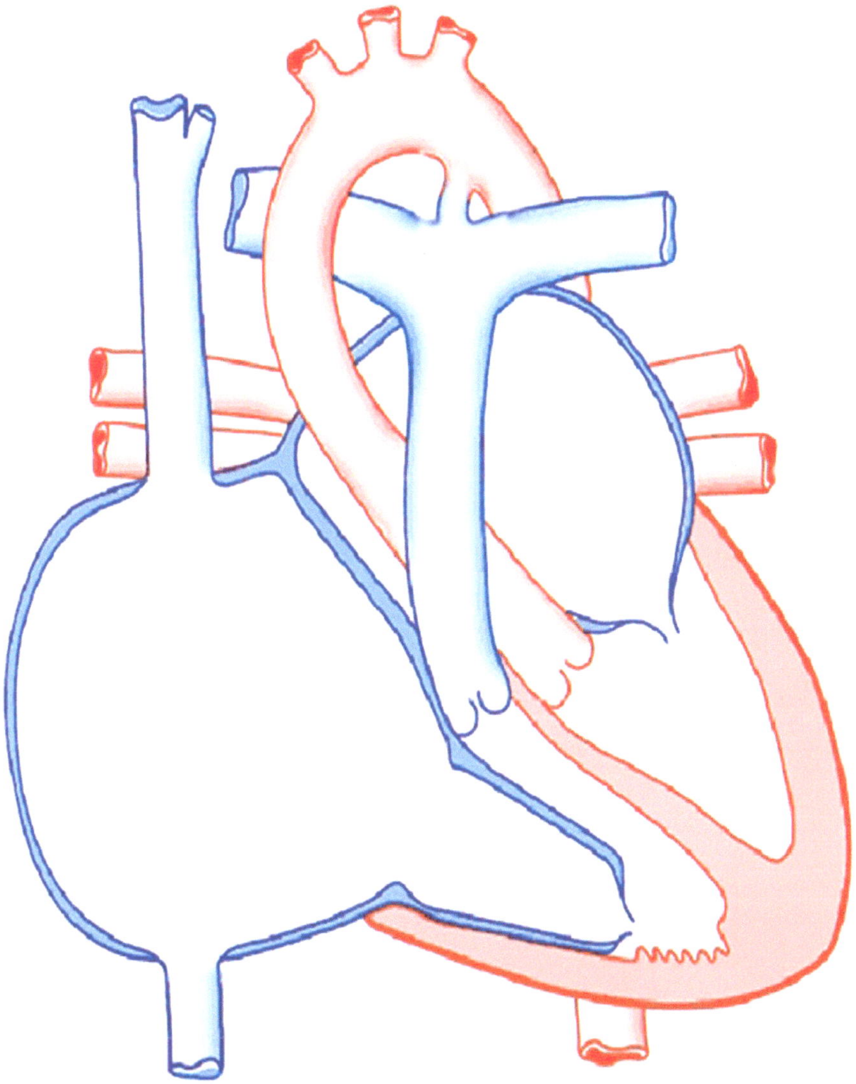

Figure 2: Ebstein anomaly (Ebstein's malformation of tricuspid valve), PDA. Ebstein malformation of tricuspid valve and congenital giant right atrium with patent arterial duct.

*Corresponding author Oran B: Medicana International Hospital, Department of Pediatric Cardiology, İzmir, Turkey
E-mail:boran@medicana.com.tr and bulentoran@hotmail.com

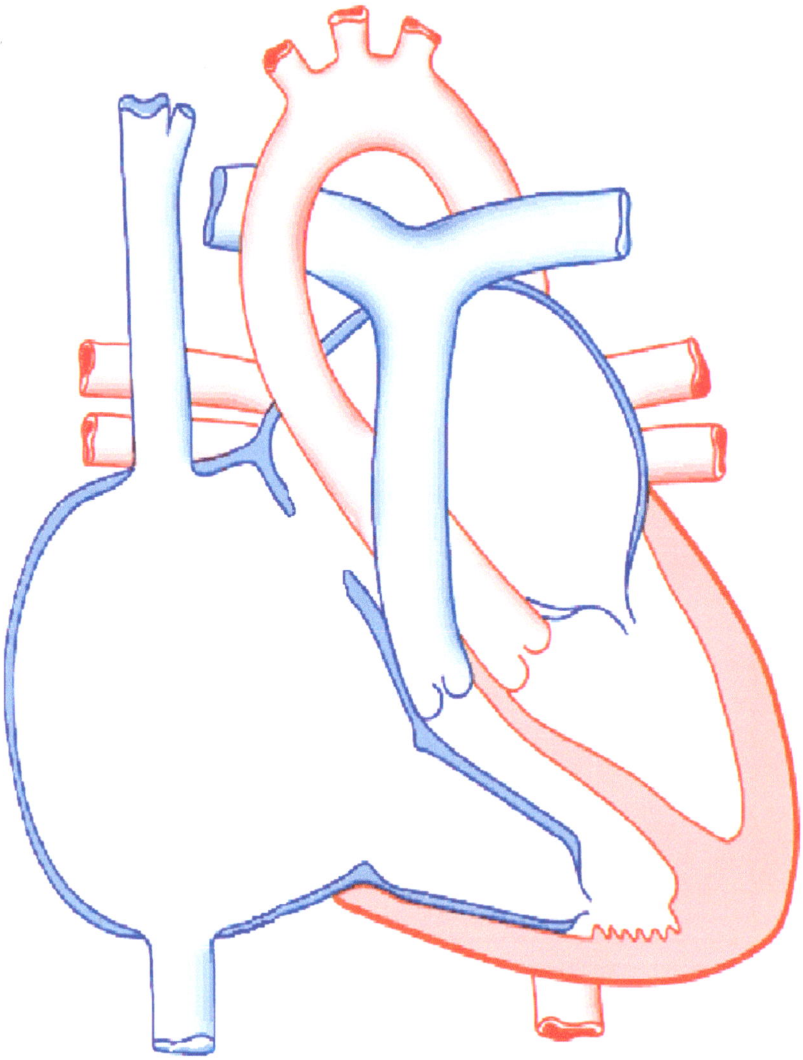

Figure 3: Ebstein anomaly (Ebstein's malformation of tricuspid valve), ASD. Ebstein malformation of tricuspid valve and congenital giant right atrium, atrial septal defect within oval fossa.

*Corresponding author Oran B: Medicana International Hospital, Department of Pediatric Cardiology, İzmir, Turkey
E-mail:boran@medicana.com.tr and bulentoran@hotmail.com

Uhl's Anomaly

Uhl's anomaly (parchment heart) is characterized by the absence of the right ventricle myocardial layer, which causes the right ventricular wall to be very thin and hypocontractile. Without the myocardial layer, the endocardium connects directly to the epicardium. It is impossible for these patients to survive into adulthood without surgery.

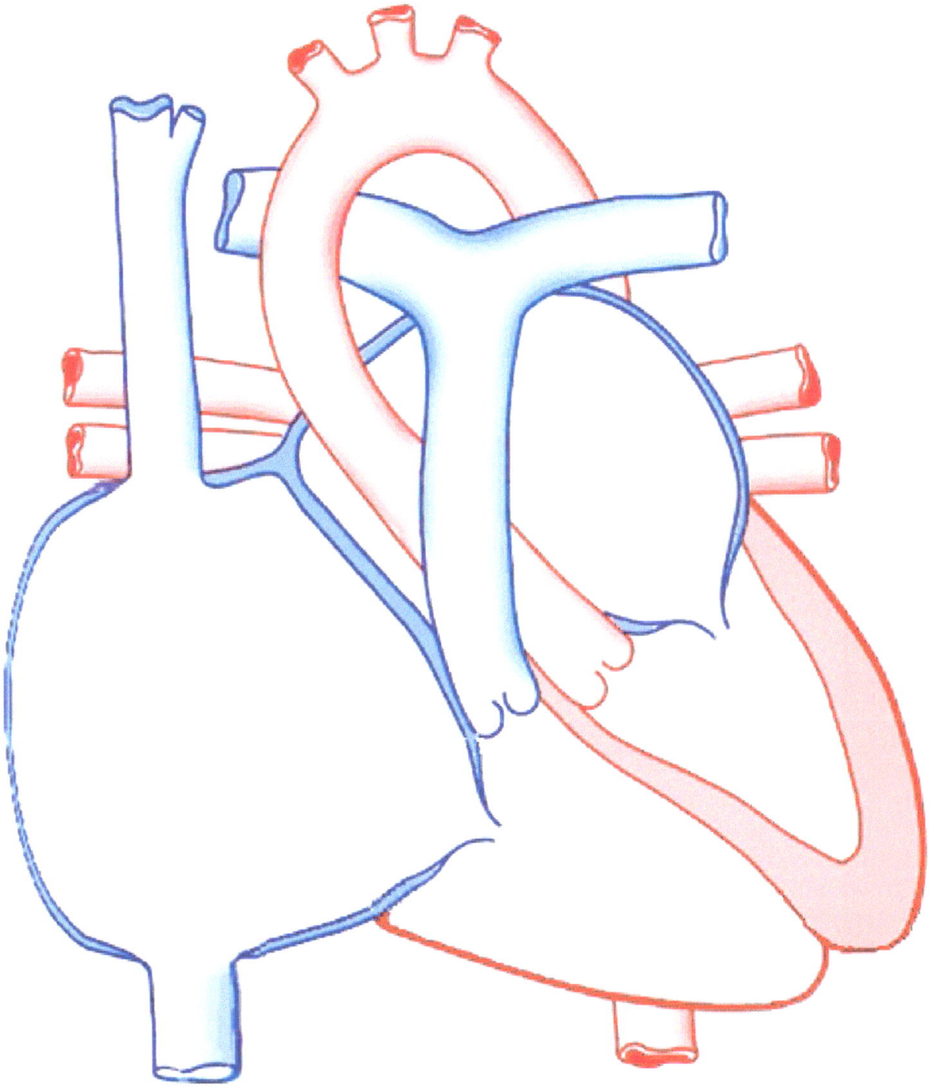

Figure 4: Uhl anomaly. Parchment right ventricle.

*Corresponding author Oran B: Medicana International Hospital, Department of Pediatric Cardiology, İzmir, Turkey
E-mail:boran@medicana.com.tr and bulentoran@hotmail.com

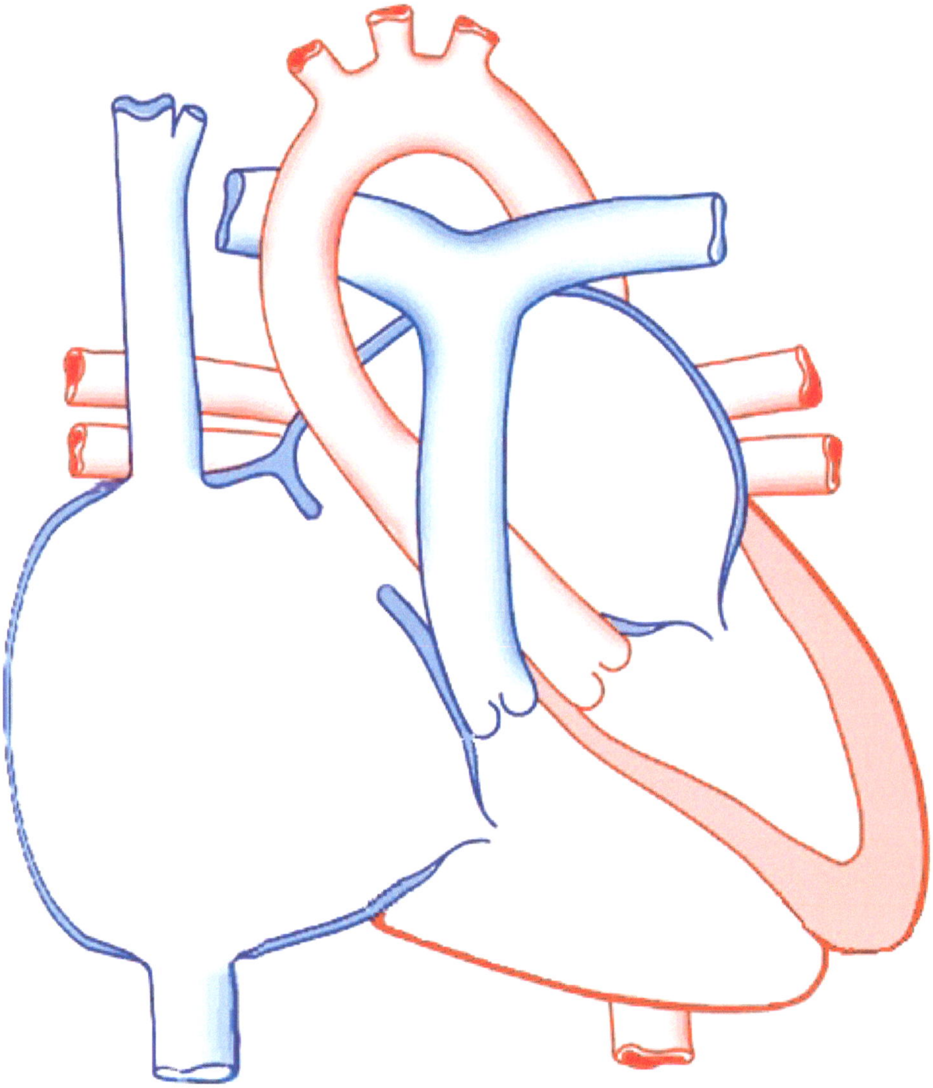

Figure 5: Uhl anomaly, ASD. Parchment right ventricle with atrial septal defect within oval fossa.

*Corresponding author Oran B: Medicana International Hospital, Department of Pediatric Cardiology, İzmir, Turkey
E-mail:boran@medicana.com.tr and bulentoran@hotmail.com

Double-Chambered Right Ventricle

Double-chambered right ventricles are characterized by large anomalous myocardial bands, which cause both infundibular and sub-infundibular stenosis. These bands divide the right ventricle into two chambers: proximal chambers (high-pressure) and distal chambers (low-pressure). A pressure gradient exists when the transition between the two separate chambers is narrow. Perimembranous VSDs typically accompany this malformation. The presence of a mild to moderate pressure gradient in childhood does not produce many symptoms, but stenosis is progressive in adulthood and may eventually lead to right ventricular hypertrophy and dilatation.

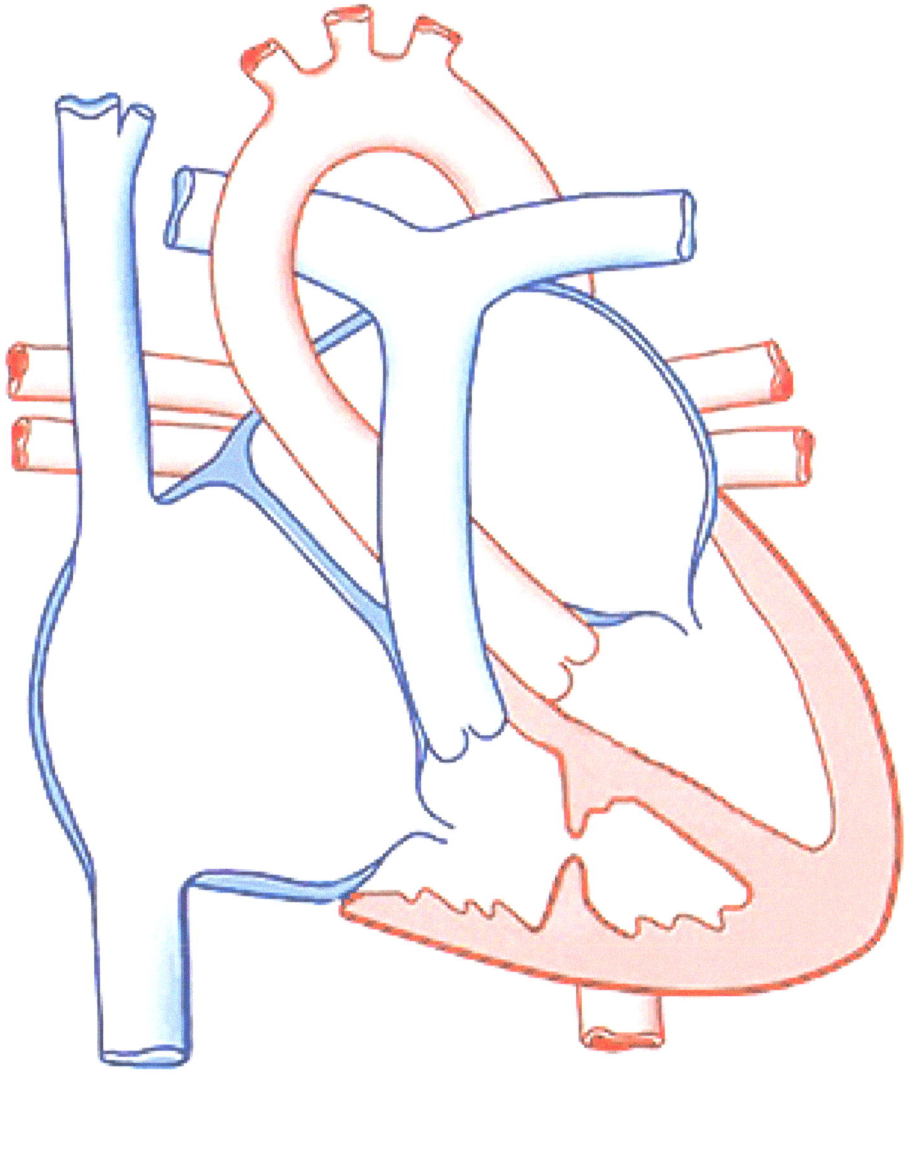

Figure 6: Double-chambered right ventricle. Double chambered right ventricle.

*Corresponding author Oran B: Medicana International Hospital, Department of Pediatric Cardiology, İzmir, Turkey
E-mail:boran@medicana.com.tr and bulentoran@hotmail.com

Double Outlet Right Ventricle

Double outlet right ventricle is a cardiac malformation in which both the aorta and pulmonary artery arise from the right ventricle. The morphological anatomy of double outlet right ventricle ranges from tetralogy of Fallot to transposition of the great arteries. The great arteries may override the ventricular septum by more than 50%, or both arteries may arise fully from the right ventricle. There are four types of double outlet right ventricle: tetralogy of Fallot, transposition of the great arteries, single ventricle, and remote VSD.

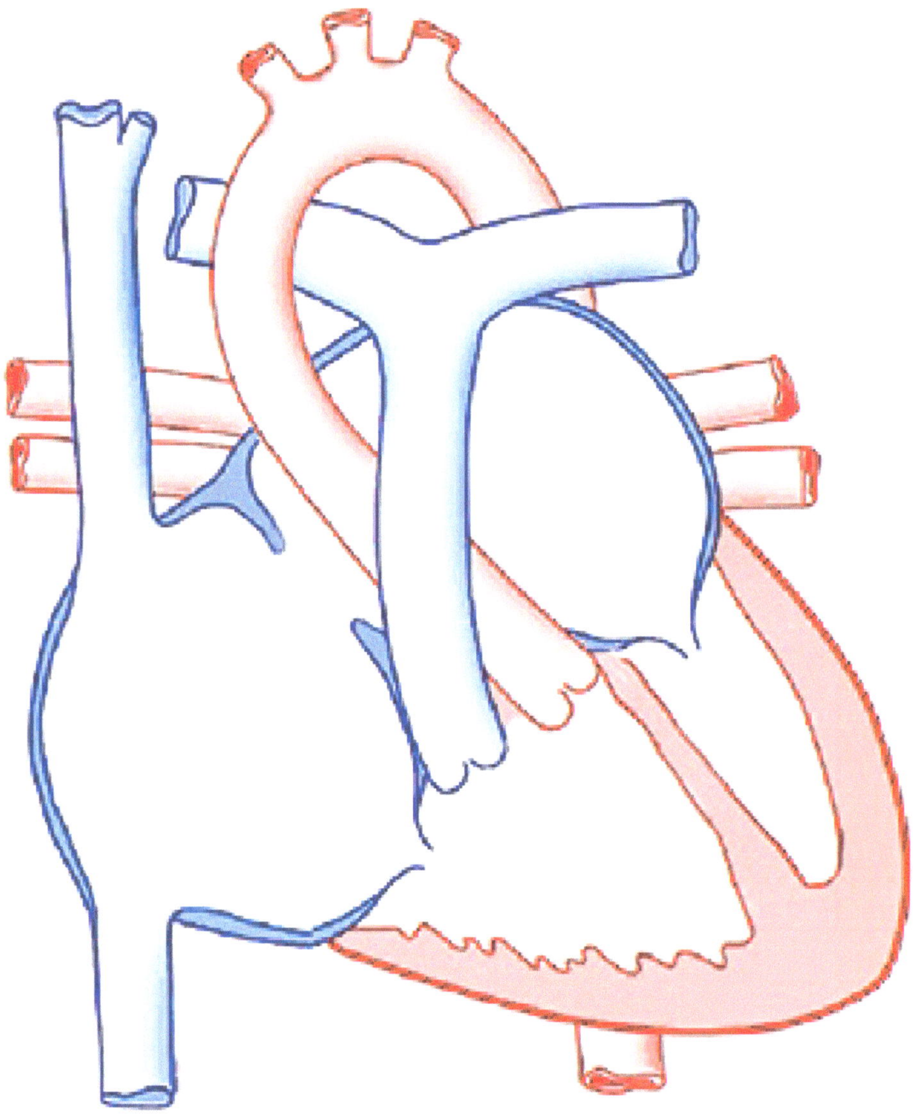

Figure 7: Double outlet right ventricle. Double outlet right ventricle without pulmonary stenosis.

*Corresponding author Oran B: Medicana International Hospital, Department of Pediatric Cardiology, İzmir, Turkey
E-mail:boran@medicana.com.tr and bulentoran@hotmail.com

Double Outlet Right Ventricle, Fallot type

The Fallot type double outlet right ventricle is characterized by ASDs, VSDs, and pulmonary infundibular stenosis. Without treatment, prognosis is poor due to severe cyanosis.

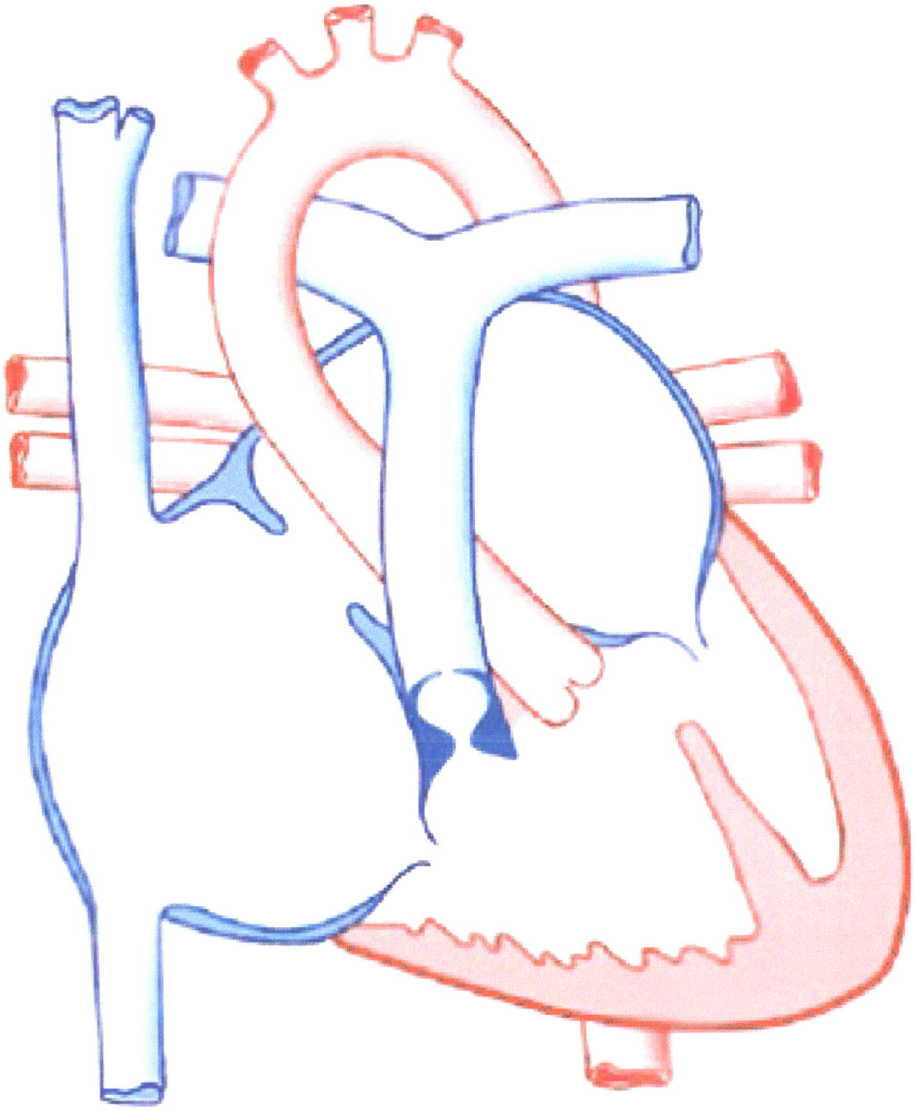

Figure 8: Double outlet right ventricle, Fallot type. Double outlet right ventricle with ventricular septal defect and pulmonary stenosis, Fallot type.

*Corresponding author Oran B: Medicana International Hospital, Department of Pediatric Cardiology, İzmir, Turkey
E-mail:boran@medicana.com.tr and bulentoran@hotmail.com

Double Outlet Right Ventricle, Transposition type (Taussig Bing type)

The Tasussig Bing heart defect is characterized by a double outlet right ventricle and an abnormal ventriculo-arterial connection with transposition of the great arteries. Hemodynamic findings are similar to those in patients with transposition of the great arteries.

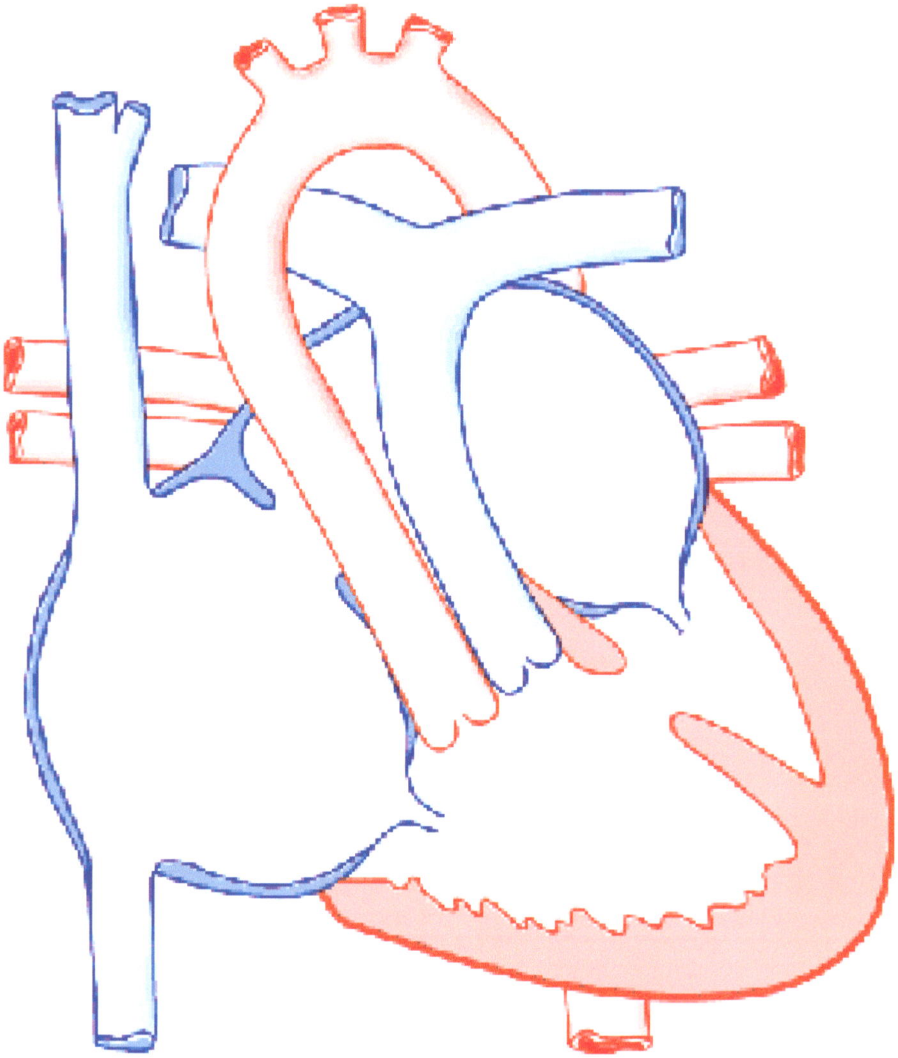

Figure 9: Double outlet right ventricle, transposition type (Taussig Bing type), ASD. Double outlet right ventricle with subpulmonary ventricular septal defect, transposition type and atrial septal defect within oval fossa.

*Corresponding author Oran B: Medicana International Hospital, Department of Pediatric Cardiology, İzmir, Turkey
E-mail:boran@medicana.com.tr and bulentoran@hotmail.com

Double Outlet Right Ventricle, Remote VSD type

Double outlet right ventricle coexists with VSDs (often, muscle VSDs).

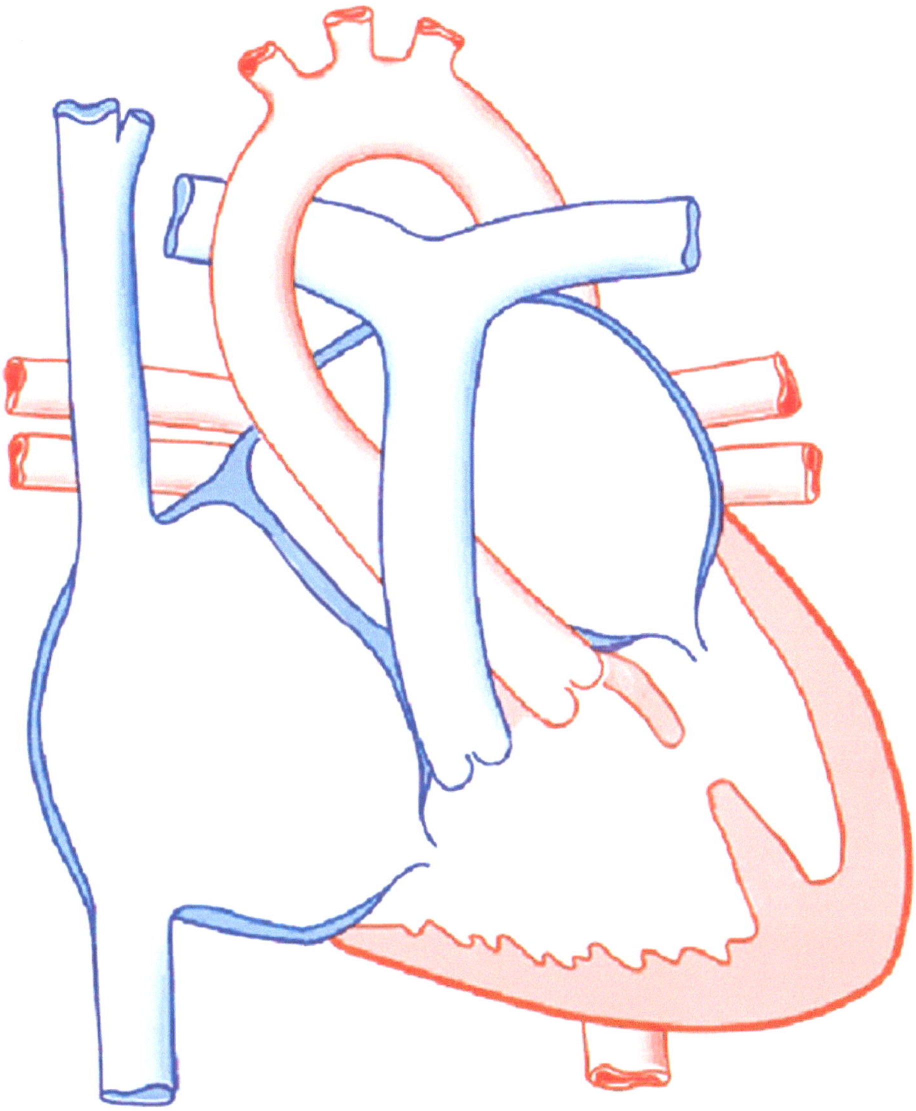

Figure 10: Double outlet right ventricle, remote VSD type.

*Corresponding author Oran B: Medicana International Hospital, Department of Pediatric Cardiology, İzmir, Turkey
E-mail:boran@medicana.com.tr and bulentoran@hotmail.com

Double Outlet Right Ventricle, Single Ventricle type

This malformation is characterized by the presence of a single ventricle. It is impossible for these patients to survive into adulthood without Interventional procedures or surgery.

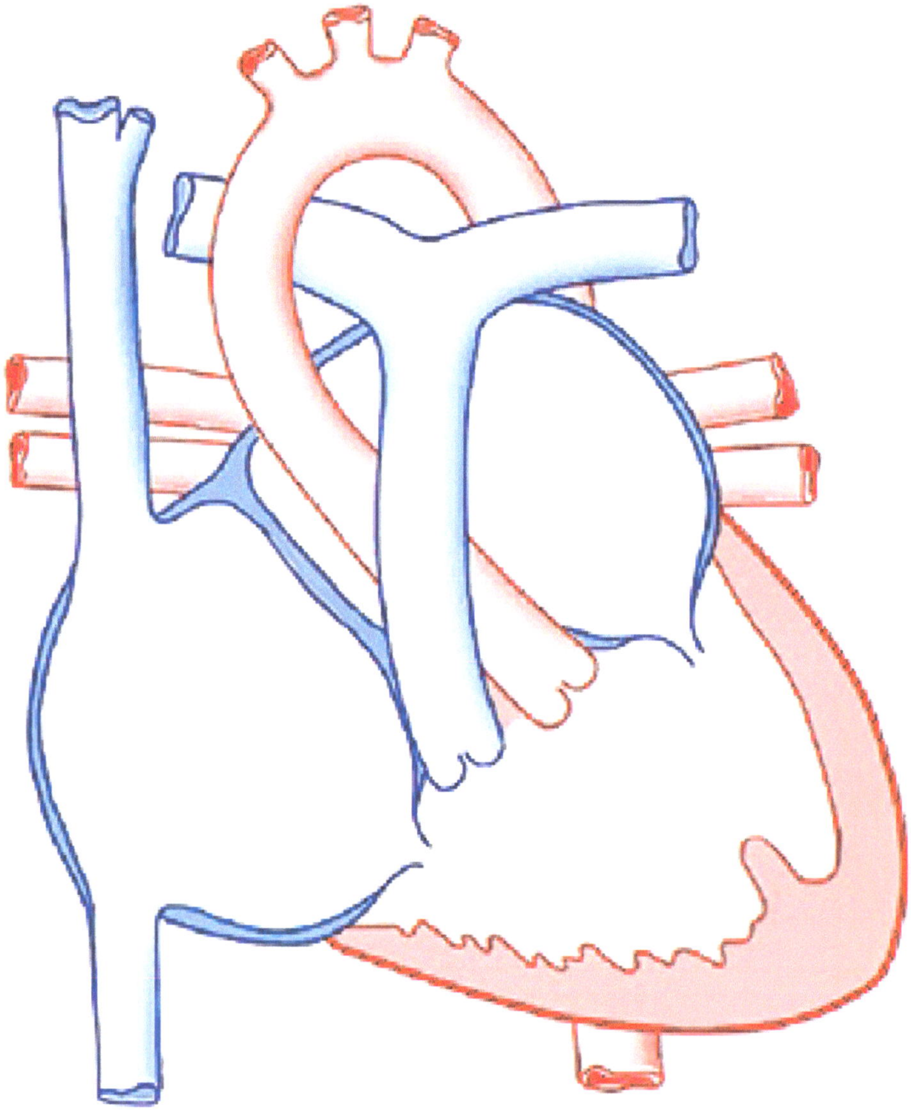

Figure 11: Double outlet right ventricle, single ventricle type.

*Corresponding author Oran B: Medicana International Hospital, Department of Pediatric Cardiology, İzmir, Turkey
E-mail:boran@medicana.com.tr and bulentoran@hotmail.com

Double Outlet Right Ventricle with Intact Ventricular Septum

A double outlet right ventricle with an intact ventricular septum is extremely rare. A VSD is necessary for survival, since it represents the only outlet of the left ventricle. The degrees of left ventricular and mitral hyperplasia influence interatrial communication. It is impossible for these patients to survive into adulthood without interventional procedures or surgery.

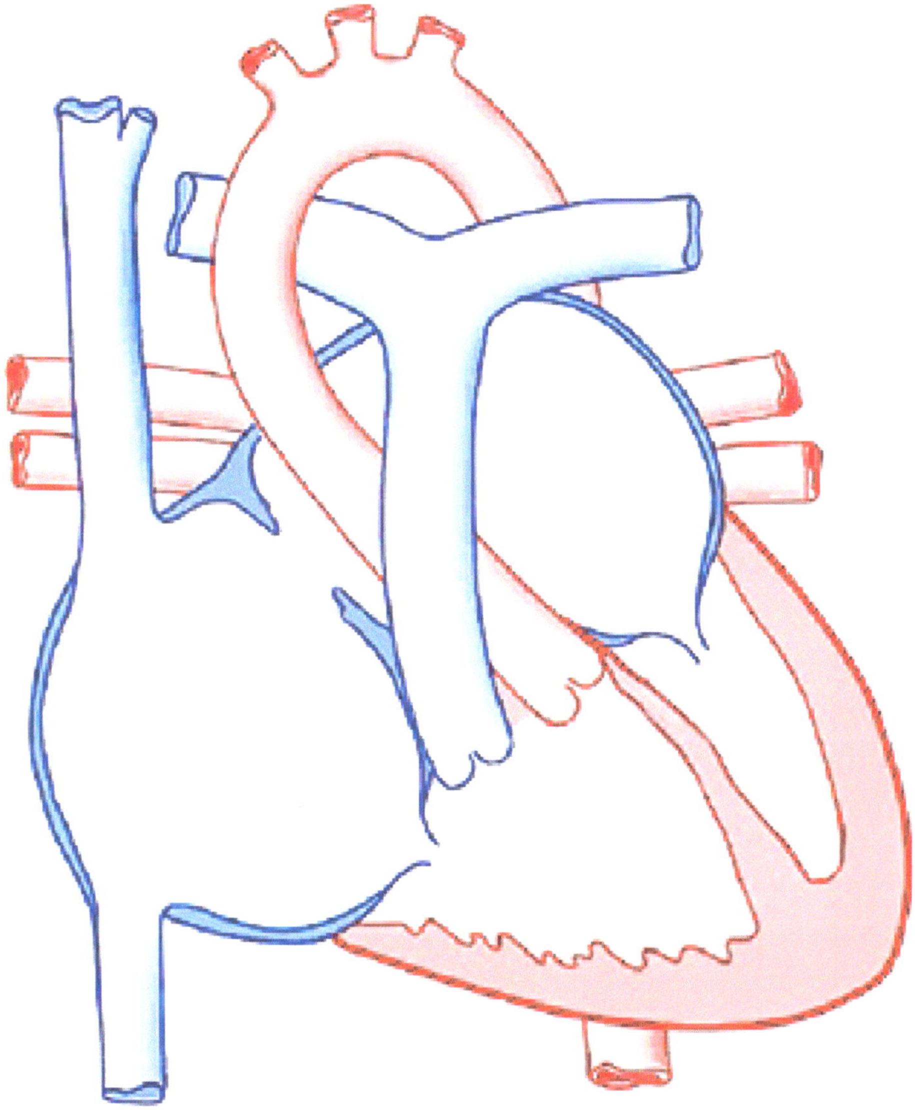

Figure 12: Double outlet right ventricle with intact ventricular septum and ASD..

*Corresponding author Oran B: Medicana International Hospital, Department of Pediatric Cardiology, İzmir, Turkey
E-mail:boran@medicana.com.tr and bulentoran@hotmail.com

Double Outlet Left Ventricle

In double outlet left ventricle, both the aorta and the pulmonary artery arise, either exclusively or predominantly, from the morphological left ventricle. This anomaly encompasses a broad spectrum of clinical and pathologic features of various physiologic entities, ranging from simple VSD to tetralogy of Fallot and complete transposition of the great arteries.

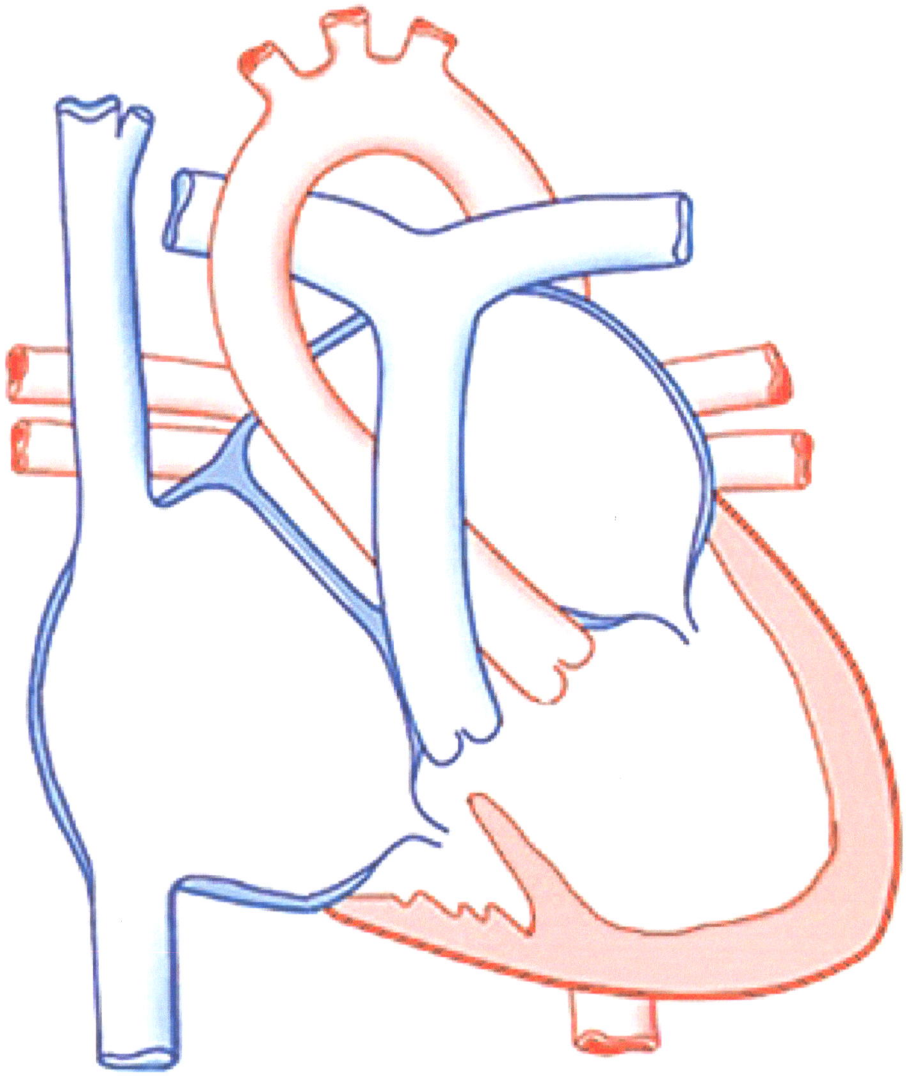

Figure 13: Double outlet left ventricle and VSD

.

*Corresponding author Oran B: Medicana International Hospital, Department of Pediatric Cardiology, İzmir, Turkey
E-mail:boran@medicana.com.tr and bulentoran@hotmail.com

Mirror Image Dextrocardi, ASD, VSD

Dextrocardia with situs inversus refers to a mirror image heart, situated on the right side. In patients with mirror image dextrocardia, the apex of the heart is located on the right side.

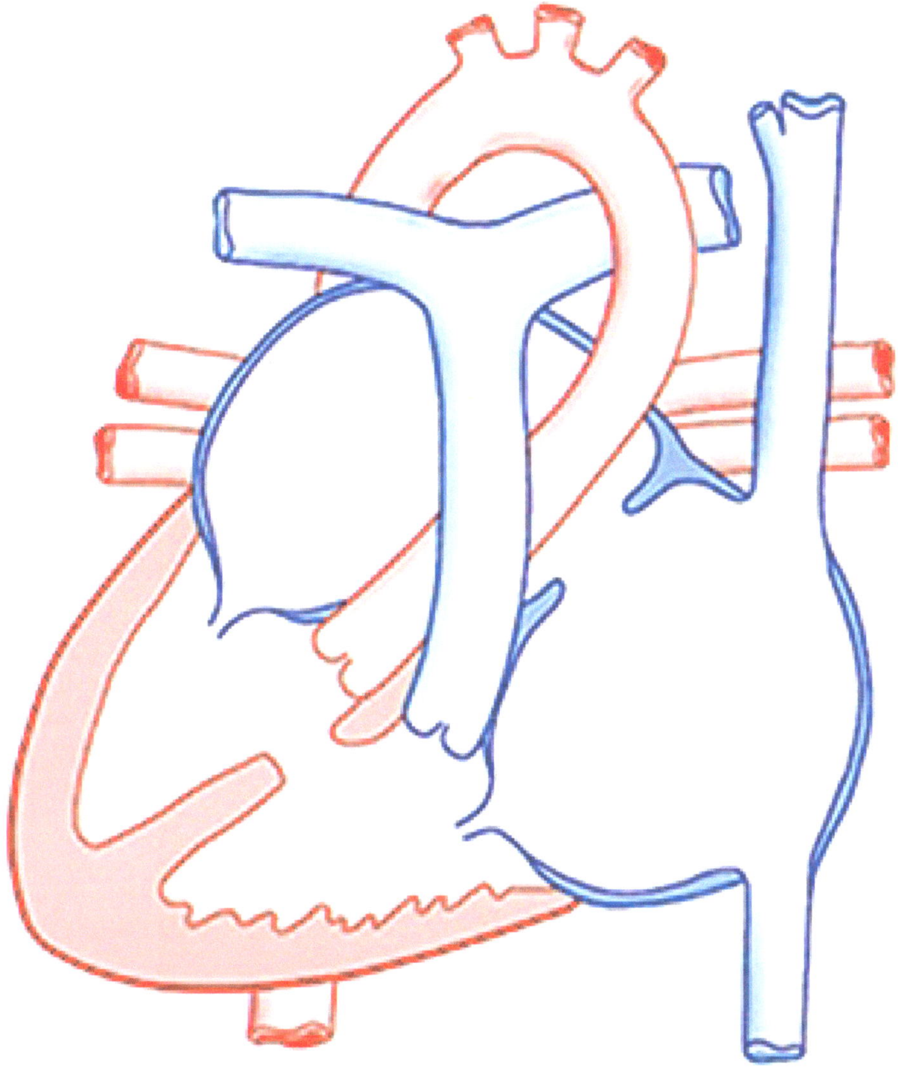

Figure 14: Mirror image dextrocardi, ASD, VSD. Total mirror imagery, ventricular septal defect, and atrial septal defect within oval fossa.

*Corresponding author Oran B: Medicana International Hospital, Department of Pediatric Cardiology, İzmir, Turkey
E-mail:boran@medicana.com.tr and bulentoran@hotmail.com

Ventricular diverticulum and aneurysm

The ventricular diverticulum is a congenital anomaly unlike aneurysms and contains all the layers (endocardium, myocardium and pericardium) of the heart. Ventricular aneurysm do not contain all layers of the heart and contain only fibrous tissue and pericardium, so they do not have contractile properties. They usually develop secondary to other diseases.

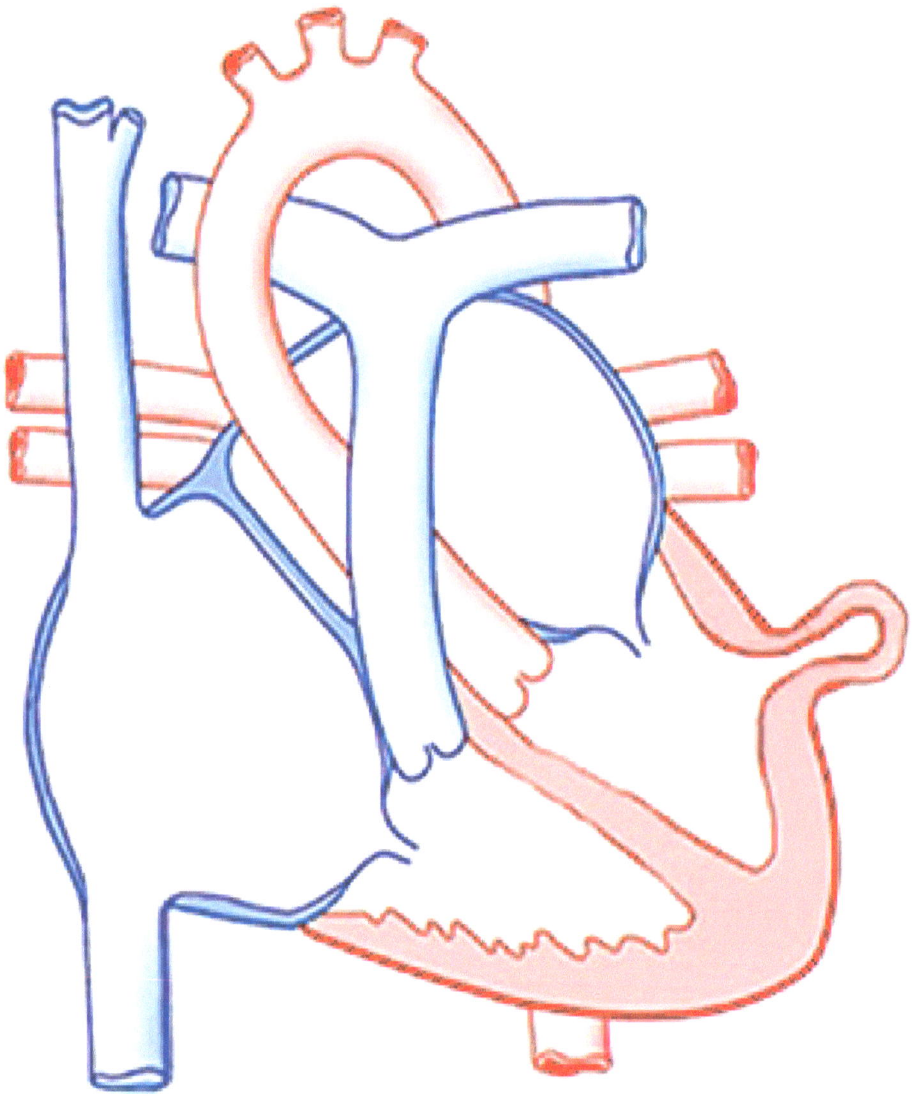

Figure 15: Left ventricular diverticulum. Congenital left ventricular diverticulum.

*Corresponding author Oran B: Medicana International Hospital, Department of Pediatric Cardiology, İzmir, Turkey
E-mail:boran@medicana.com.tr and bulentoran@hotmail.com

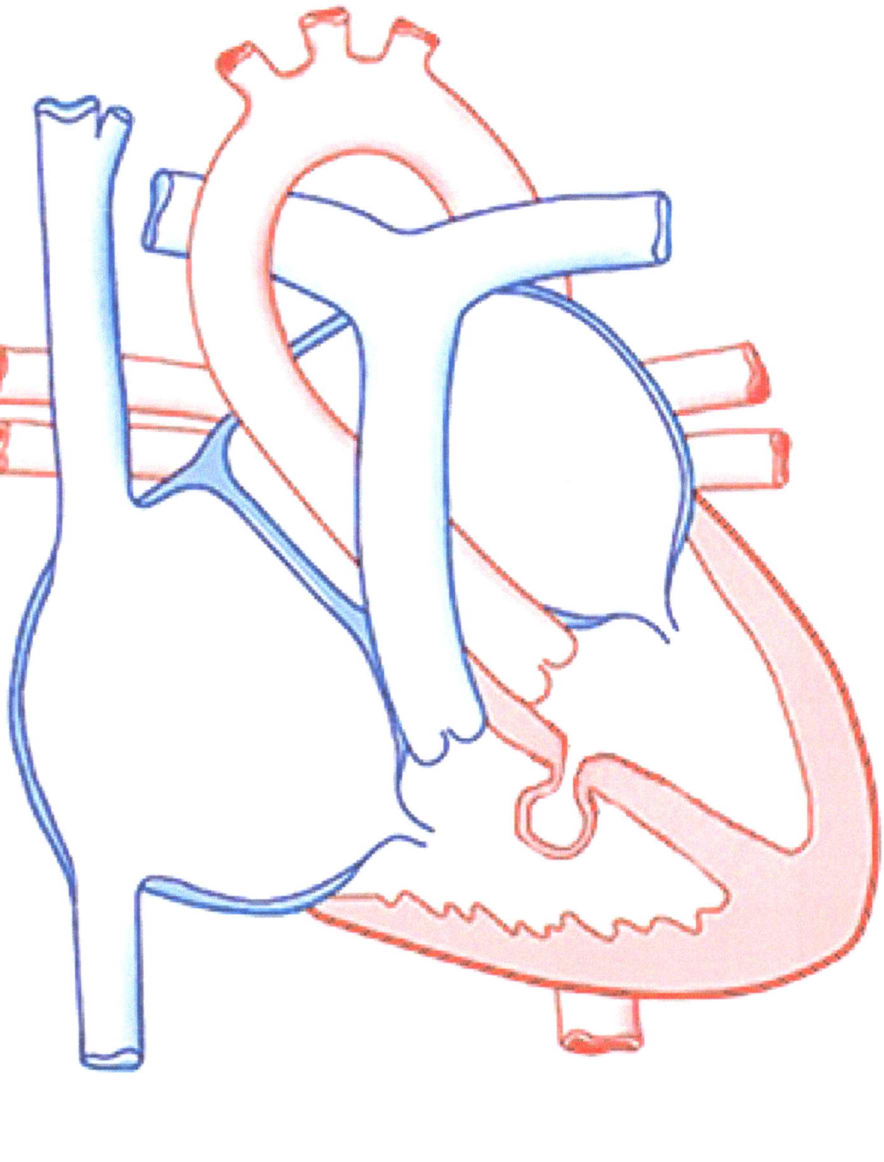

Figure 16: Left ventricular diverticulum. Congenital left ventricular diverticulum.

*Corresponding author Oran B: Medicana International Hospital, Department of Pediatric Cardiology, İzmir, Turkey
E-mail:boran@medicana.com.tr and bulentoran@hotmail.com

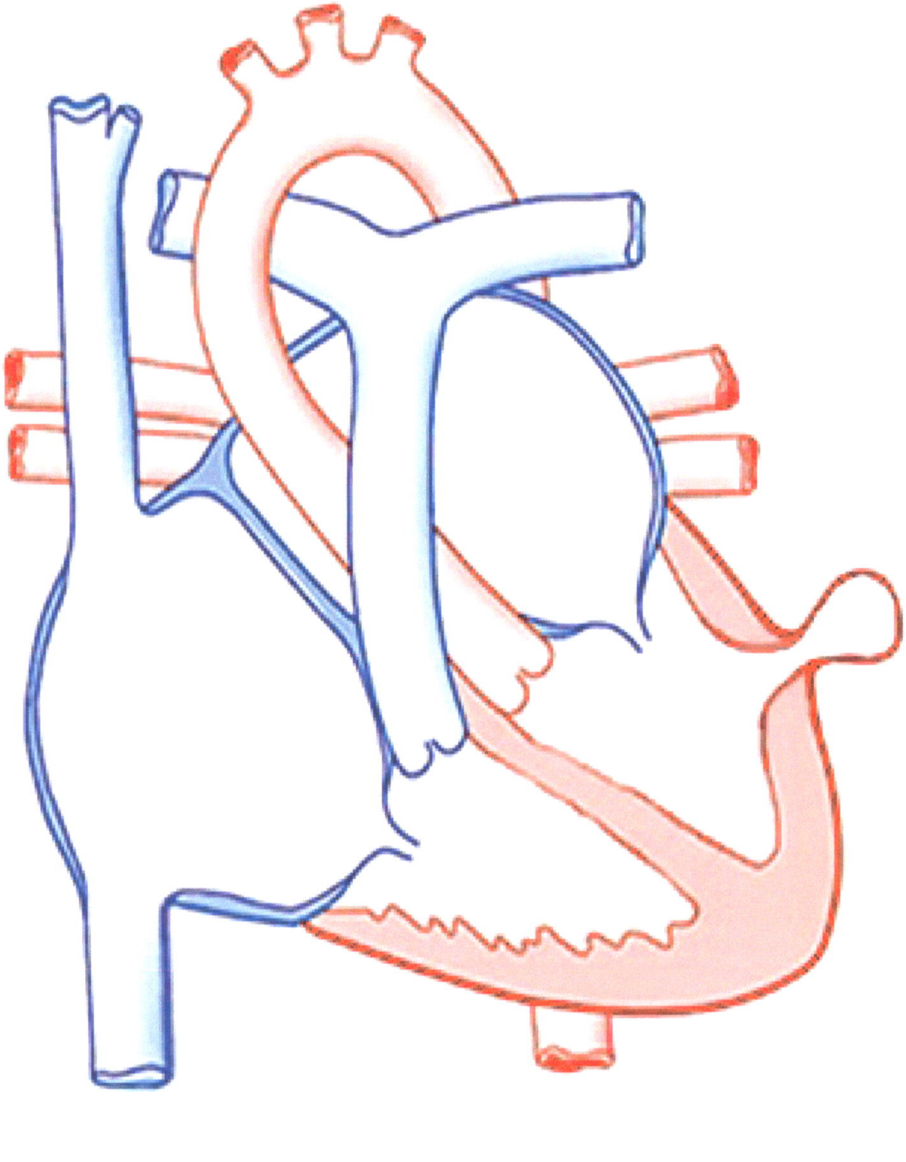

Figure 17: Left ventricular aneurysm. Congenital left ventricular aneurysm.

*Corresponding author Oran B: Medicana International Hospital, Department of Pediatric Cardiology, İzmir, Turkey
E-mail:boran@medicana.com.tr and bulentoran@hotmail.com

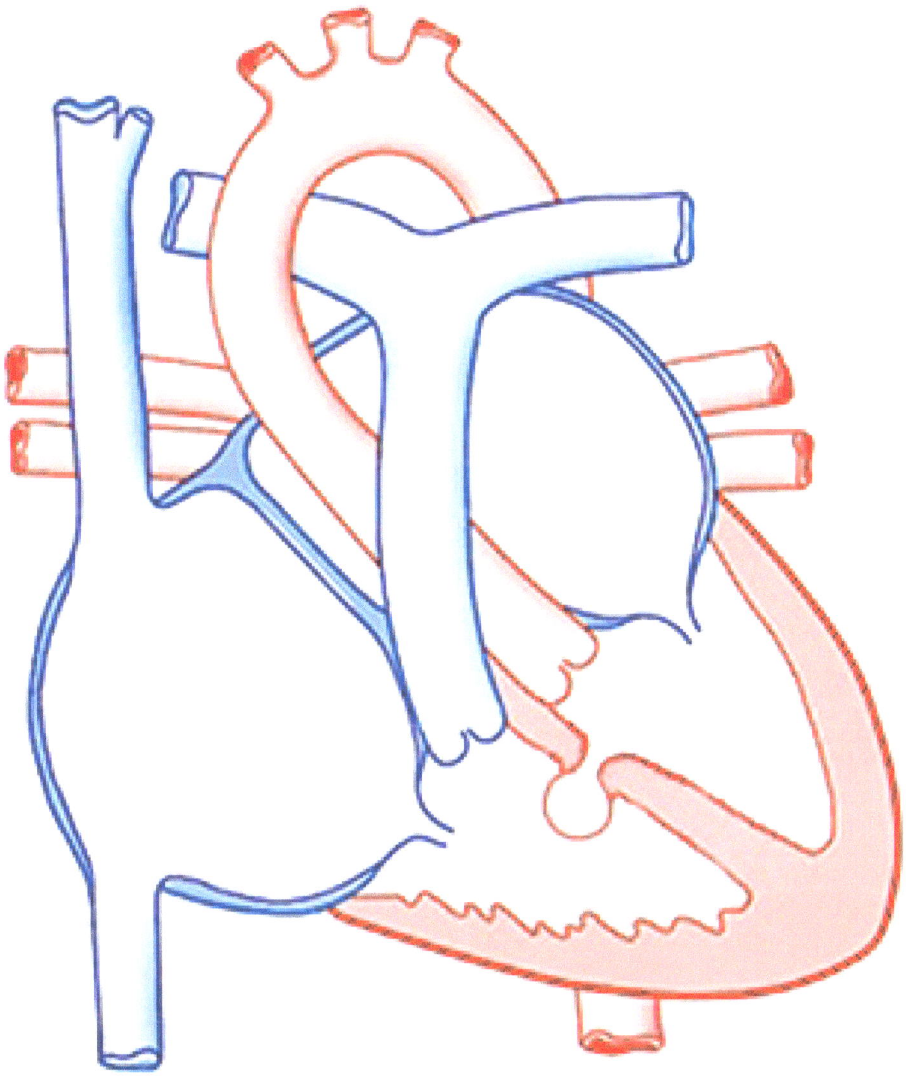

Figure 18: Left ventricular aneurysm. Congenital left ventricular aneurysm.

*Corresponding author Oran B: Medicana International Hospital, Department of Pediatric Cardiology, İzmir, Turkey
E-mail:boran@medicana.com.tr and bulentoran@hotmail.com

Single Ventricle

It is impossible for these patients to survive into adulthood without Interventional procedures or surgery.

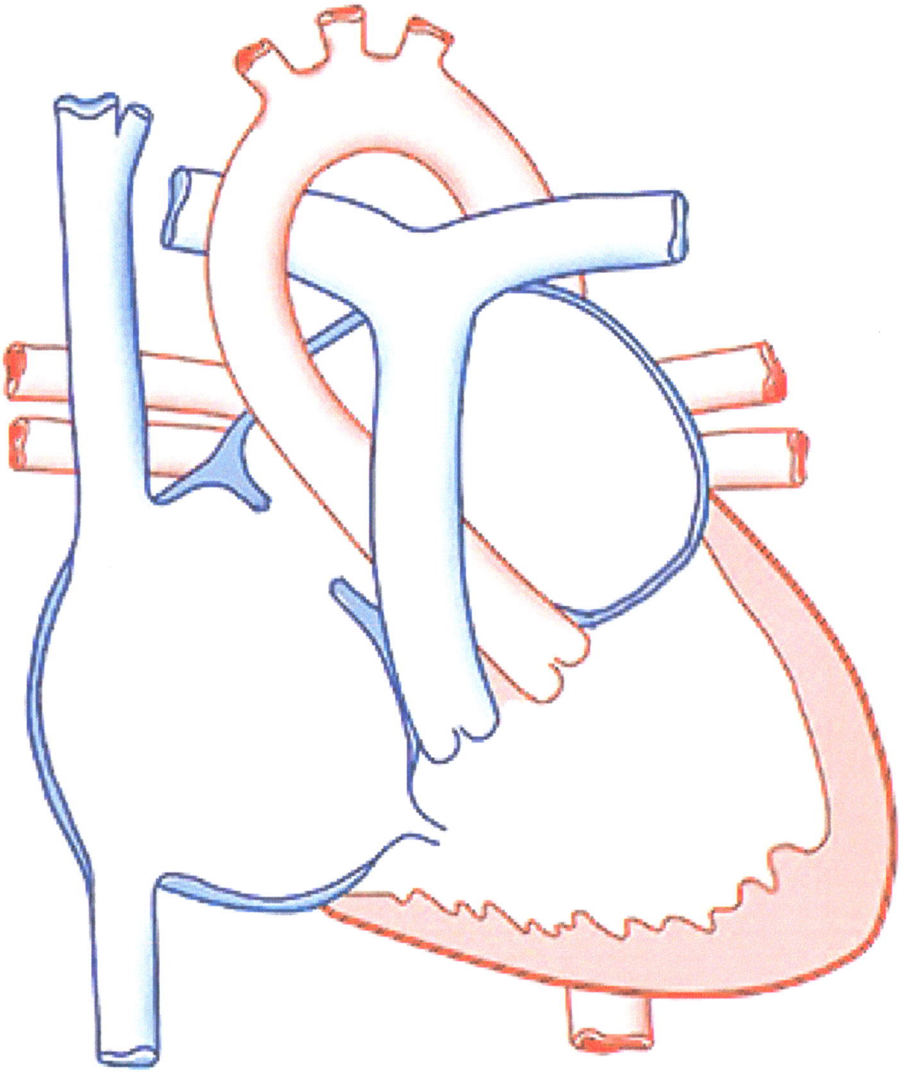

Figure 19: Single ventricle, mitral atresia, ASD. Functionally univentricular heart, atrial septal defects within oval fossa.

*Corresponding author Oran B: Medicana International Hospital, Department of Pediatric Cardiology, İzmir, Turkey
E-mail:boran@medicana.com.tr and bulentoran@hotmail.com

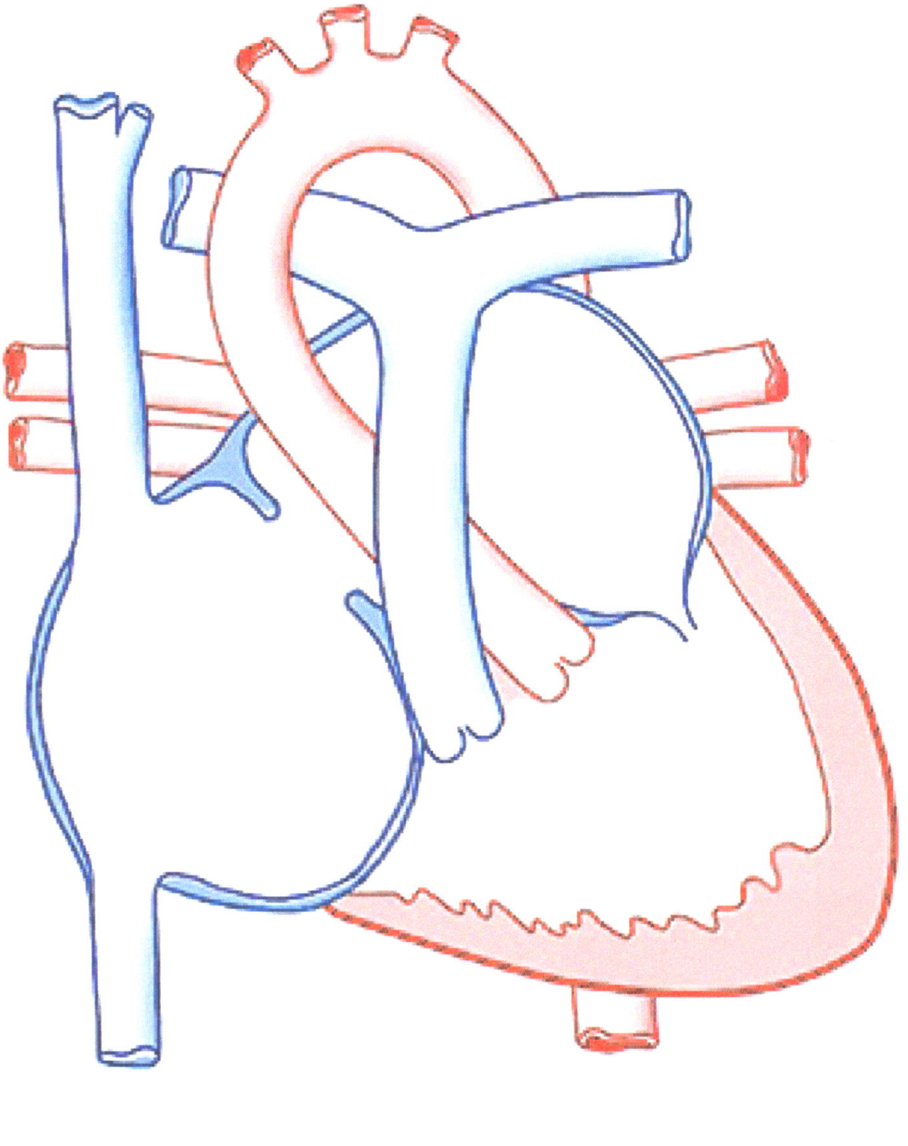

Figure 20: Single ventricle, Tricuspid atresia, ASD. Functionally univentricular heart, atrial septal defects within oval fossa.

*Corresponding author Oran B: Medicana International Hospital, Department of Pediatric Cardiology, İzmir, Turkey
E-mail:boran@medicana.com.tr and bulentoran@hotmail.com

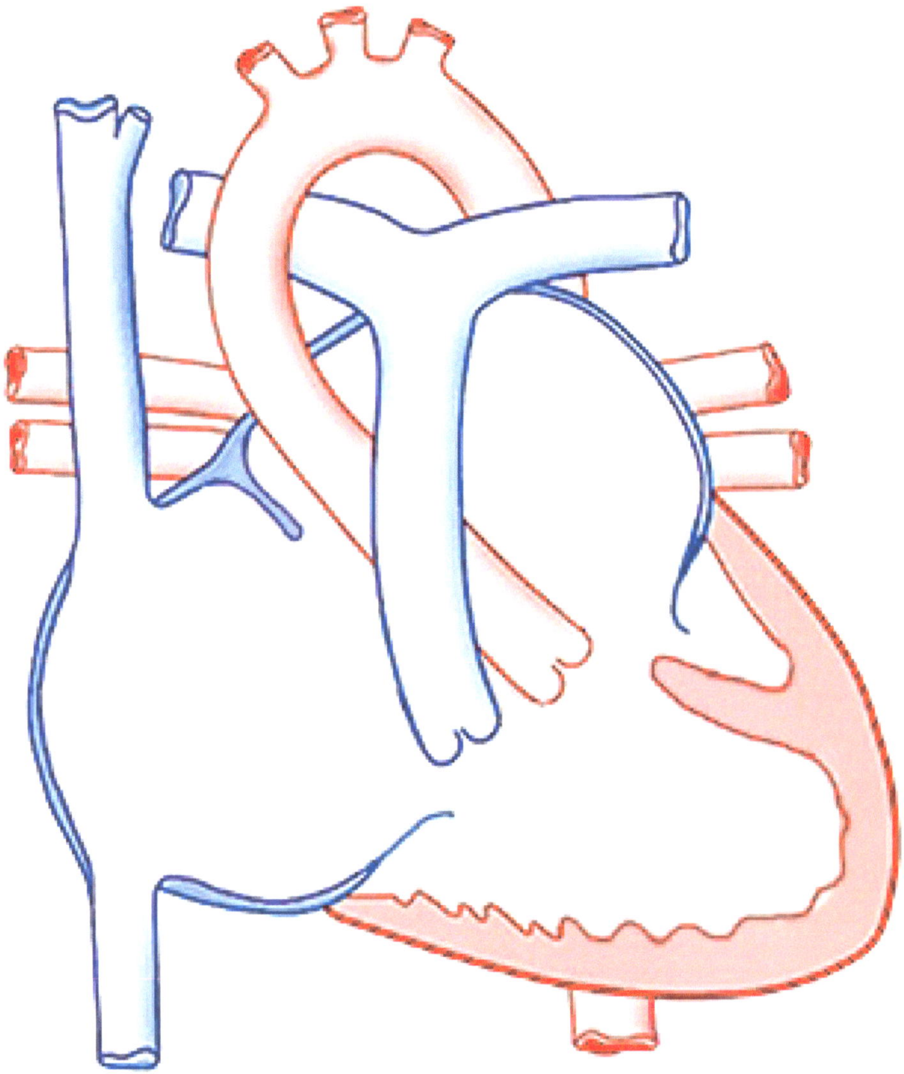

Figure 21: Atrioventricular septal defect with ventricular imbalance, single ventricle. Common atrioventricular valve with unbalanced commitment of valve to right ventricle.

*Corresponding author Oran B: Medicana International Hospital, Department of Pediatric Cardiology, İzmir, Turkey
E-mail:boran@medicana.com.tr and bulentoran@hotmail.com

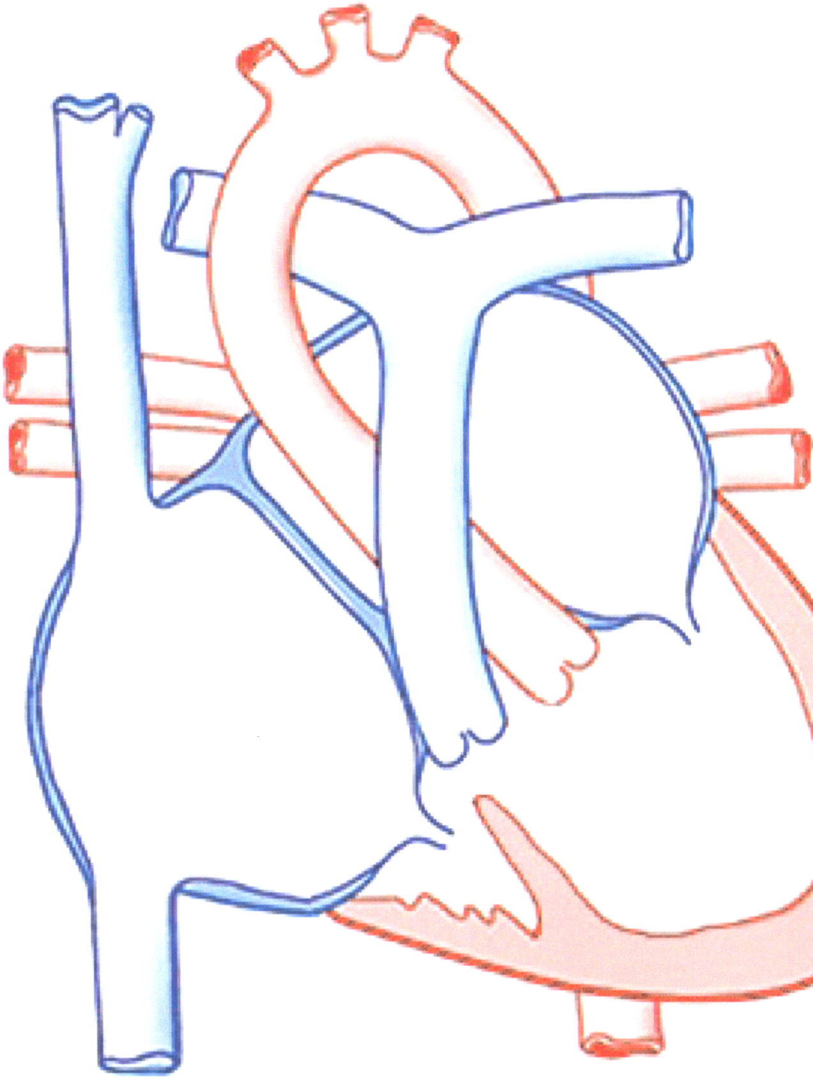

Figure 22: Atrioventricular septal defect with ventricular imbalance, single ventricle. Common atrioventricular valve with unbalanced commitment of valve to left ventricle.

*Corresponding author Oran B: Medicana International Hospital, Department of Pediatric Cardiology, İzmir, Turkey
E-mail:boran@medicana.com.tr and bulentoran@hotmail.com

*Corresponding author Oran B: Medicana International Hospital, Department of Pediatric Cardiology, İzmir, Turkey
E-mail:boran@medicana.com.tr and bulentoran@hotmail.com

CHAPTER 7

Transpositions of the Great Arteries

Oran B.

Medicana International Hospital, Department of Pediatric Cardiology, İzmir, Turkey

*Corresponding author Oran B: Medicana International Hospital, Department of Pediatric Cardiology, İzmir, Turkey
E-mail:boran@medicana.com.tr and bulentoran@hotmail.com

Transposition of the Great Arteries

Transposition of the great arteries is characterized by the combination of cardiac situs solitus, concordant atrioventricular connection, and discordant ventriculoarterial connection. The aorta originates from the morphological right ventricle, while the pulmonary artery originates from the morphological left ventricle. The aorta is located anterior to the pulmonary artery and on the right side. Affected patients cannot reach adulthood without intervention. Transposition of the great arteries is associated with VSDs, pulmonary stenosis, aortic stenosis, coarctation of the aorta, and the Taussig-Bing anomaly.

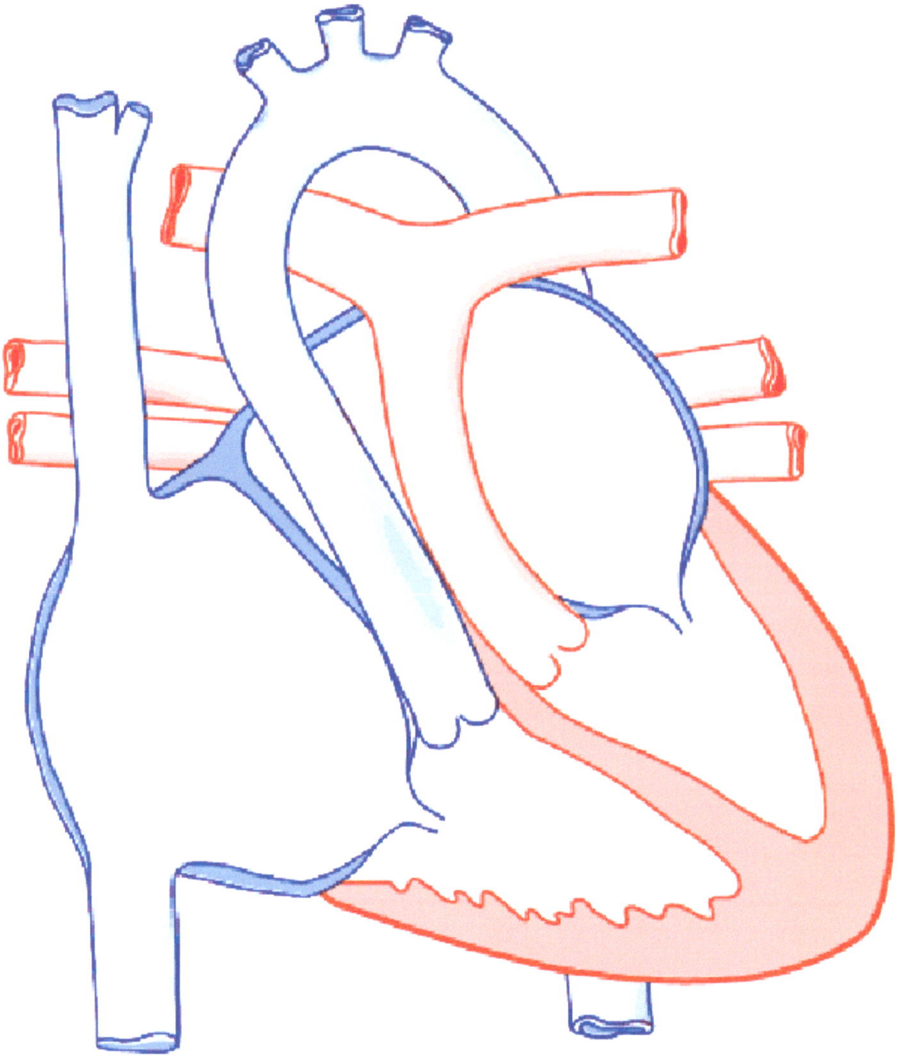

Figure 1: Transposition of the great arteries (d-TGA). Transposition of the great arteries, and intact ventricular septum. Discordant ventriculoarterial connections.

*Corresponding author Oran B: Medicana International Hospital, Department of Pediatric Cardiology, İzmir, Turkey
E-mail:boran@medicana.com.tr and bulentoran@hotmail.com

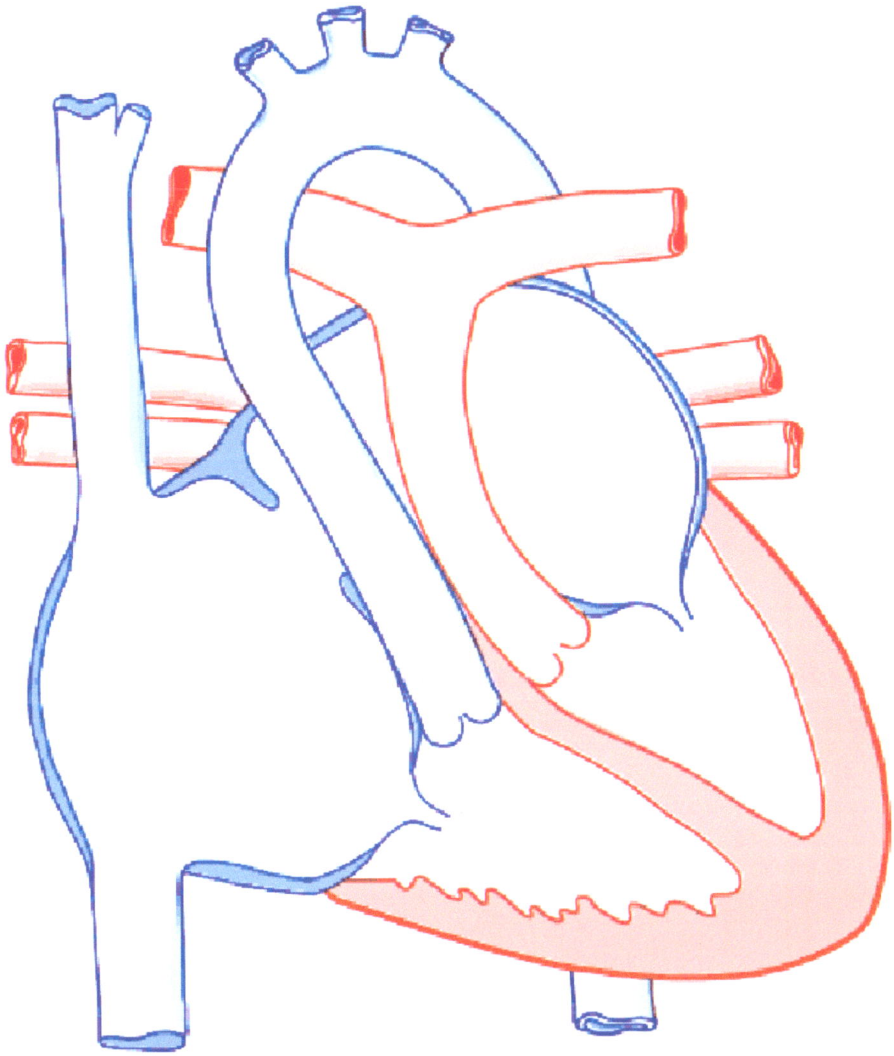

Figure 2: Transposition of the great arteries, ASD. Transposition of the great arteries, and intact ventricular septum. Discordant ventriculoarterial connections, with atrial septal defect within oval fossa.

*Corresponding author Oran B: Medicana International Hospital, Department of Pediatric Cardiology, İzmir, Turkey
E-mail:boran@medicana.com.tr and bulentoran@hotmail.com

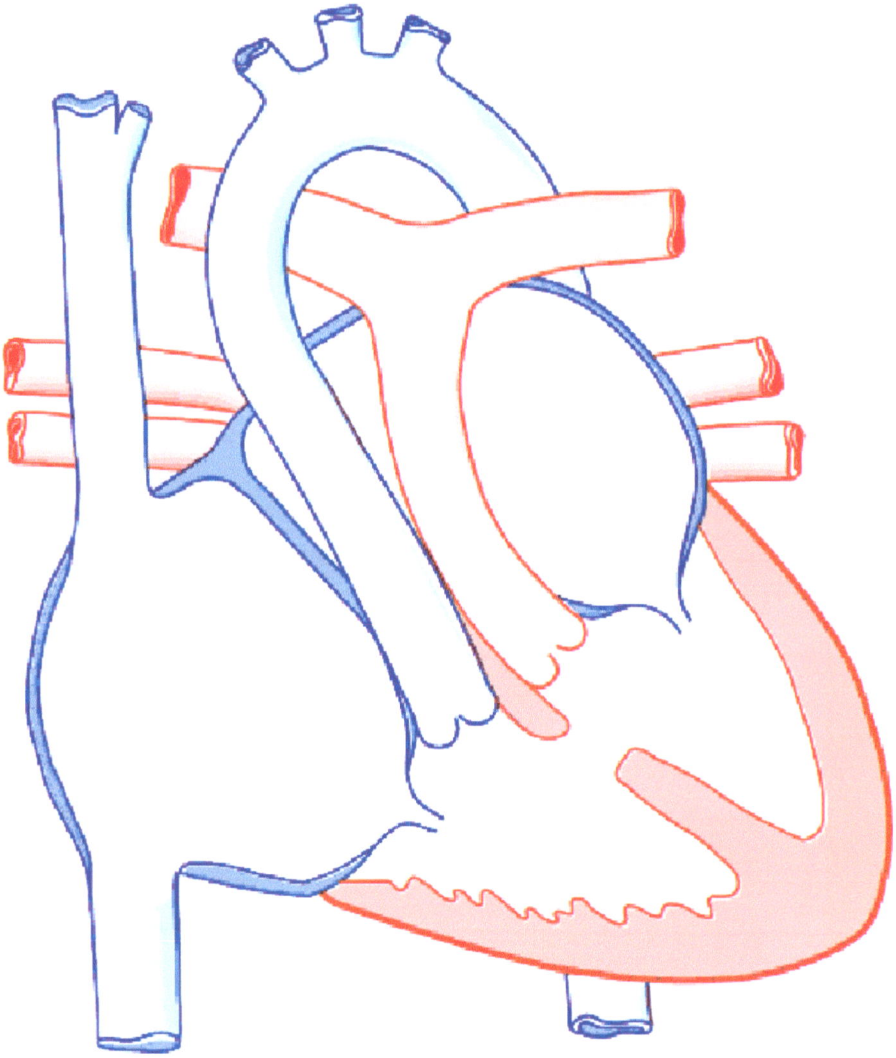

Figure 3: Transposition of the great arteries, VSD. Transposition of the great arteries. Discordant ventriculoarterial connections, with ventricular septal defect.

*Corresponding author Oran B: Medicana International Hospital, Department of Pediatric Cardiology, İzmir, Turkey
E-mail:boran@medicana.com.tr and bulentoran@hotmail.com

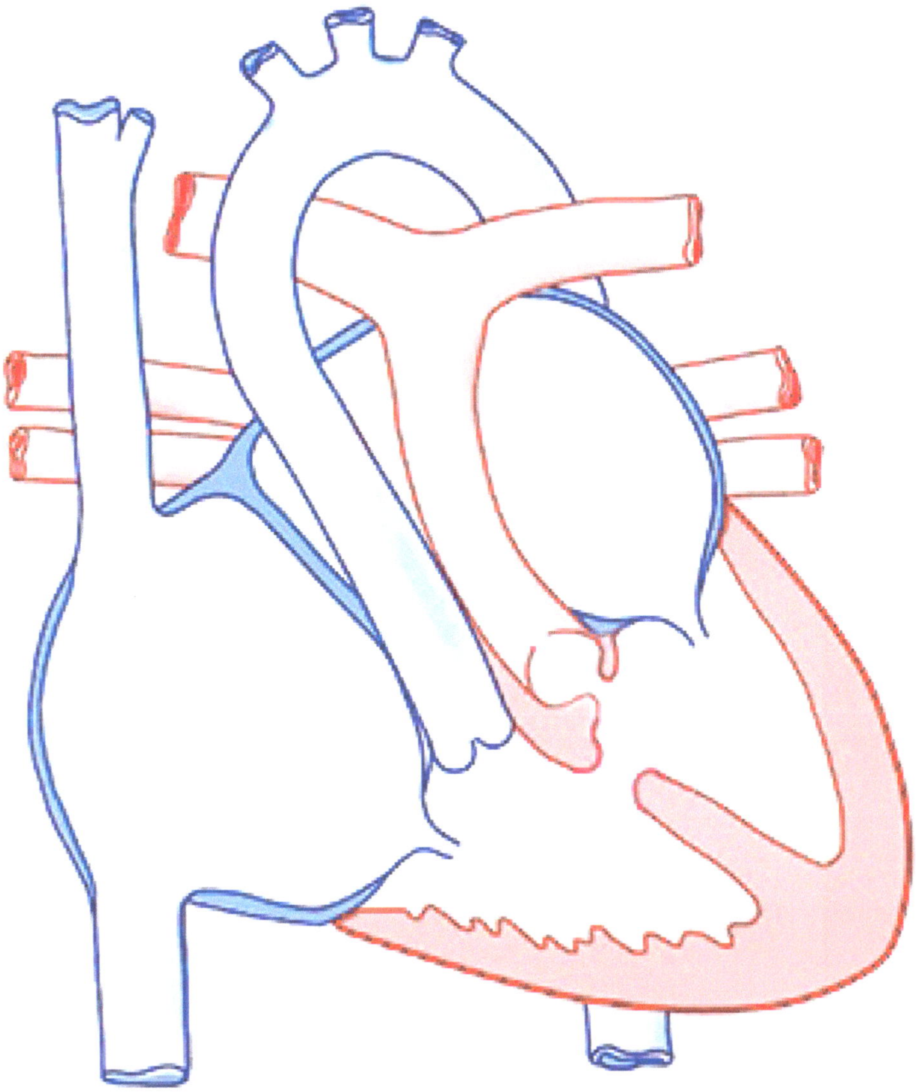

Figure 4: Transposition of the great arteries, VSD, left ventricular outflow tract obstruction. Transposition of the great arteries and ventricular septal defect with left ventricular outflow tract obstruction.

*Corresponding author Oran B: Medicana International Hospital, Department of Pediatric Cardiology, İzmir, Turkey
E-mail:boran@medicana.com.tr and bulentoran@hotmail.com

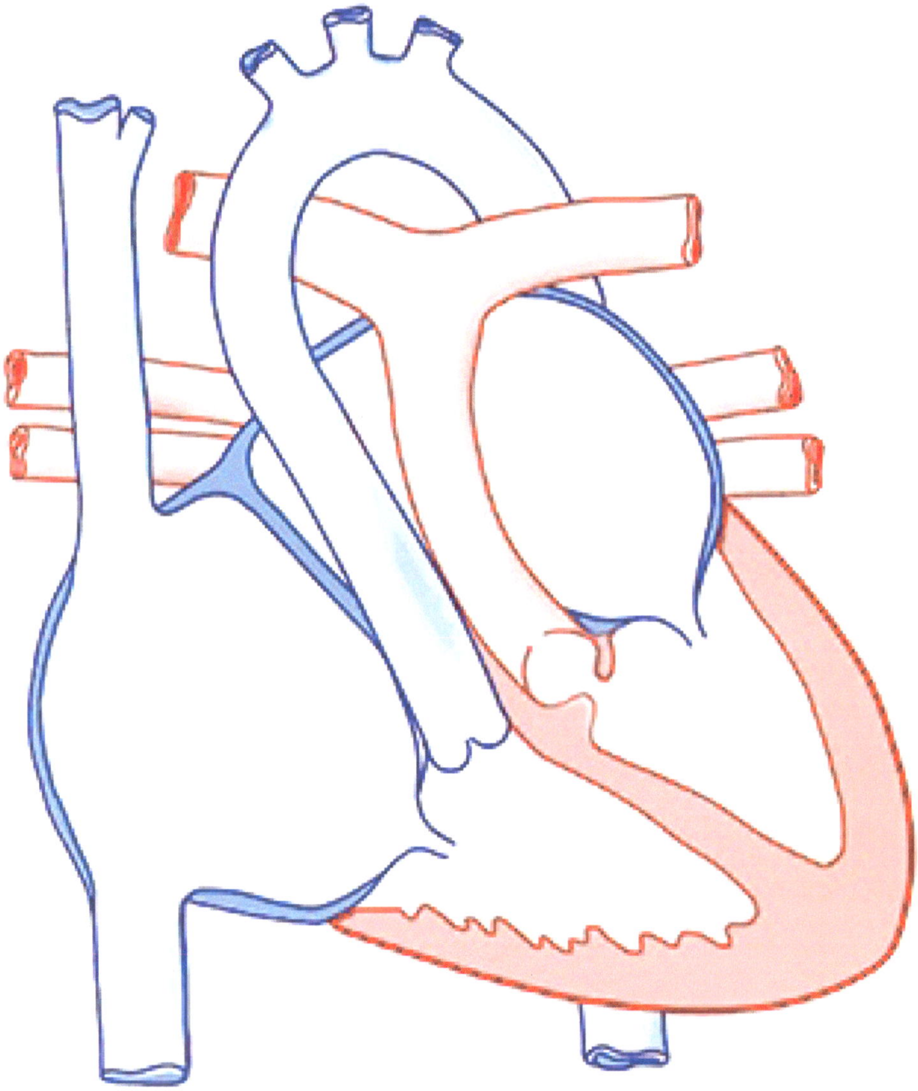

Figure 5: Transposition of the great arteries, intact interventricular septum, left ventricular outflow tract obstruction.

*Corresponding author Oran B: Medicana International Hospital, Department of Pediatric Cardiology, İzmir, Turkey
E-mail:boran@medicana.com.tr and bulentoran@hotmail.com

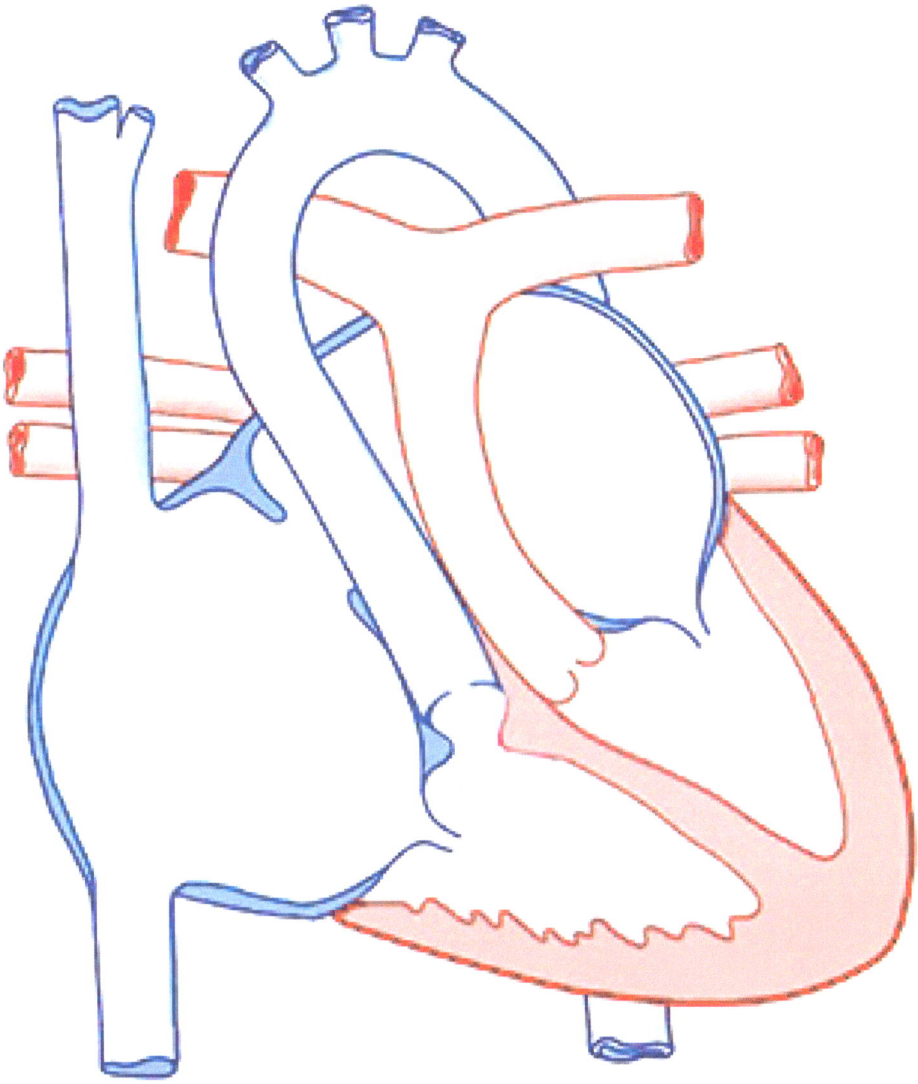

Figure 6: Transposition of the great arteries, ASD, right ventricular outflow tract obstruction. Transposition of the great arteries and atrial septal defect within oval fossa and right ventricular outflow tract obstruction.

*Corresponding author Oran B: Medicana International Hospital, Department of Pediatric Cardiology, İzmir, Turkey
E-mail:boran@medicana.com.tr and bulentoran@hotmail.com

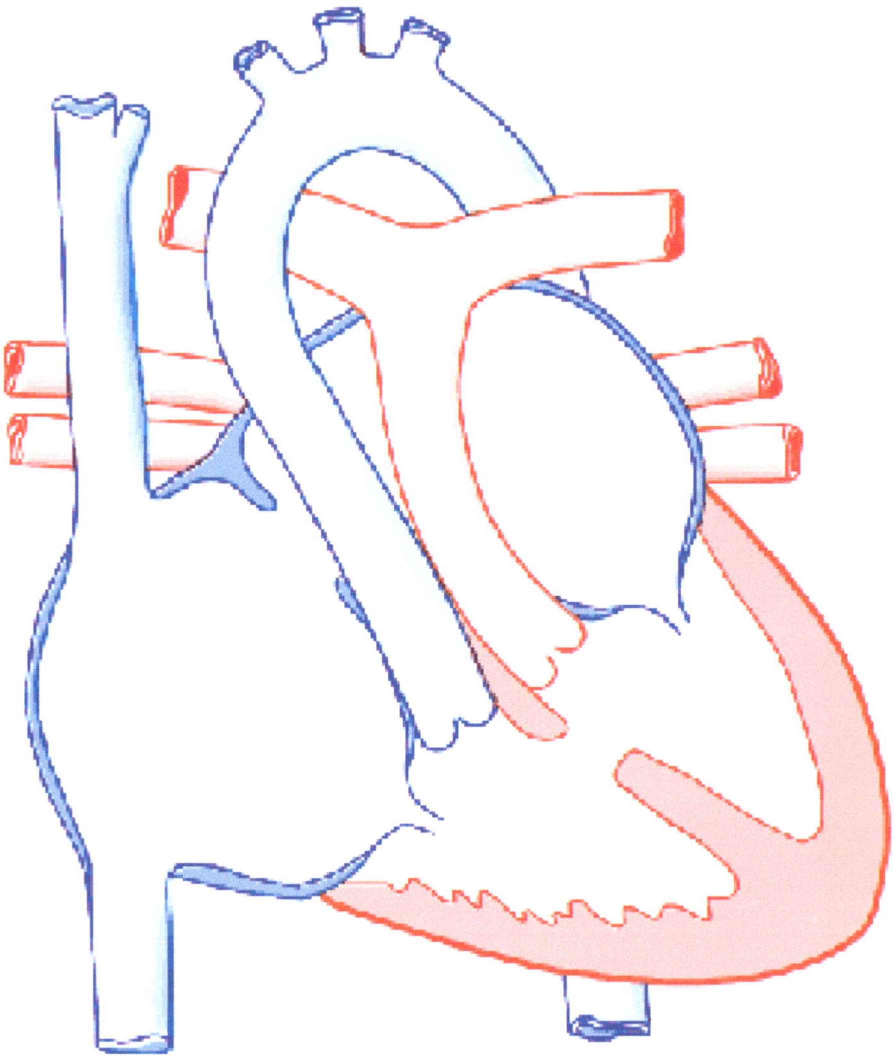

Figure 7: Transposition of the great arteries, ASD, VSD. Transposition of the great arteries with ventricular septal defect and atrial septal defects within oval fossa.

*Corresponding author Oran B: Medicana International Hospital, Department of Pediatric Cardiology, İzmir, Turkey
E-mail:boran@medicana.com.tr and bulentoran@hotmail.com

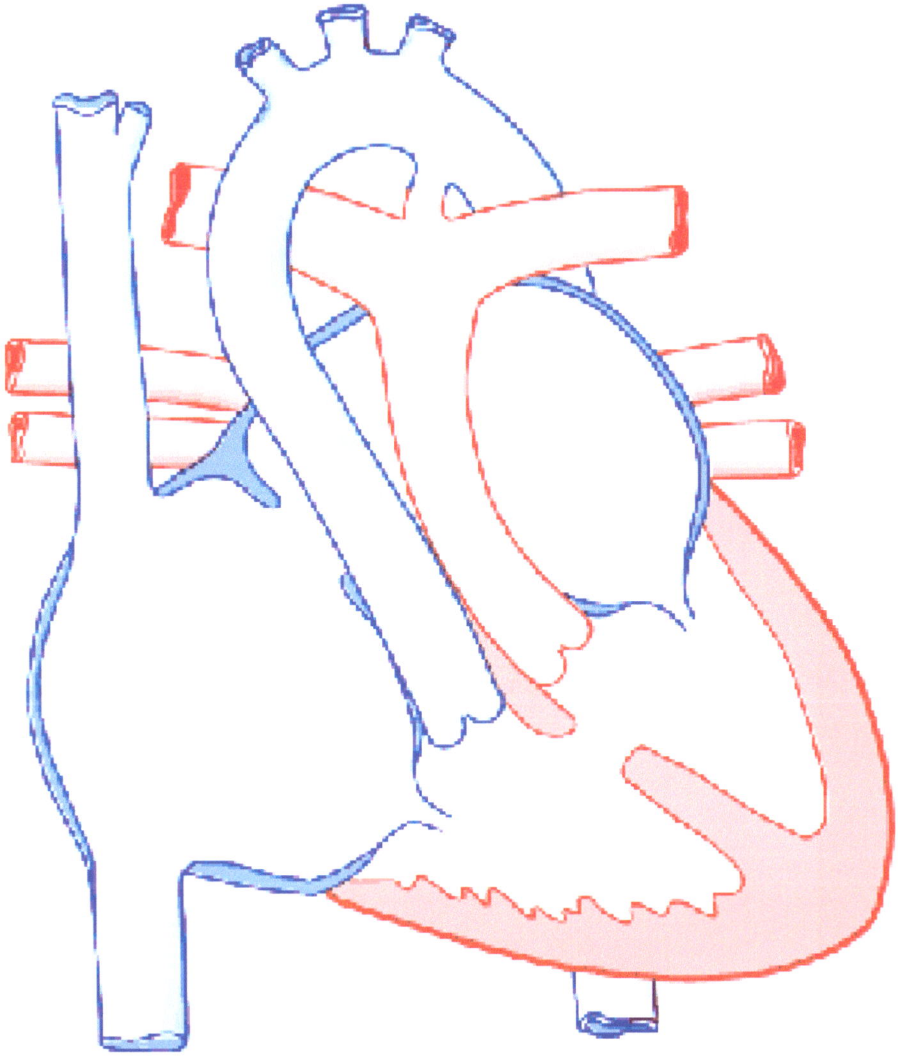

Figure 8: Transposition of the great arteries, ASD, VSD and PDA. Transposition of the great arteries with ventricular septal defect, patent arterial duct and atrial septal defects within oval foss

*Corresponding author Oran B: Medicana International Hospital, Department of Pediatric Cardiology, İzmir, Turkey
E-mail:boran@medicana.com.tr and bulentoran@hotmail.com

Congenitally Corrected Transposition of Great Arteries

Congenitally corrected transposition of the great arteries is characterized by discordant atrioventricular and ventriculoarterial connections. This malformation is also known as corrected transposition of the great arteries or L-transposition of the great arteries. With ventricular inversion, the morphological right ventricle is located on the left side and the morphological left ventricle is located on the right side. It is rare for these patients to survive into adulthood without interventional procedures or surgery.

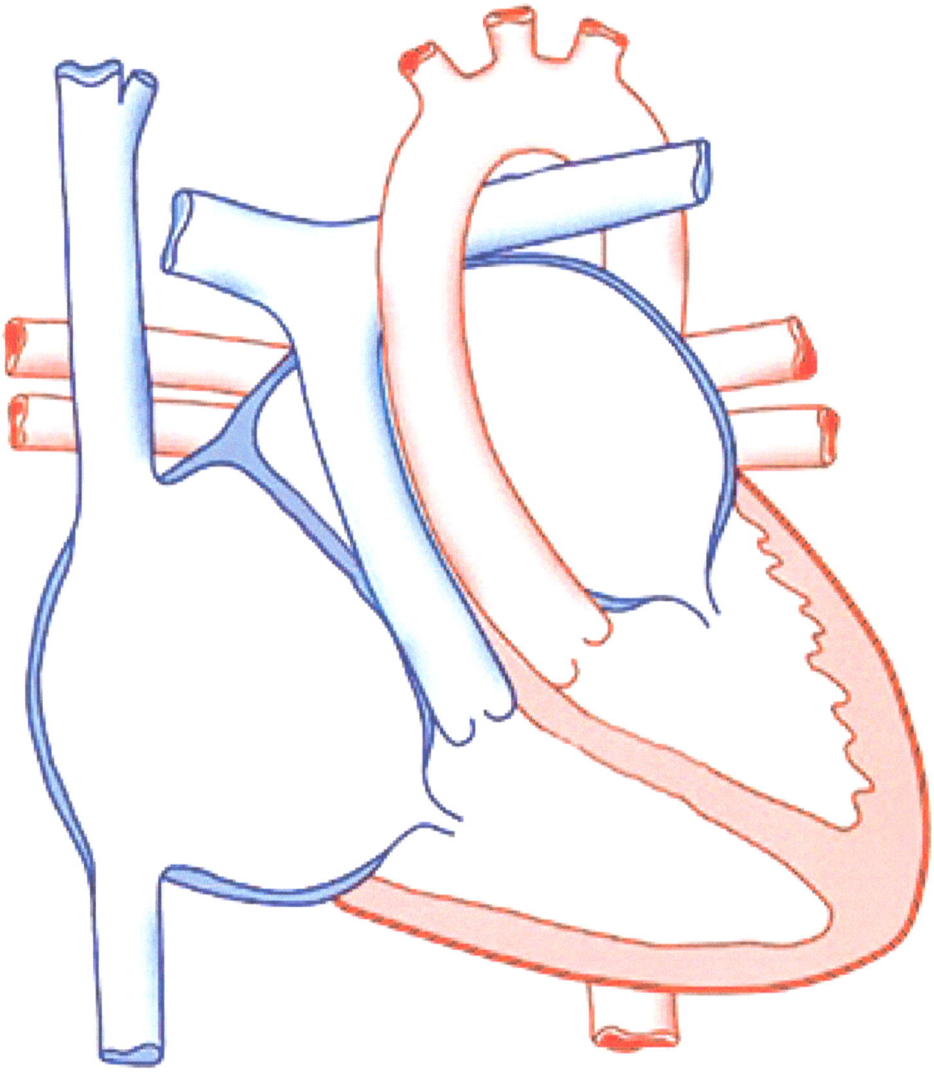

Figure 9: Congenitally corrected transposition of great arteries (L-TGA).

*Corresponding author Oran B: Medicana International Hospital, Department of Pediatric Cardiology, İzmir, Turkey
E-mail:boran@medicana.com.tr and bulentoran@hotmail.com

Congenitally Corrected Transposition of Great Arteries (continue)

Patients are typically situs solitus (95%). The aorta is located anterior to the pulmonary artery and on the left side. Because the infundibulum is located in the right ventricle, mitral pulmonary valve continuity is observed, instead of mitral aortic continuity. This malformation is associated with VSDs, ASDs, pulmonary stenosis, aortic stenosis, tricuspid valve anomaly or insufficiency, PDA, Ebstein's anomaly, and dysrhythmias (e.g., heart blocks, Wolff-Parkinson-White syndrome, or supraventricular tachycardia).

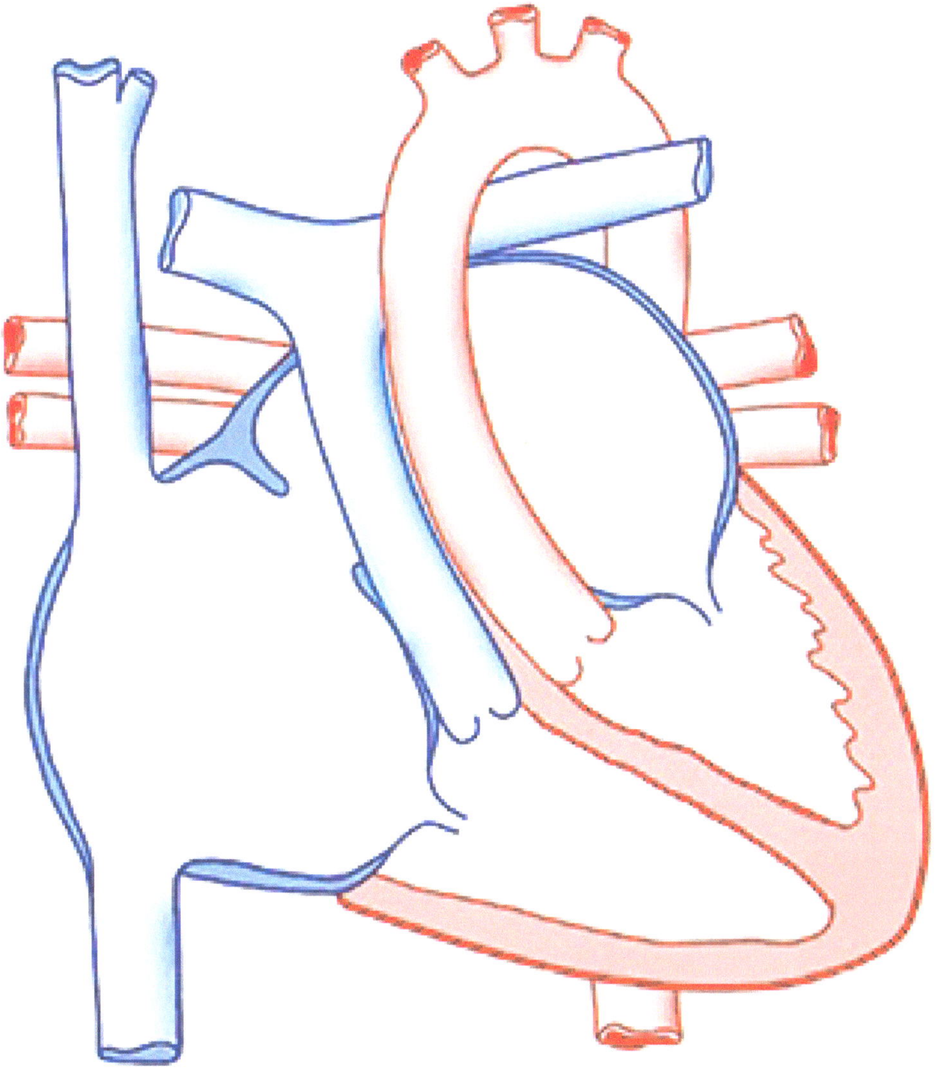

Figure 10: Congenitally corrected transposition of the great arteries with atrial septal defect within oval fossa.

*Corresponding author Oran B: Medicana International Hospital, Department of Pediatric Cardiology, İzmir, Turkey
E-mail:boran@medicana.com.tr and bulentoran@hotmail.com

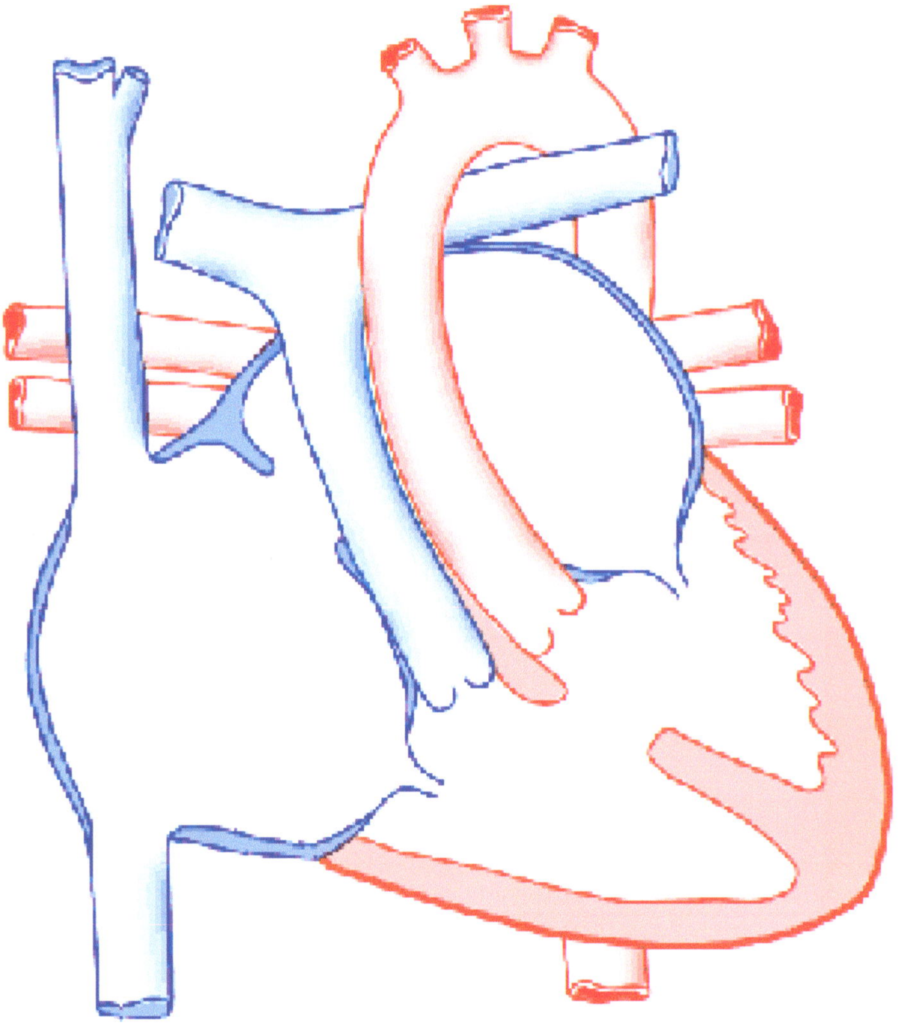

Figure 11: Congenitally corrected transposition of the great arteries, ventricular septal defect, atrial septal defect within oval fossa.

*Corresponding author Oran B: Medicana International Hospital, Department of Pediatric Cardiology, İzmir, Turkey
E-mail:boran@medicana.com.tr and bulentoran@hotmail.com

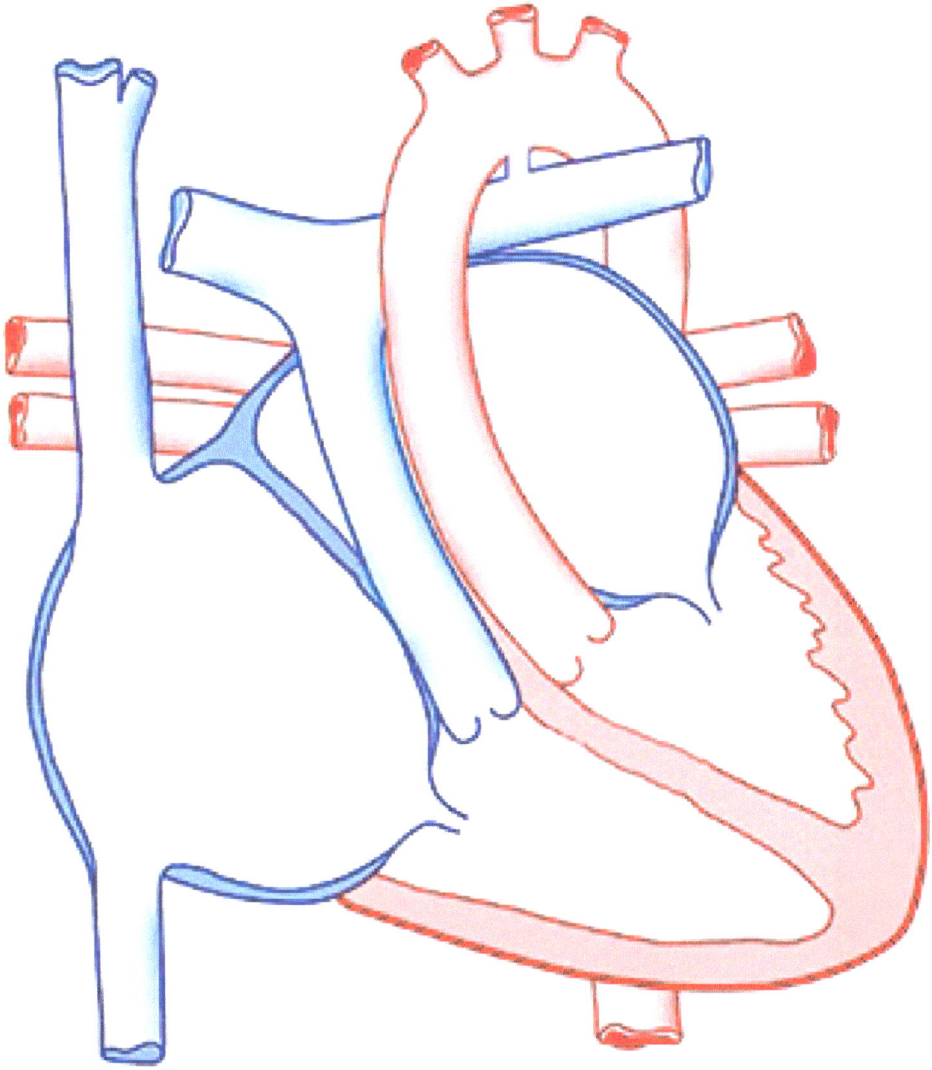

Figure 12: Congenitally corrected transposition of the great arteries, patent arterial duct.

*Corresponding author Oran B: Medicana International Hospital, Department of Pediatric Cardiology, İzmir, Turkey
E-mail:boran@medicana.com.tr and bulentoran@hotmail.com

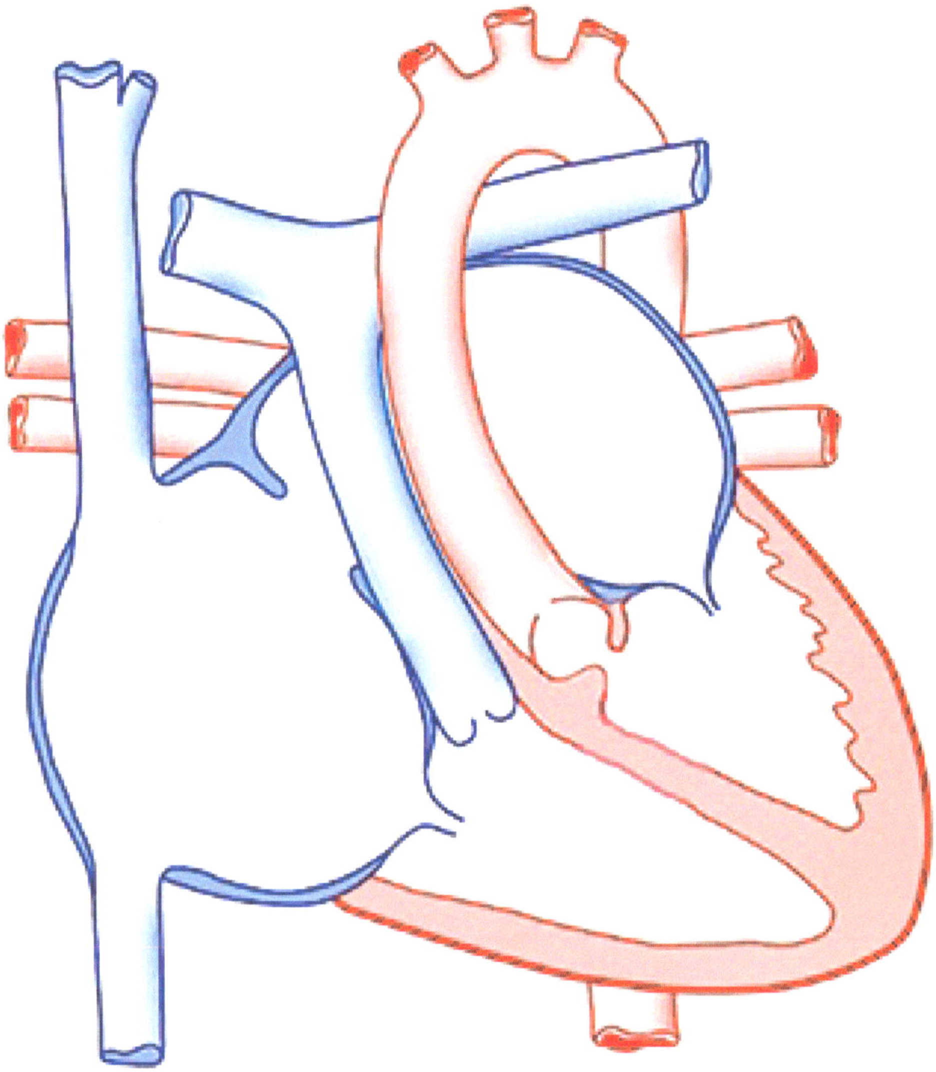

Figure 13: Congenitally corrected transposition of the great arteries, atrial septal defect within oval fossa with aortic stenosis.

*Corresponding author Oran B: Medicana International Hospital, Department of Pediatric Cardiology, İzmir, Turkey
E-mail:boran@medicana.com.tr and bulentoran@hotmail.com

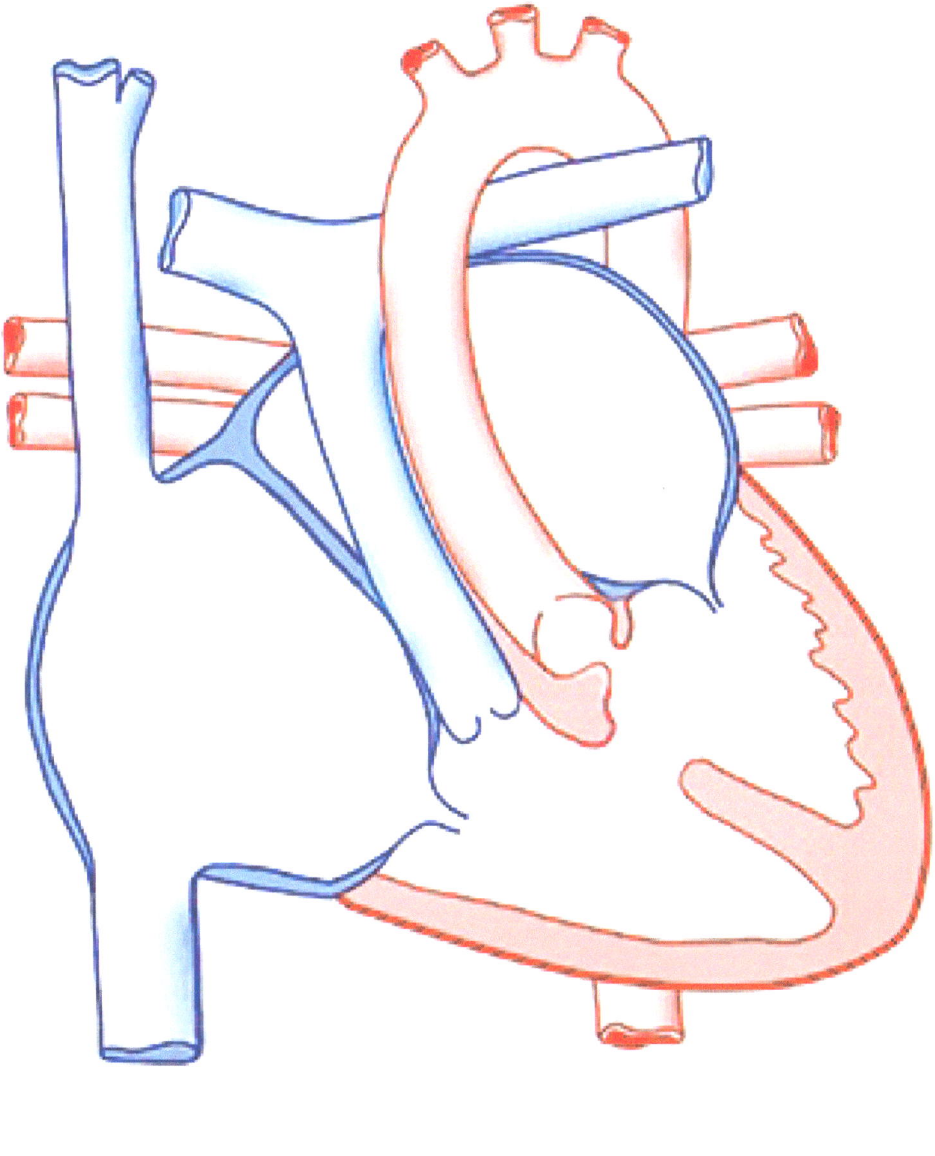

Figure 14: Congenitally corrected transposition of the great arteries, ventricular septal defect with aortic stenosis.

*Corresponding author Oran B: Medicana International Hospital, Department of Pediatric Cardiology, İzmir, Turkey
E-mail:boran@medicana.com.tr and bulentoran@hotmail.com

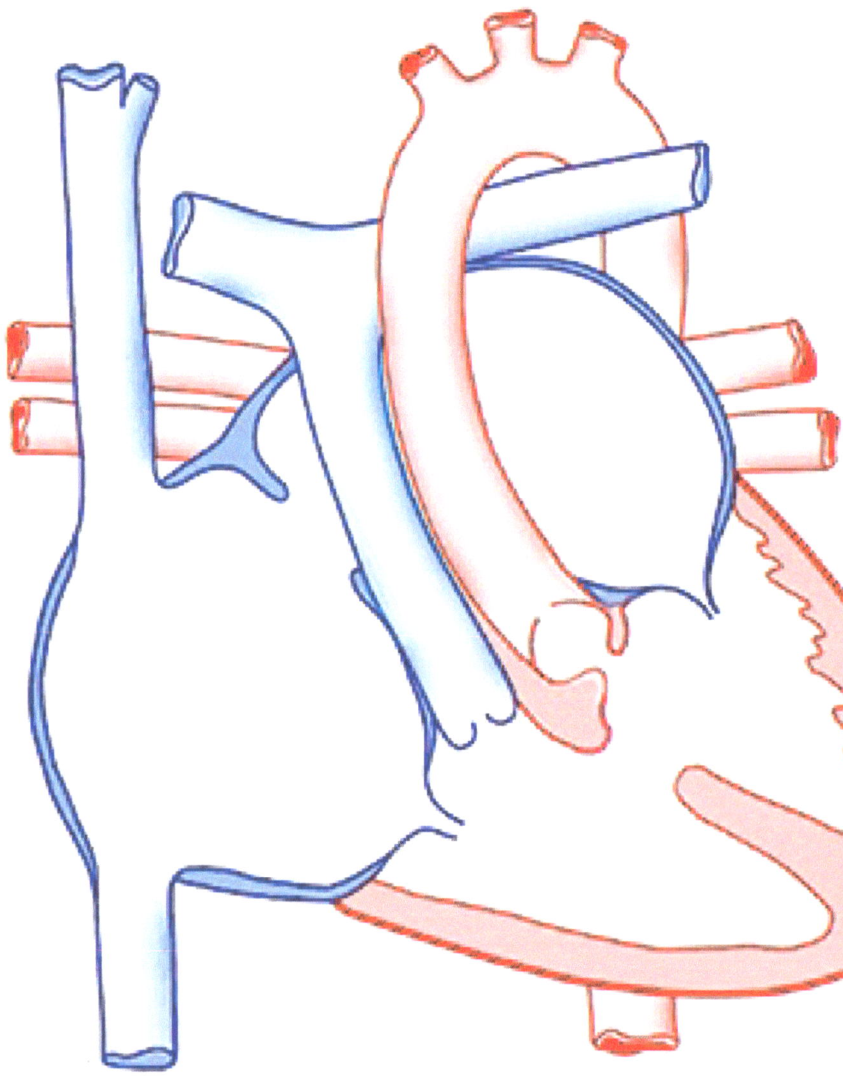

Figure 15: Congenitally corrected transposition of the great arteries, ventricular septal defect, atrial septal defect within oval fossa with aortic stenosis

*Corresponding author Oran B: Medicana International Hospital, Department of Pediatric Cardiology, İzmir, Turkey
E-mail:boran@medicana.com.tr and bulentoran@hotmail.com

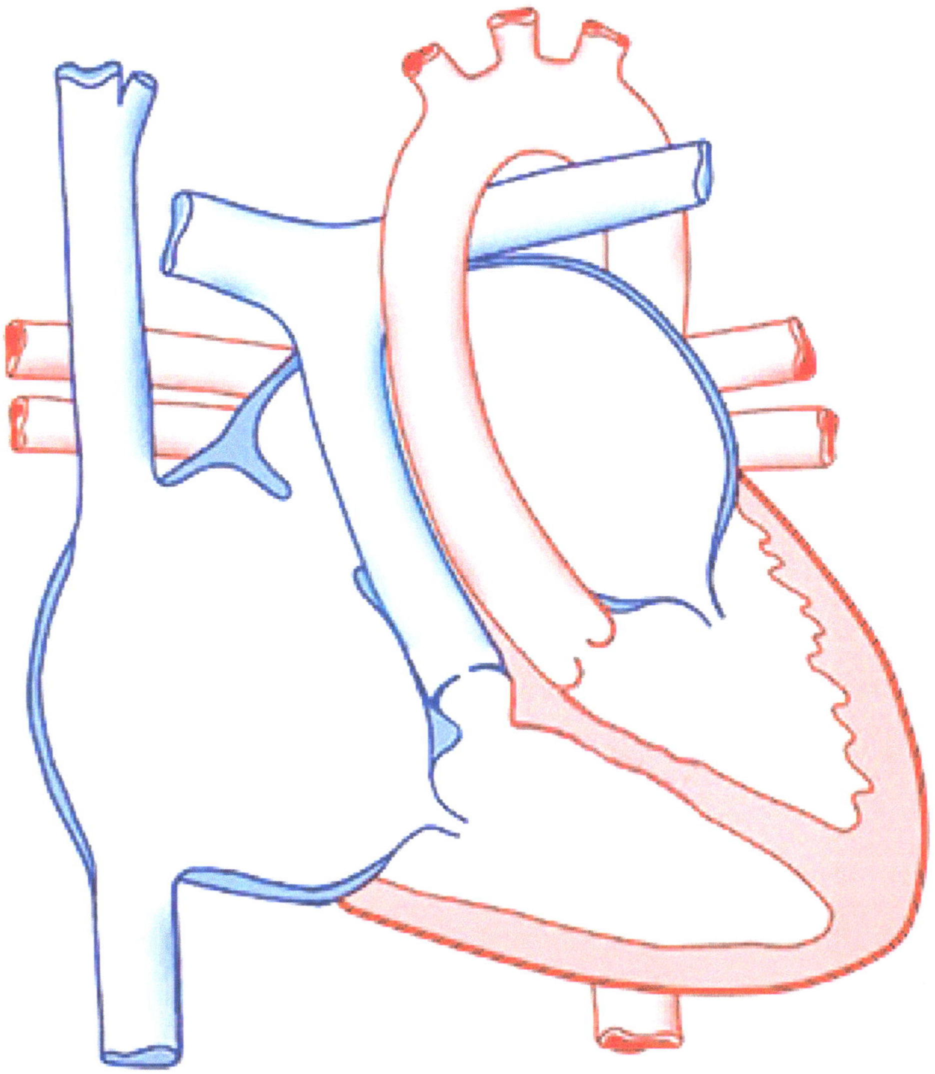

Figure 16: Congenitally corrected transposition of the great arteries, atrial septal defect within oval fossa with pulmonary stenosis.

*Corresponding author Oran B: Medicana International Hospital, Department of Pediatric Cardiology, İzmir, Turkey
E-mail:boran@medicana.com.tr and bulentoran@hotmail.com

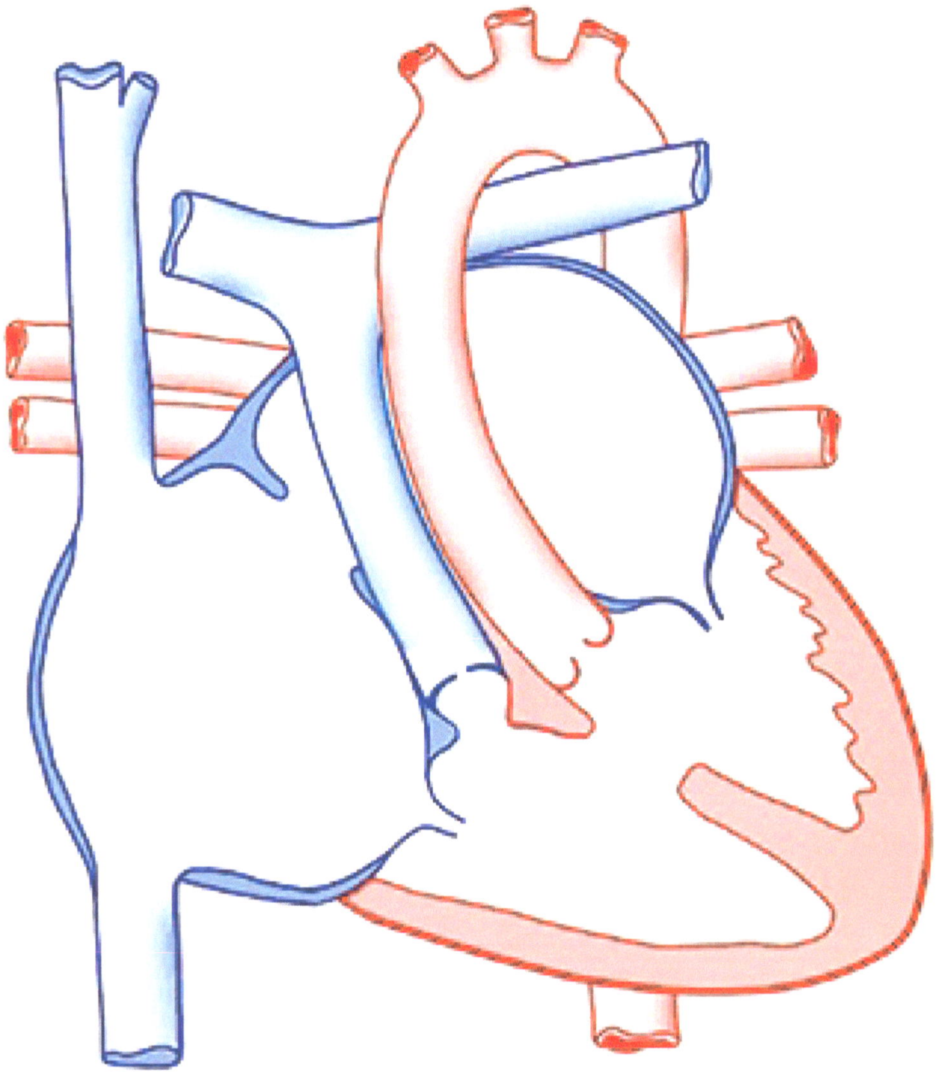

Figure 17: Congenitally corrected transposition of the great arteries, ventricular septal defect, atrial septal defect within oval fossa with pulmonary stenosis.

*Corresponding author Oran B: Medicana International Hospital, Department of Pediatric Cardiology, İzmir, Turkey
E-mail:boran@medicana.com.tr and bulentoran@hotmail.com

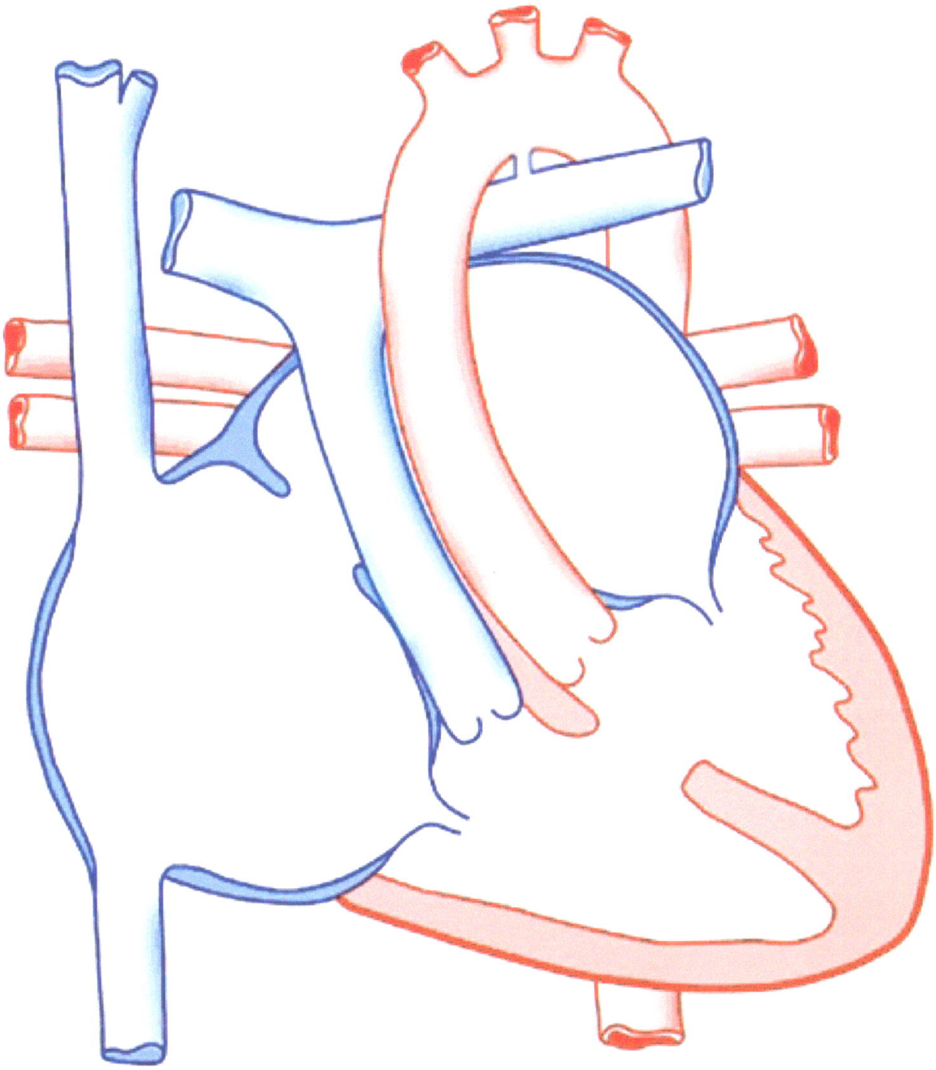

Figure 18: Congenitally corrected transposition of the great arteries, ventricular septal defect, atrial septal defect within oval fossa and patent arterial duct.

*Corresponding author Oran B: Medicana International Hospital, Department of Pediatric Cardiology, İzmir, Turkey
E-mail:boran@medicana.com.tr and bulentoran@hotmail.com

*Corresponding author Oran B: Medicana International Hospital, Department of Pediatric Cardiology, İzmir, Turkey
E-mail:boran@medicana.com.tr and bulentoran@hotmail.com

CHAPTER 8

Single Ventricular Morphology

Oran B.

Medicana International Hospital, Department of Pediatric Cardiology, İzmir, Turkey

*Corresponding author Oran B: Medicana International Hospital, Department of Pediatric Cardiology, İzmir, Turkey
E-mail:boran@medicana.com.tr and bulentoran@hotmail.com

Single Ventricle

Single ventricle is a rare and highly complex form of cyanotic congenital heart disease. Affected patients have either a single functioning ventricular cavity or two separate ventricular configurations, but one constitutes the non-functioning hypoplastic ventricle. In practice, designation of the right or left ventricle is made by observation of the other functioning ventricle. Single ventricle is associated with valve stenosis or insufficiency. Affected patients cannot survive until adulthood without intervention.

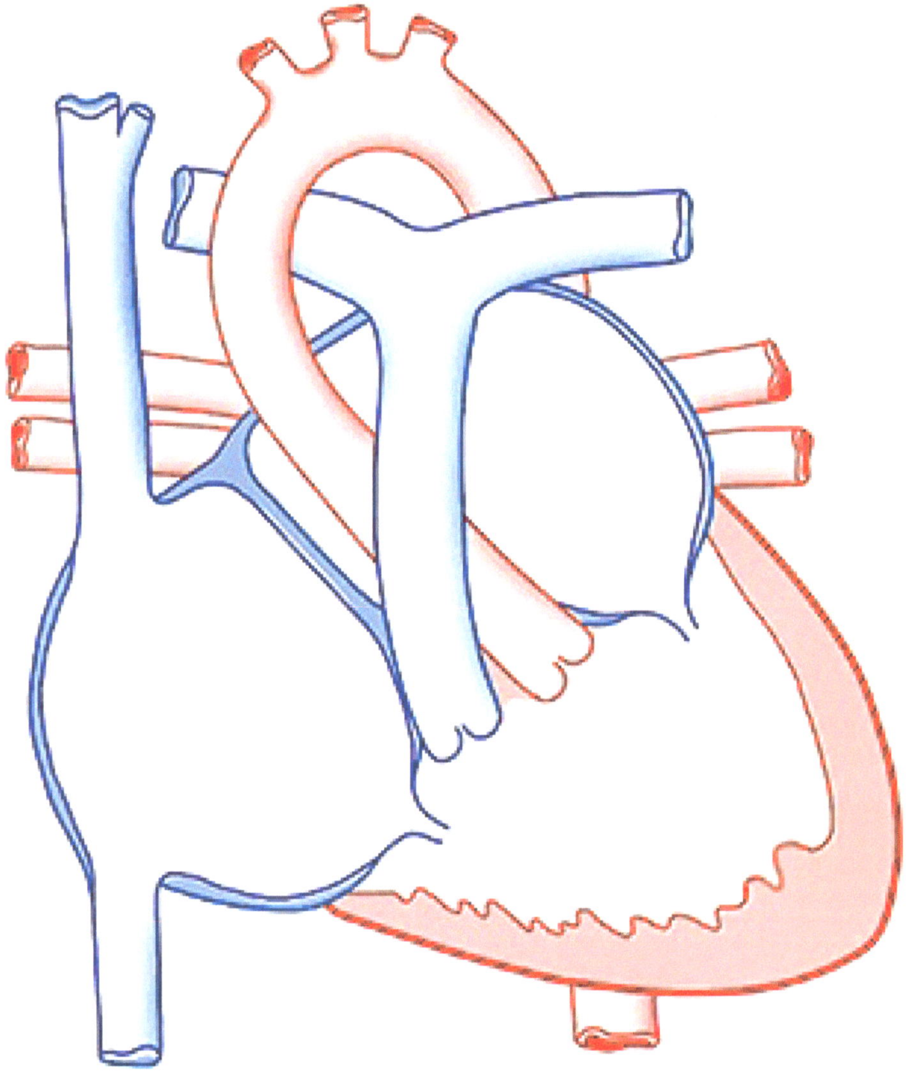

Figure 1: Single ventricle.

*Corresponding author Oran B: Medicana International Hospital, Department of Pediatric Cardiology, İzmir, Turkey
E-mail:boran@medicana.com.tr and bulentoran@hotmail.com

Single Ventricle, Double Inlet Left Ventricle

A double inlet left ventricle is either a single ventricle with two separate entrances or two separate atrioventricular valves that drain into a single ventricle. The right ventricle is typically the hypoplastic ventricle. Atrioventricular valve chordae tendineae are often in the straddling, overriding position. This malformation is associated with transposition of the great arteries, pulmonary stenosis, subaortic aortic stenosis, and coarctation of the aorta.

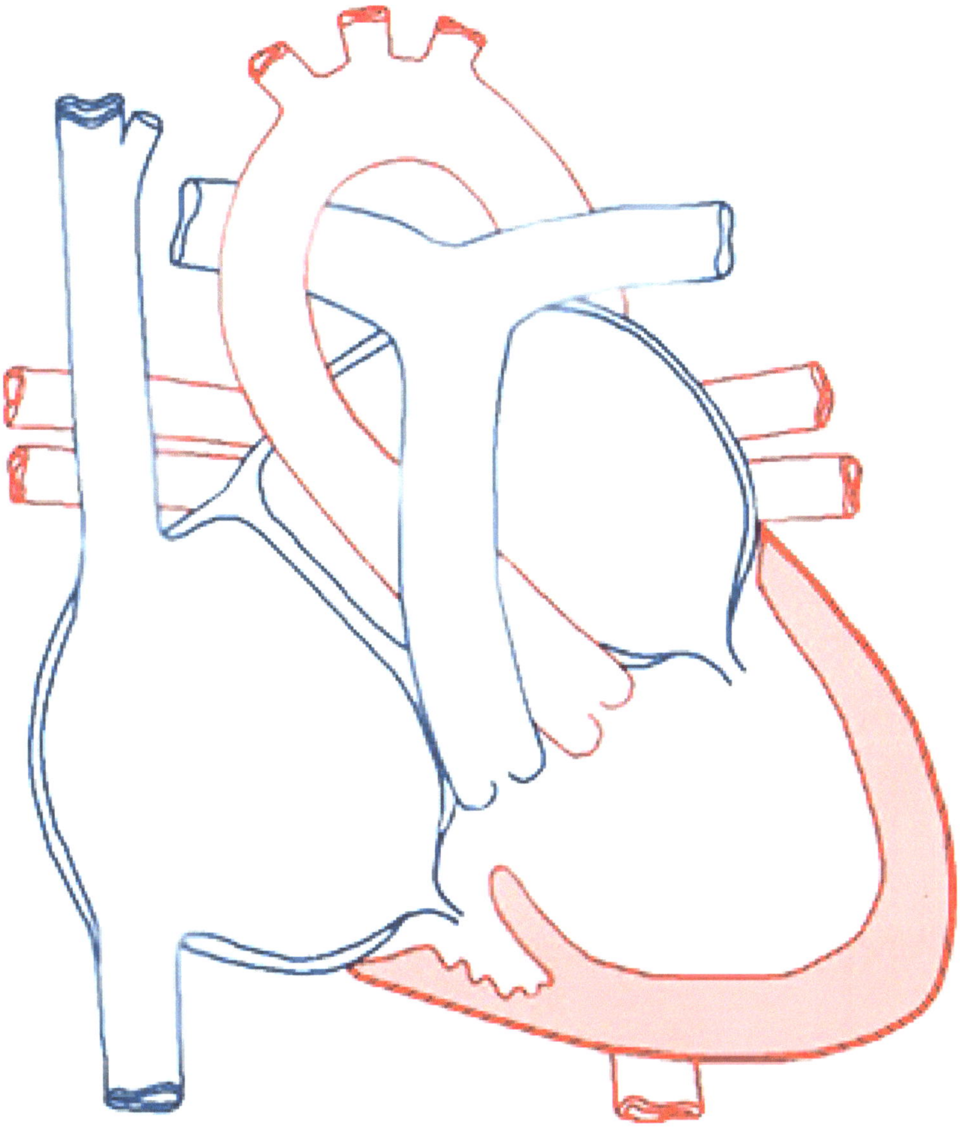

Figure 2: Single ventricle, double inlet left ventricle (functionally univentricular heart).

*Corresponding author Oran B: Medicana International Hospital, Department of Pediatric Cardiology, İzmir, Turkey
E-mail:boran@medicana.com.tr and bulentoran@hotmail.com

Single Ventricle, Double İnlet Right Ventricle

A double inlet right ventricle is a very complex heart defect. The atria connect to the right ventricle and the left ventricle is absent or very small.

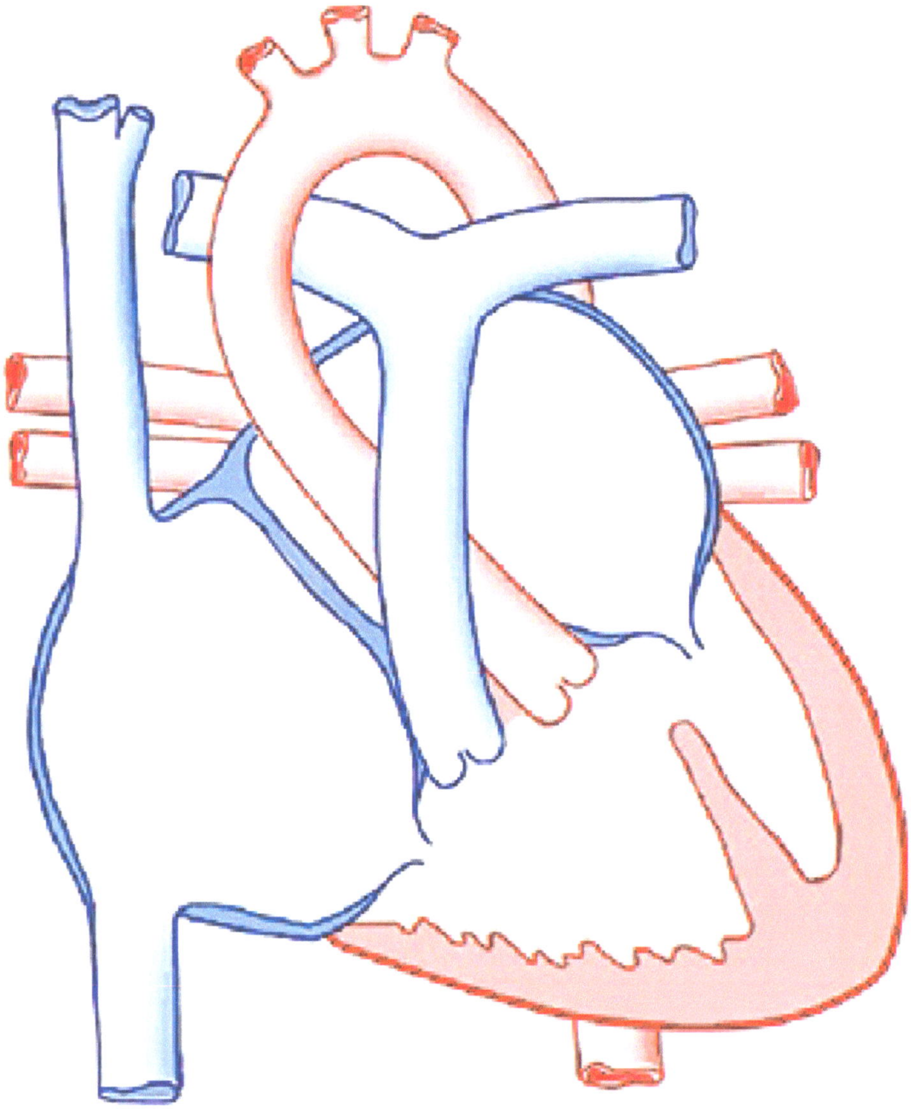

Figure 3: Single ventricle, double inlet right ventricle (functionally univentricular heart).

*Corresponding author Oran B: Medicana International Hospital, Department of Pediatric Cardiology, İzmir, Turkey
E-mail:boran@medicana.com.tr and bulentoran@hotmail.com

Single Ventricle, Mitral Atresia, ASD

Mitral atresia and an ASD are associated with the single ventricle malformation. Affected patients cannot survive until adulthood without intervention.

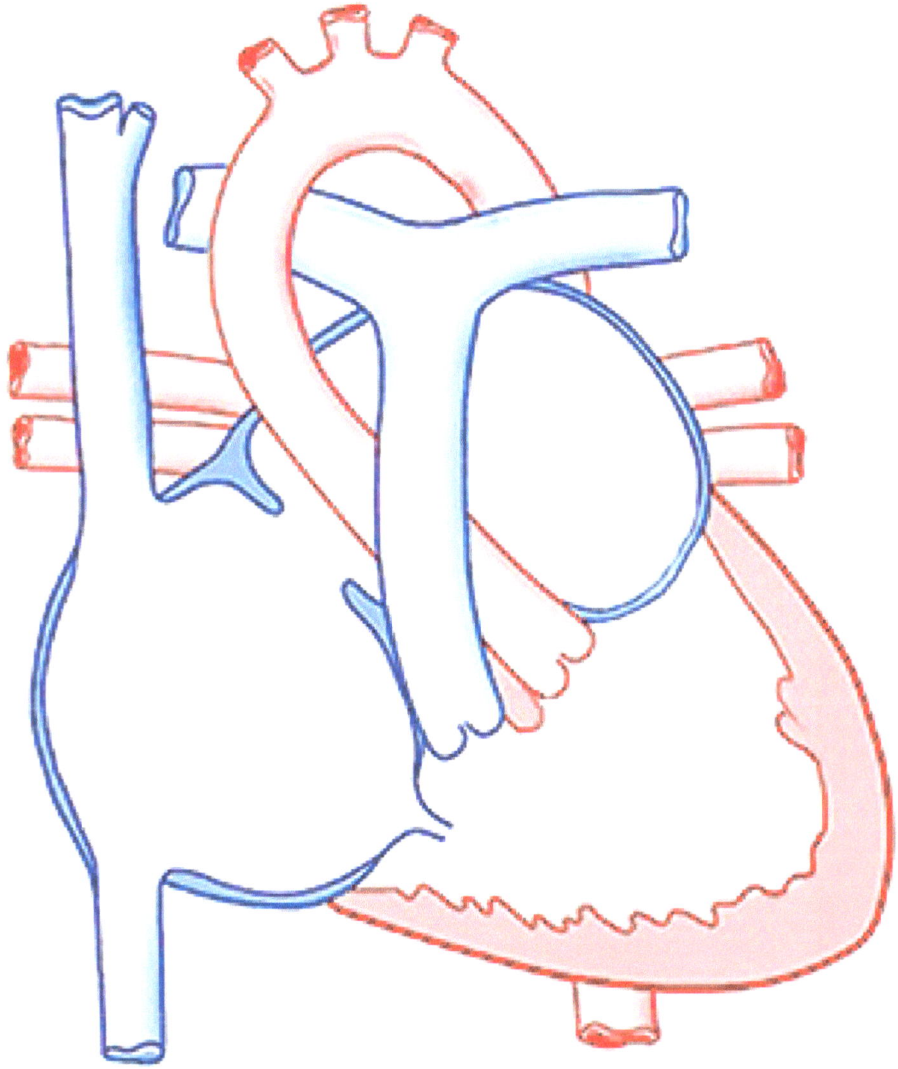

Figure 4: Single ventricle, mitral atresia, atrial septal defect within oval fossa.

*Corresponding author Oran B: Medicana International Hospital, Department of Pediatric Cardiology, İzmir, Turkey
E-mail:boran@medicana.com.tr and bulentoran@hotmail.com

Single Ventricle, Tricuspid Atresia, ASD

Tricuspid atresia is the absence of a tricuspid valve and lack of a connection between the right ventricle and right atrium. Together with an ASD or foramen ovale opening, a right-to-left shunt must be present. The right ventricle is hypoplastic and the left ventricle is dominant. The right ventricle and pulmonary valve are undeveloped. This malformation is associated with VSDs, pulmonary atresia, and pulmonary stenosis.

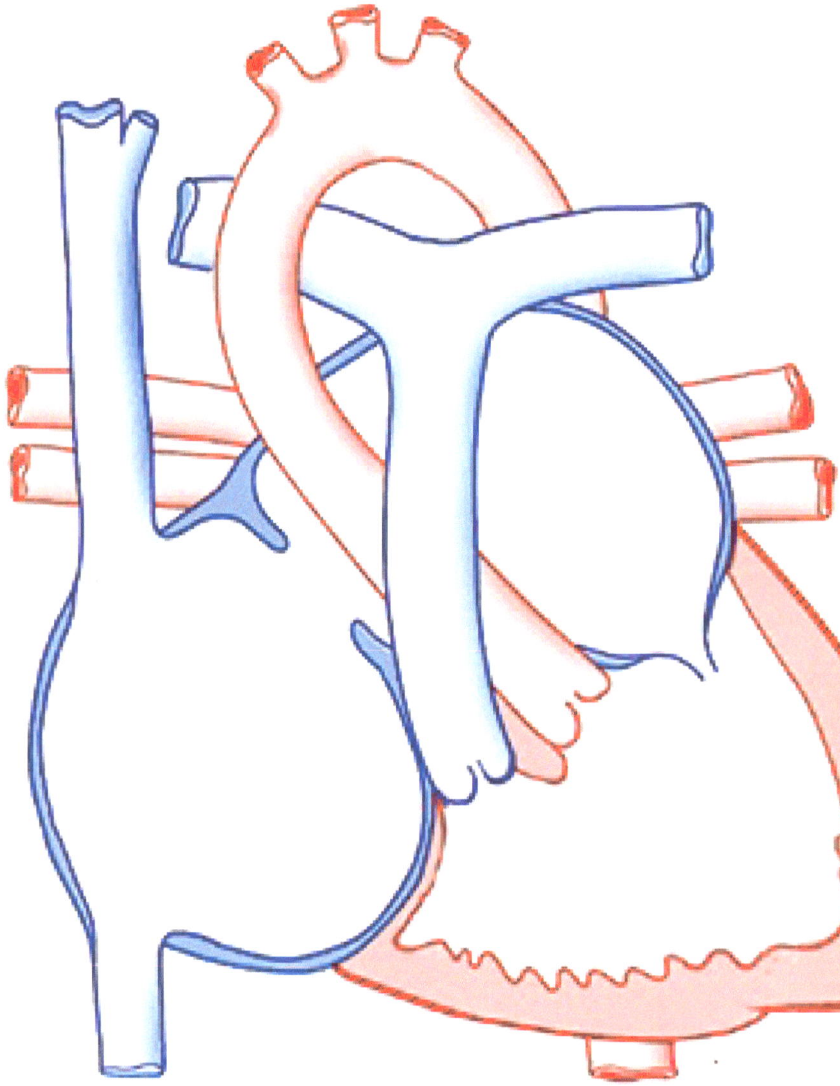

Figure 5: Single ventricle, tricuspid atresia with atrial septal defect within oval fossa.

*Corresponding author Oran B: Medicana International Hospital, Department of Pediatric Cardiology, İzmir, Turkey
E-mail:boran@medicana.com.tr and bulentoran@hotmail.com

Single Ventricle, AVSD with Ventricular Imbalance

Complete AVSDs are typically characterized by equally divided right and left valve components. However, in ventricular imbalance AVSD, right or left ventricle dominance occurs. When the imbalance is severe, patients display single ventricle hemodynamic features. Affected patients cannot survive until adulthood without intervention.

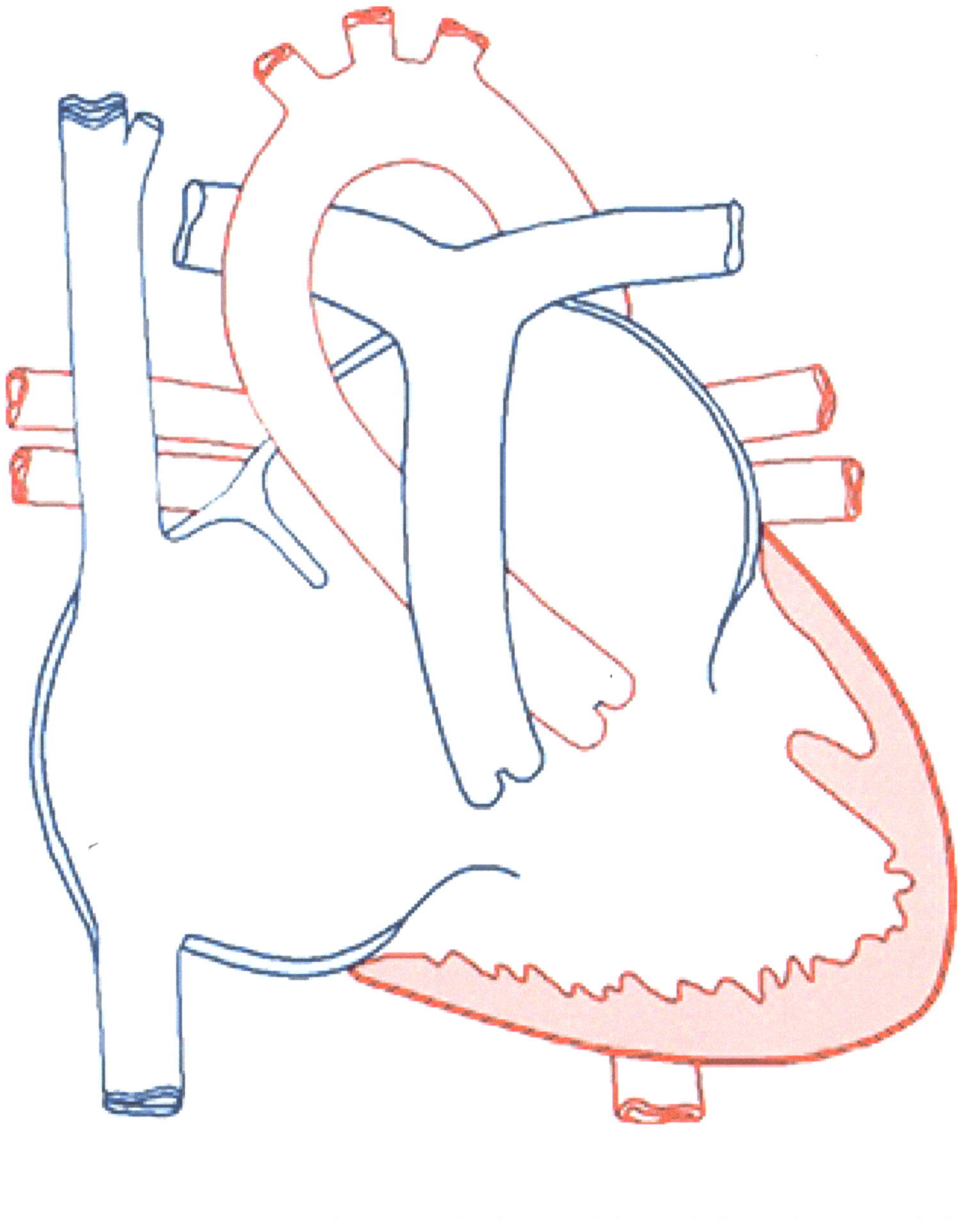

Figure 6: AVSD with ventricular imbalance, single ventricle. Unbalanced AV Canal, functionally univentricular heart.

*Corresponding auțhor Oran B: Medicana International Hospital, Department of Pediatric Cardiology, İzmir, Turkey
E-mail:boran@medicana.com.tr and bulentoran@hotmail.com

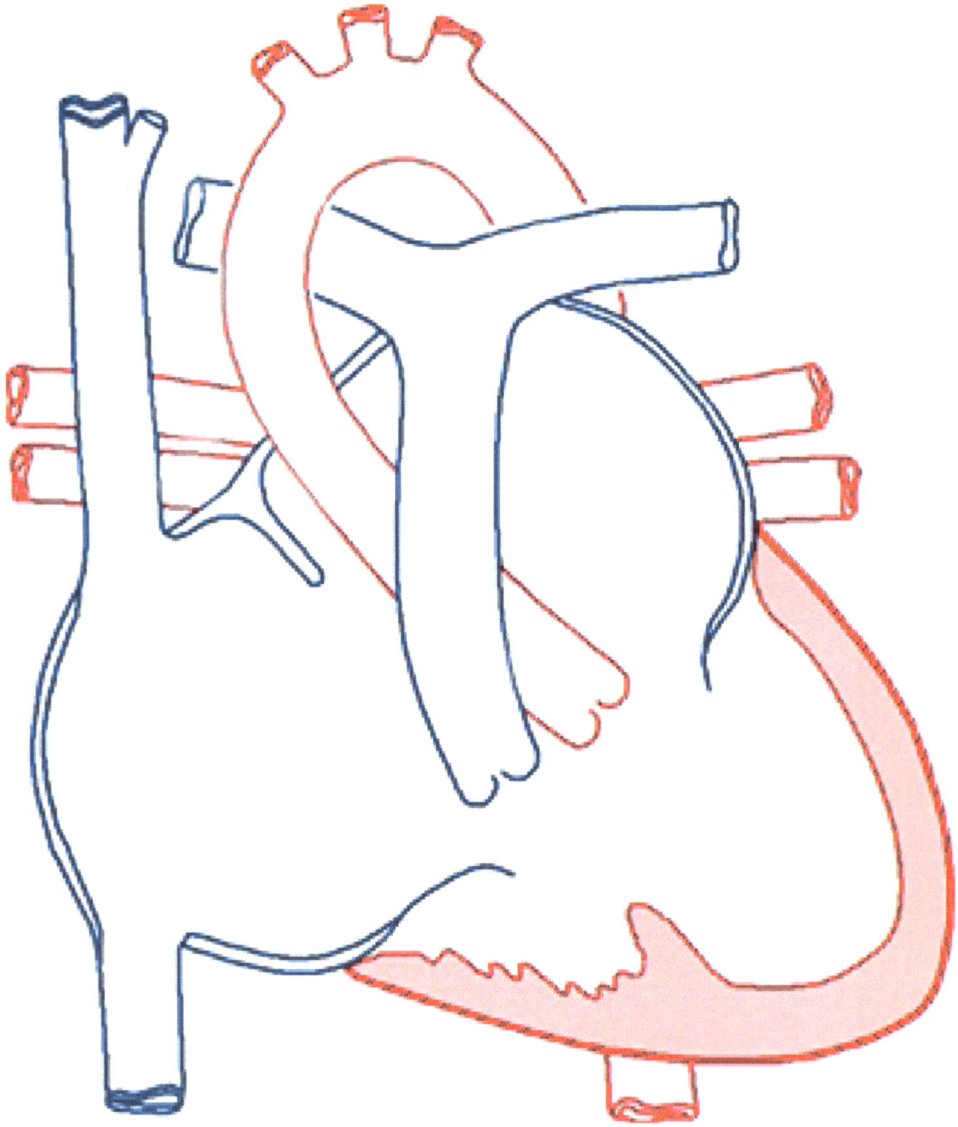

Figure 7: AVSD with ventricular imbalance, single ventricle. Unbalanced AV Canal, functionally univentricular heart.

*Corresponding author Oran B: Medicana International Hospital, Department of Pediatric Cardiology, İzmir, Turkey
E-mail:boran@medicana.com.tr and bulentoran@hotmail.com

Hypoplastic Left Heart Syndrome

Hypoplastic left heart syndrome, the most common lethal single ventricle anomaly, involves left ventricular and ascending aortic hypoplasia, as well as mitral and aortic valve stenosis or atresia. The ascending aorta is always hypoplastic; coarctation of the aorta and tricuspid valve anomalies are common. Systemic circulation is provided by the right ventricle. The survival of affected infants is only possible through a series of surgical procedures or heart transplantation.

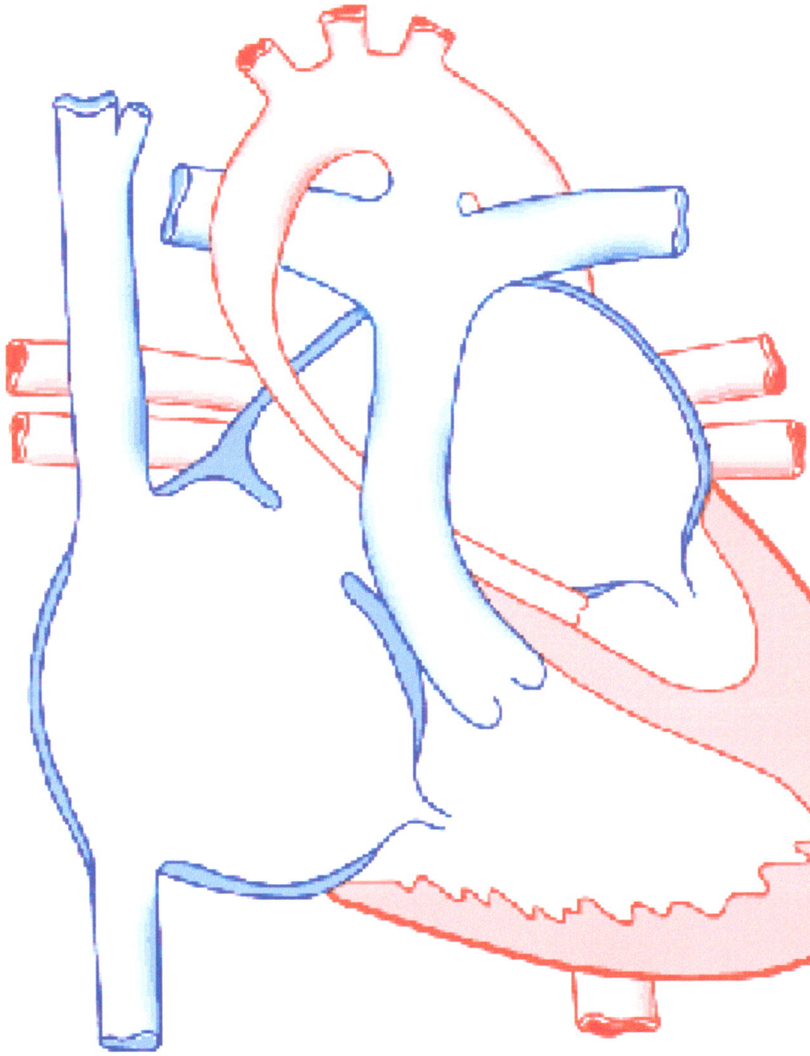

Figure 8: Hypoplastic left heart syndrome, ASD and PDA. Hypoplastic left heart syndrome, ascending aortic hypoplasia, aortic arch hypoplasia, patent arterial duct, atrial septal defect within oval fossa.

*Corresponding author Oran B: Medicana International Hospital, Department of Pediatric Cardiology, İzmir, Turkey
E-mail:boran@medicana.com.tr and bulentoran@hotmail.com

Tricuspid Atresia

Tricuspid atresia is defined as congenital absence or agenesis of the tricuspid valve. Tricuspid atresia is one of the three most common cyanotic congenital heart defects (others include tetralogy of Fallot and transposition of the great arteries). Intervention is important for survival to adulthood. A right-to-left shunt with an ASD or patent foramen ovale is necessary for diagnosis. The right ventricle is hypoplastic and underdeveloped; in addition, the right pulmonary valve is underdeveloped. Affected patients may also exhibit pulmonary stenosis or varying levels of atresia. The left ventricle is dominant. Ventriculoarterial situs is common (70-80%). This severe heart disease requires surgical intervention for survival to adulthood. This malformation is associated with VSDs, pulmonary atresia, pulmonary stenosis, coarctation of the aorta, right aortic arch, and left persistent superior vena cava.

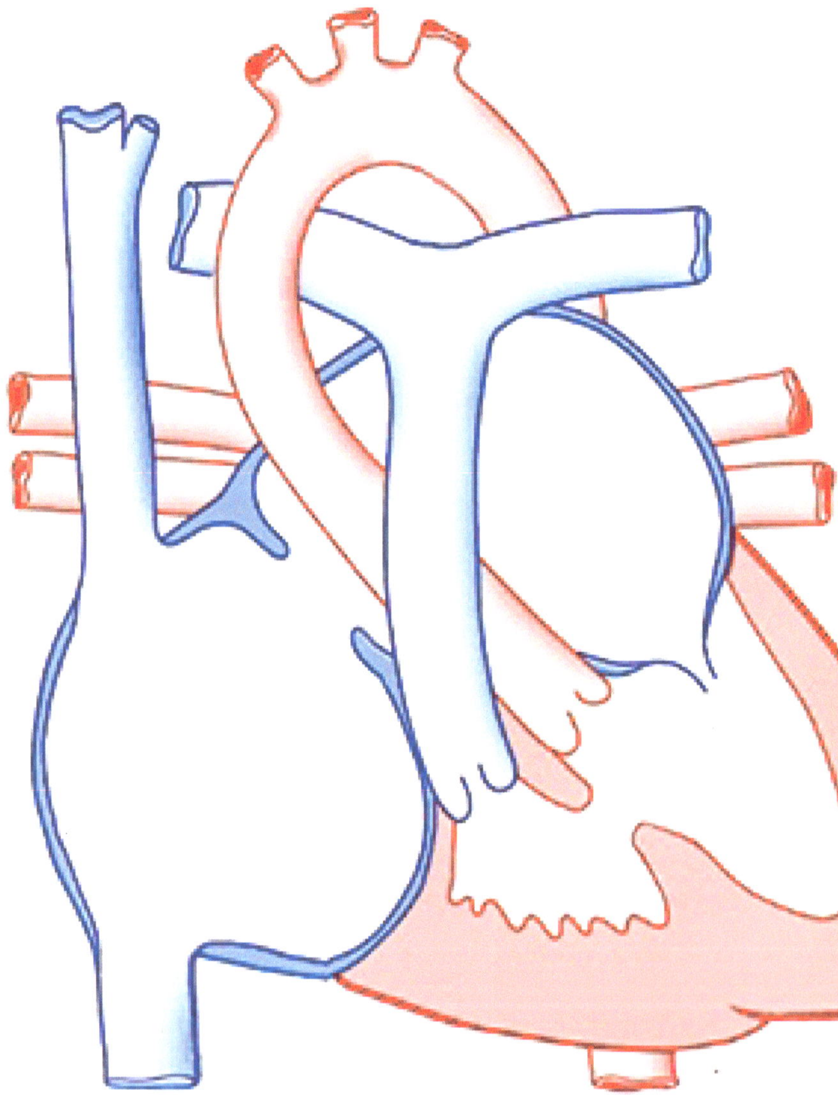

Figure 9: Tricuspid atresia with ventricular septal defect and atrial septal defect within oval fossa.

*Corresponding author Oran B: Medicana International Hospital, Department of Pediatric Cardiology, İzmir, Turkey
E-mail:boran@medicana.com.tr and bulentoran@hotmail.com

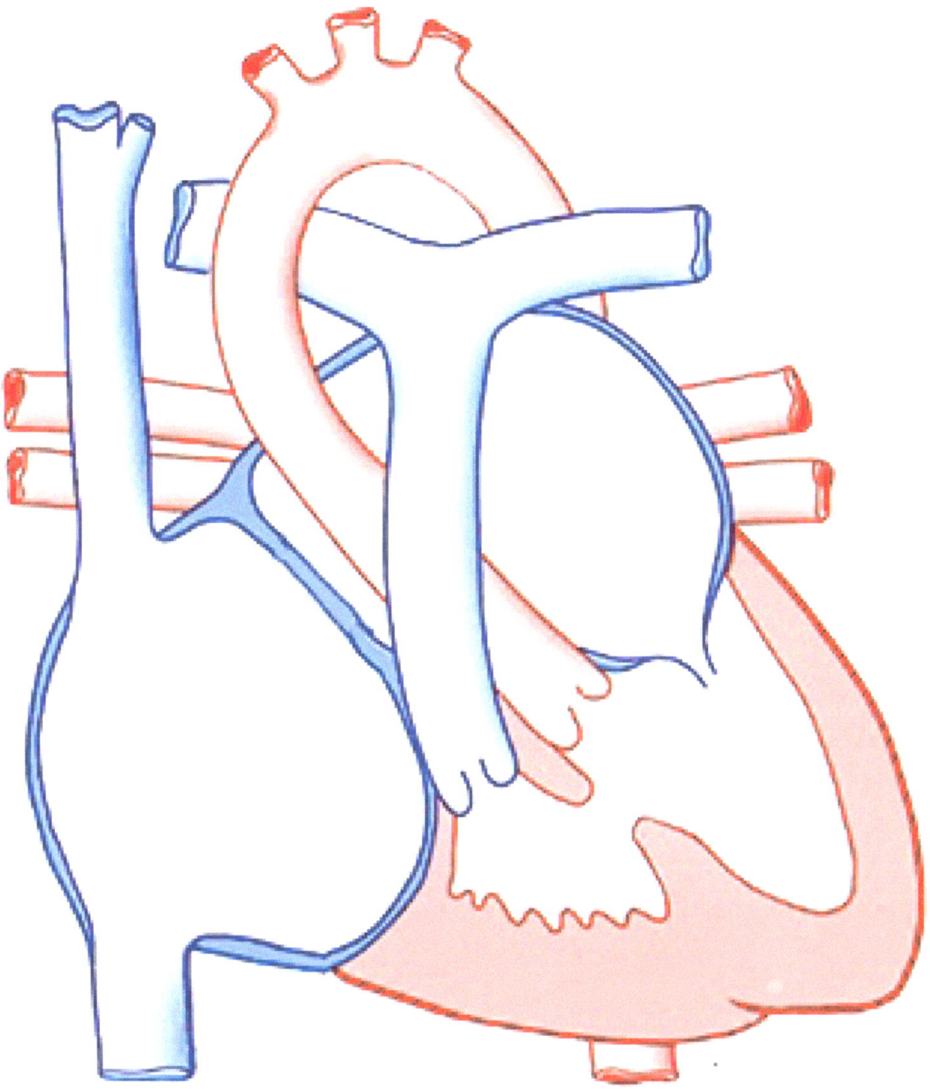

Figure 10: Tricuspid atresia with ventricular septal defect.

*Corresponding author Oran B: Medicana International Hospital, Department of Pediatric Cardiology, İzmir, Turkey
E-mail:boran@medicana.com.tr and bulentoran@hotmail.com

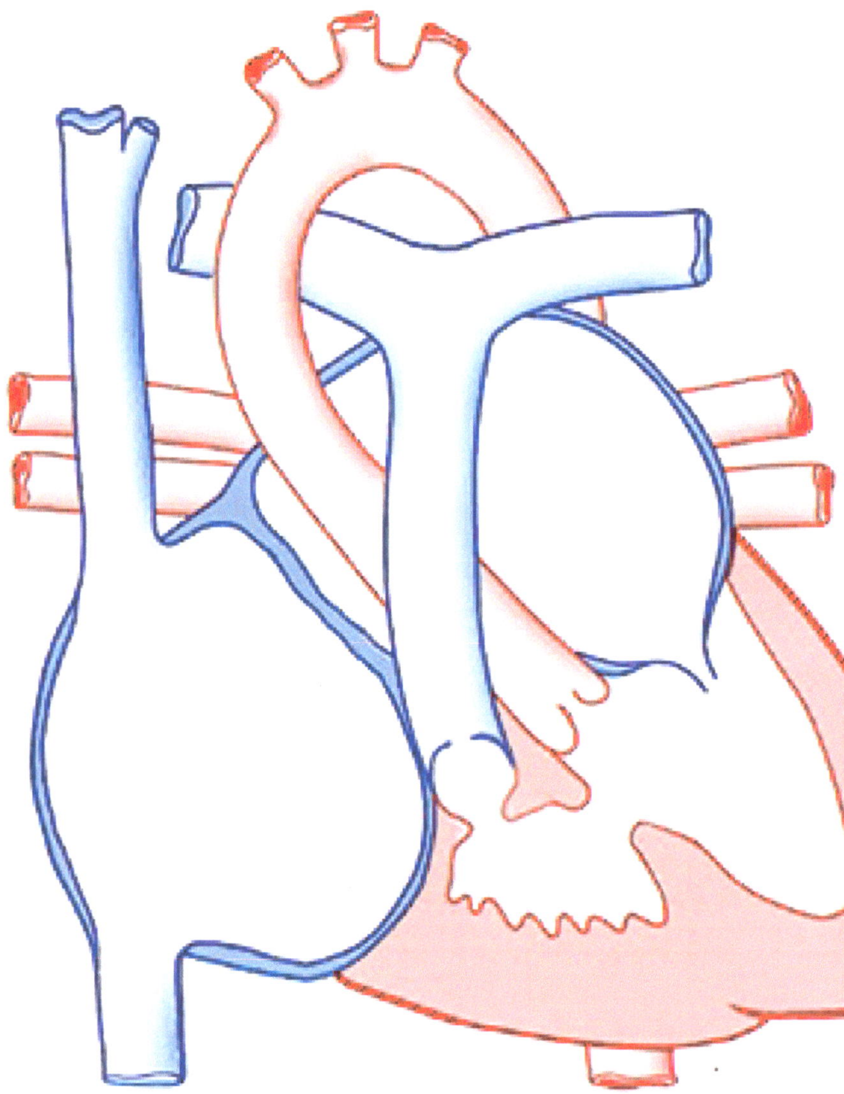

Figure 11: Tricuspid atresia with ventricular septal defect and pulmonary stenosis.

*Corresponding author Oran B: Medicana International Hospital, Department of Pediatric Cardiology, İzmir, Turkey
E-mail:boran@medicana.com.tr and bulentoran@hotmail.com

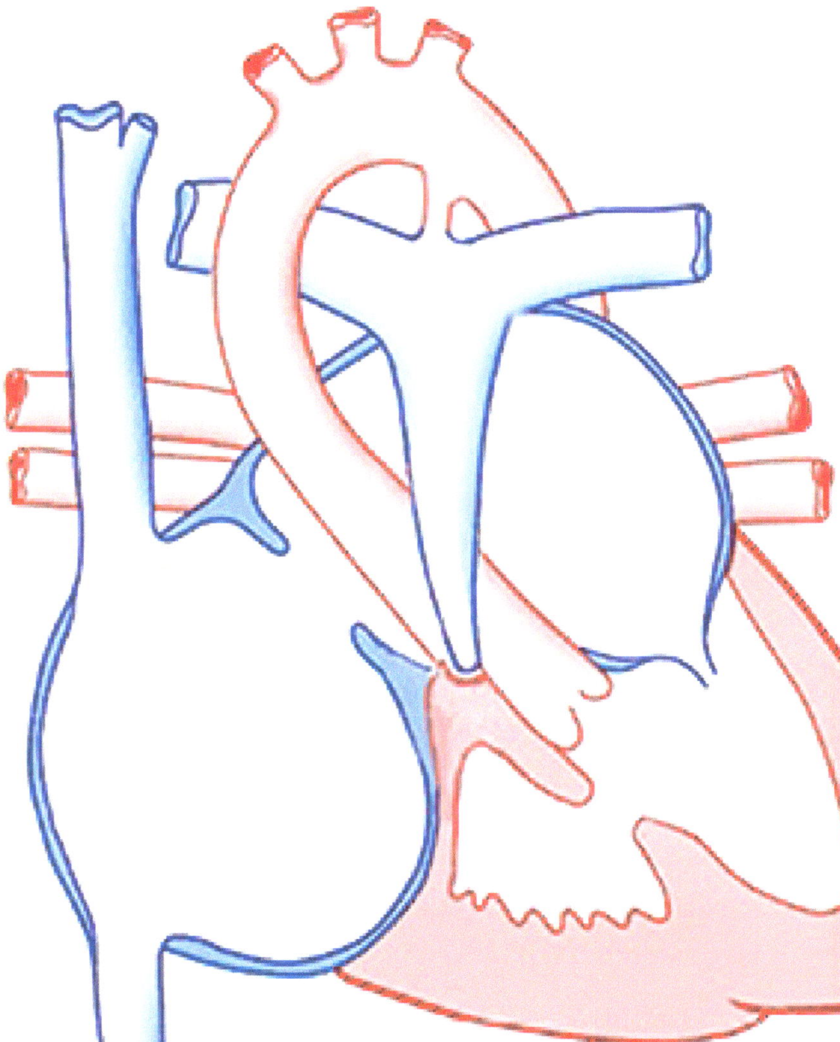

Figure 12: Tricuspid atresia with ventricular septal defect, patent arterial duct, atrial septal defect within oval fossa, and pulmonary atresia.

*Corresponding author Oran B: Medicana International Hospital, Department of Pediatric Cardiology, İzmir, Turkey
E-mail:boran@medicana.com.tr and bulentoran@hotmail.com

Pulmonary Atresia

The term pulmonary atresia has been used to describe a wide spectrum of pathologies ranging from simple valvar atresia to the absence of true pulmonary arteries. The number of affected patients who reach adulthood without any intervention is extremely limited. Pulmonary atresia involves a right-to-left shunt with VSDs, ASDs, PDA, or MAPCAs.

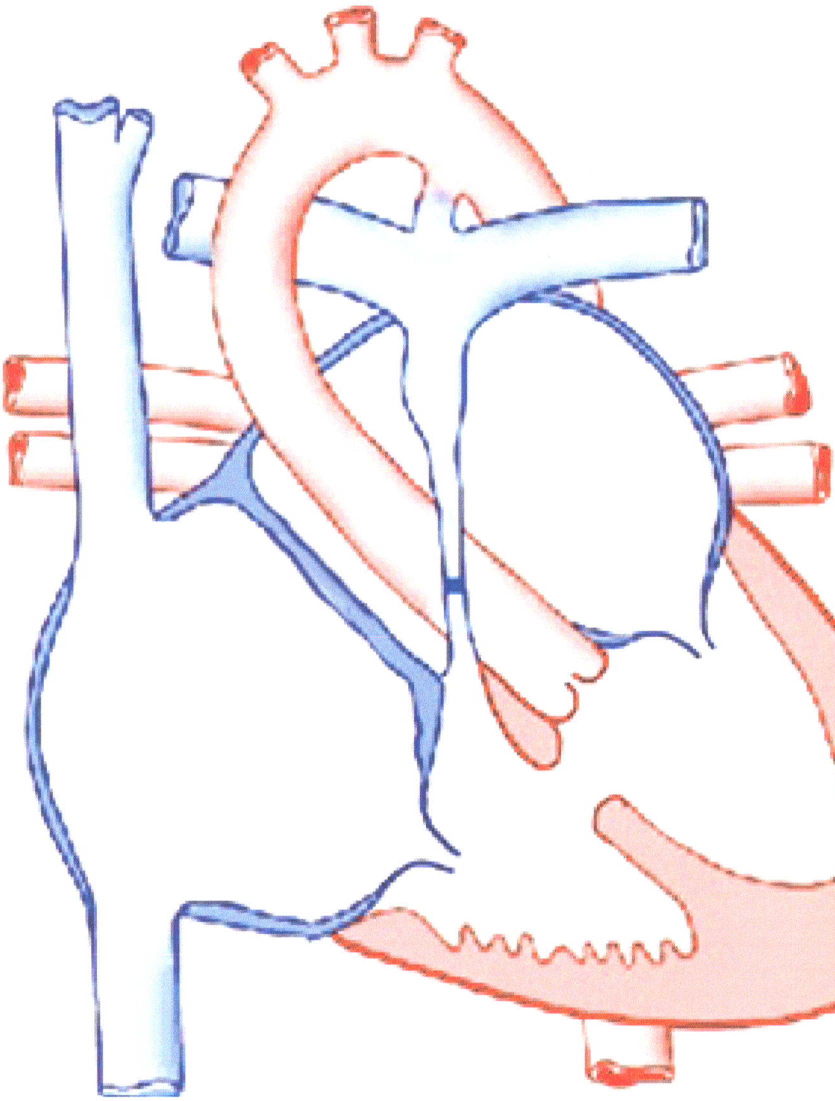

Figure 13: Pulmonary atresia, ventricular septal defect and patent arterial duct.

*Corresponding author Oran B: Medicana International Hospital, Department of Pediatric Cardiology, İzmir, Turkey
E-mail:boran@medicana.com.tr and bulentoran@hotmail.com

Pulmonary Atresia with Intact Ventricular Septum

Pulmonary atresia with intact ventricular septum is an extremely serious pediatric condition. Affected patients require intervention to reach adulthood. This defect is characterized by the absence of direct communication between the right ventricular cavity and the pulmonary trunk. Pulmonary vascular blood flow displays unifocal or multifocal circulation patterns. This malformation is characterized by a right-to-left shunt with ASDs, PDA, or MAPCAs.

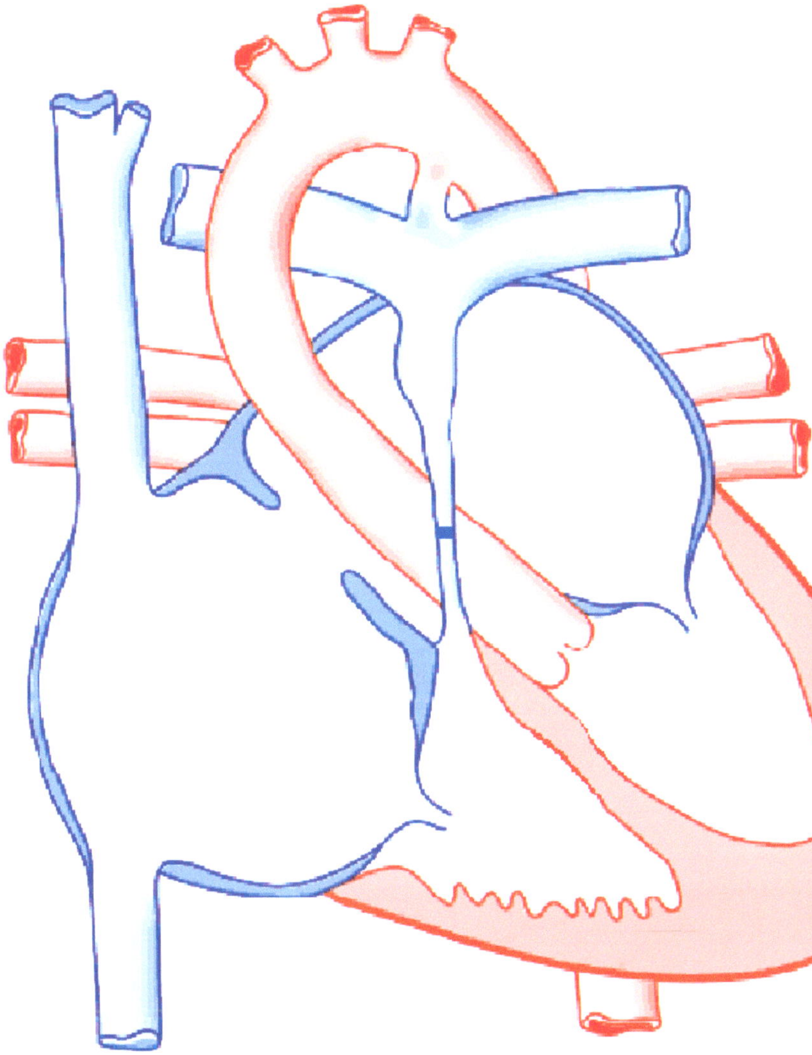

Figure 14: Pulmonary atresia with intact ventricular septum, atrial septal defect, patent arterial duct.

*Corresponding author Oran B: Medicana International Hospital, Department of Pediatric Cardiology, İzmir, Turkey
E-mail:boran@medicana.com.tr and bulentoran@hotmail.com

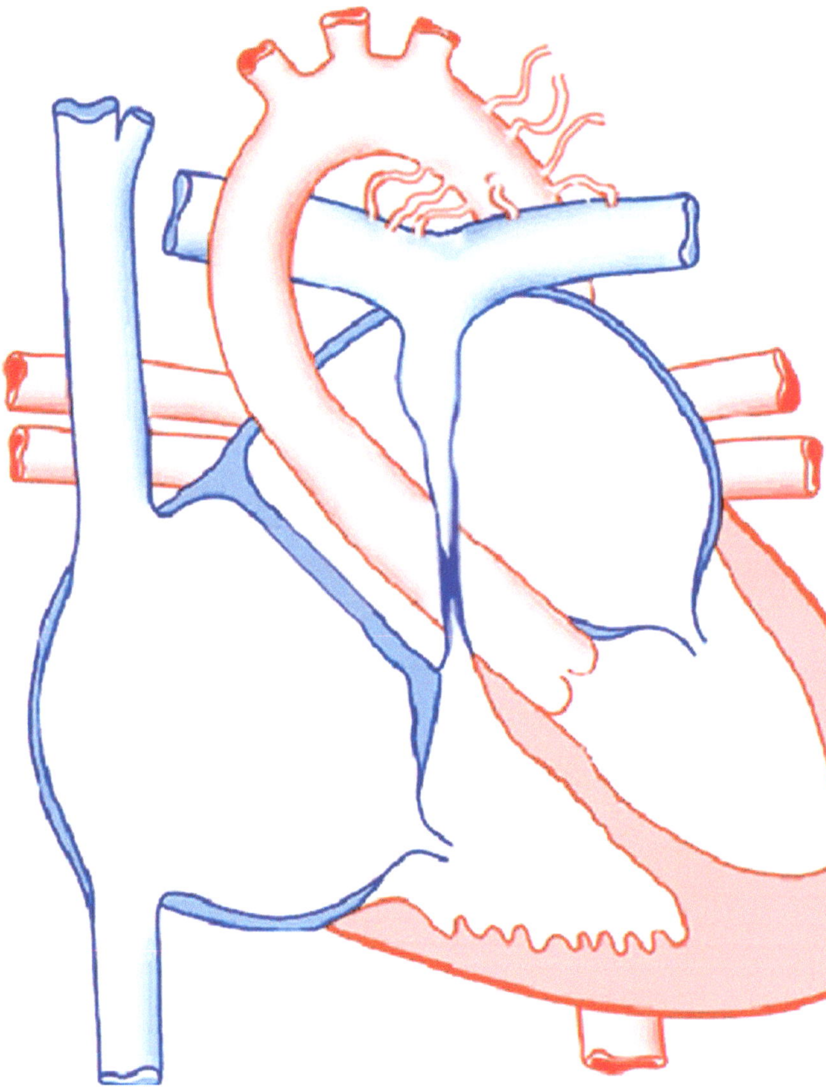

Figure 15: Pulmonary atresia with MAPCA.

*Corresponding author Oran B: Medicana International Hospital, Department of Pediatric Cardiology, İzmir, Turkey
E-mail:boran@medicana.com.tr and bulentoran@hotmail.com

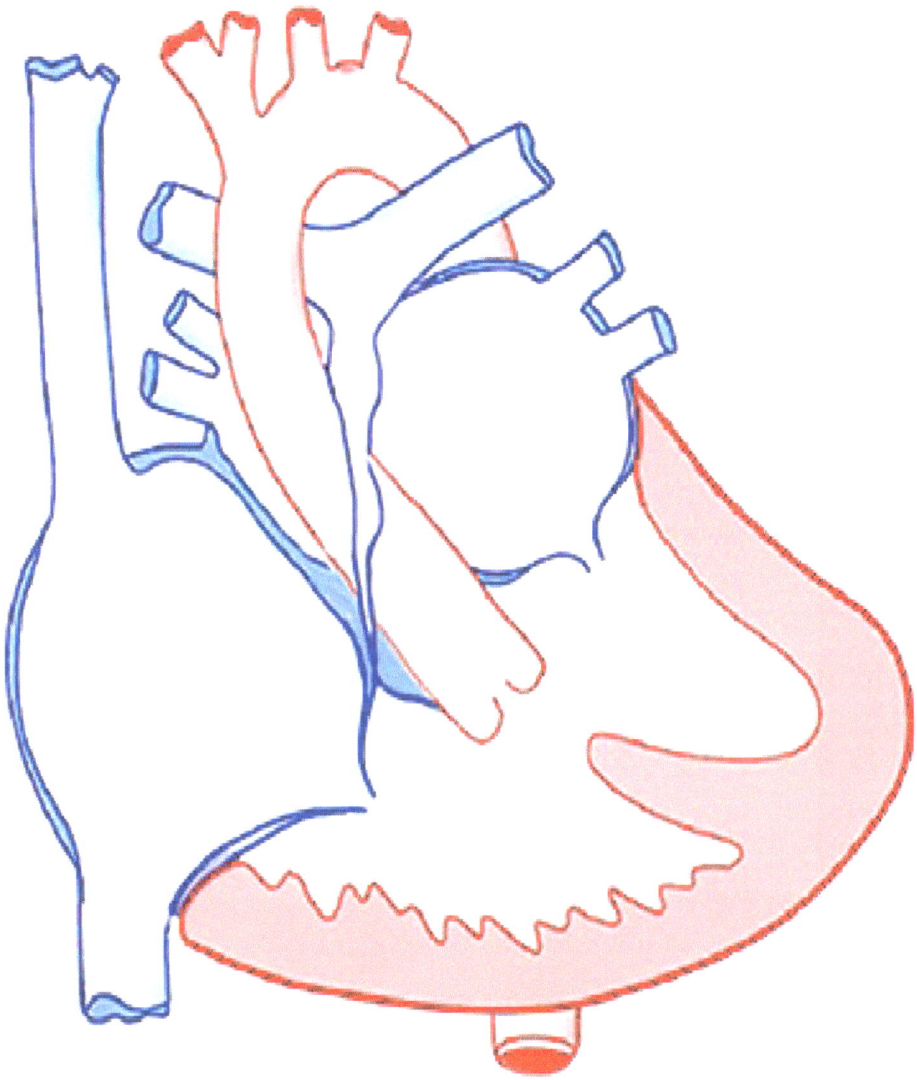

Figure 16: Pulmonary atresia with VSD (including Fallot type). Pulmonary atresia, tetralogy of Fallot type.

*Corresponding author Oran B: Medicana International Hospital, Department of Pediatric Cardiology, İzmir, Turkey
E-mail:boran@medicana.com.tr and bulentoran@hotmail.com

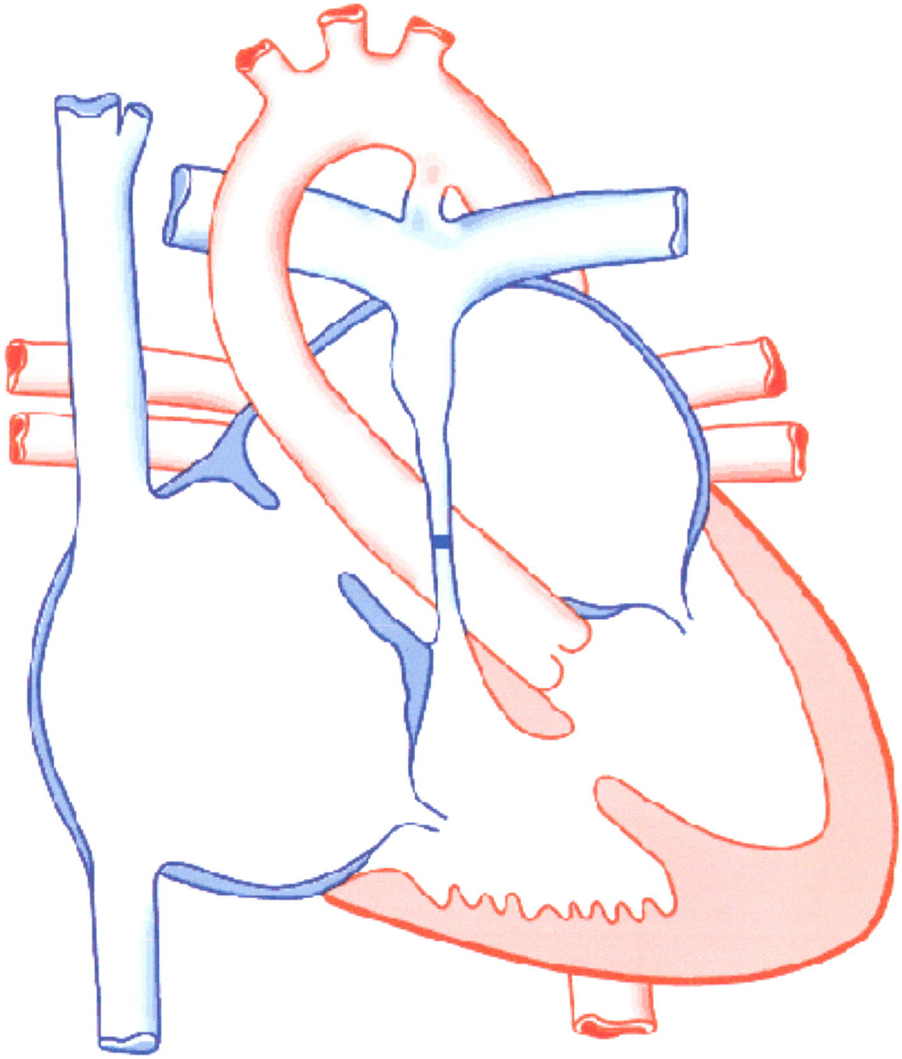

Figure 17: Pulmonary atresia with ventricular septal defect, atrial septal defect within oval fossa, patent arterial duct.

*Corresponding author Oran B: Medicana International Hospital, Department of Pediatric Cardiology, İzmir, Turkey
E-mail:boran@medicana.com.tr and bulentoran@hotmail.com

CHAPTER 9
Interventional Procedures

Oran B.

Medicana International Hospital, Department of Pediatric Cardiology, İzmir, Turkey

*Corresponding author Oran B: Medicana International Hospital, Department of Pediatric Cardiology, İzmir, Turkey
E-mail:boran@medicana.com.tr and bulentoran@hotmail.com

Balloon Atrial Septostomy

Balloon atrial septostomy is an interventional procedure in which a hole is created between the left and right atria. Access occurs via the umbilical or femoral vein. Typical femoral vein puncture is performed and a balloon septostomy catheter is advanced into the right atrium. The foramen ovale is crossed and the catheter is positioned in the left atrium.

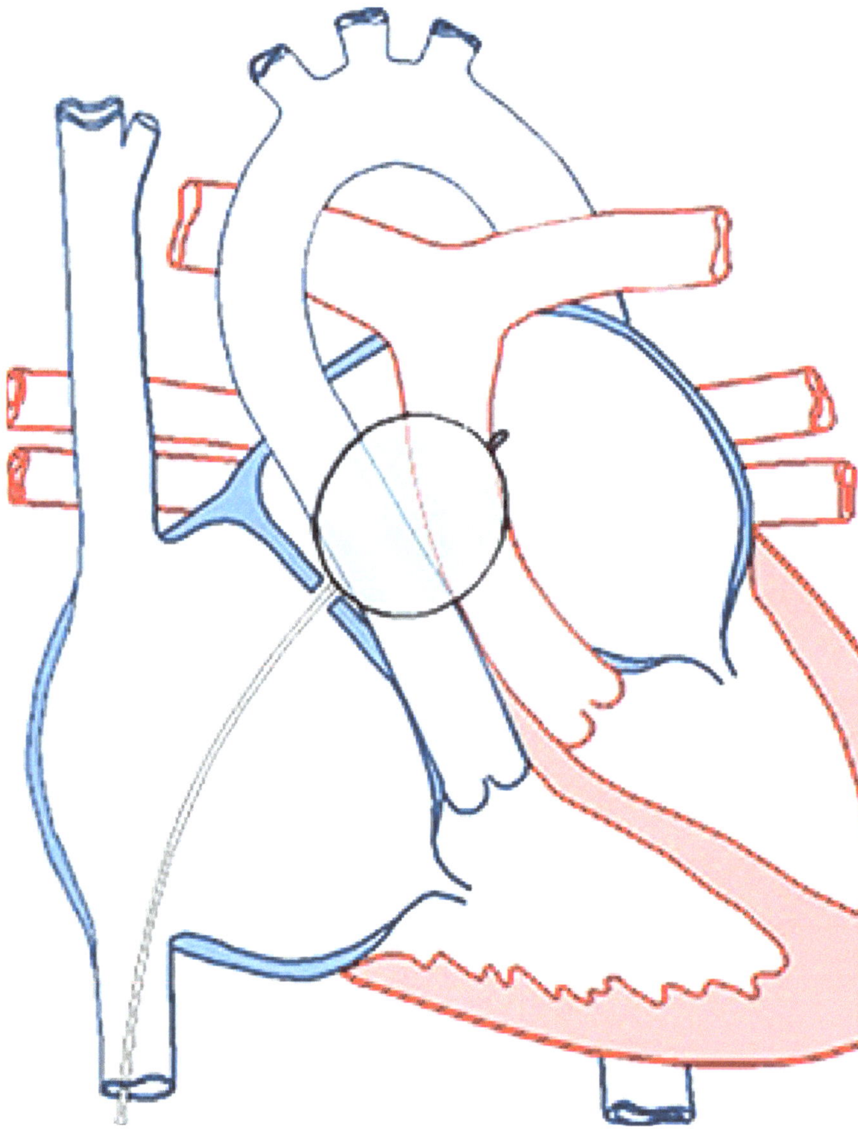

Figure 1: Balloon atrial septostomy in patient with transposition of the great arteries.

*Corresponding author Oran B: Medicana International Hospital, Department of Pediatric Cardiology, İzmir, Turkey
E-mail:boran@medicana.com.tr and bulentoran@hotmail.com

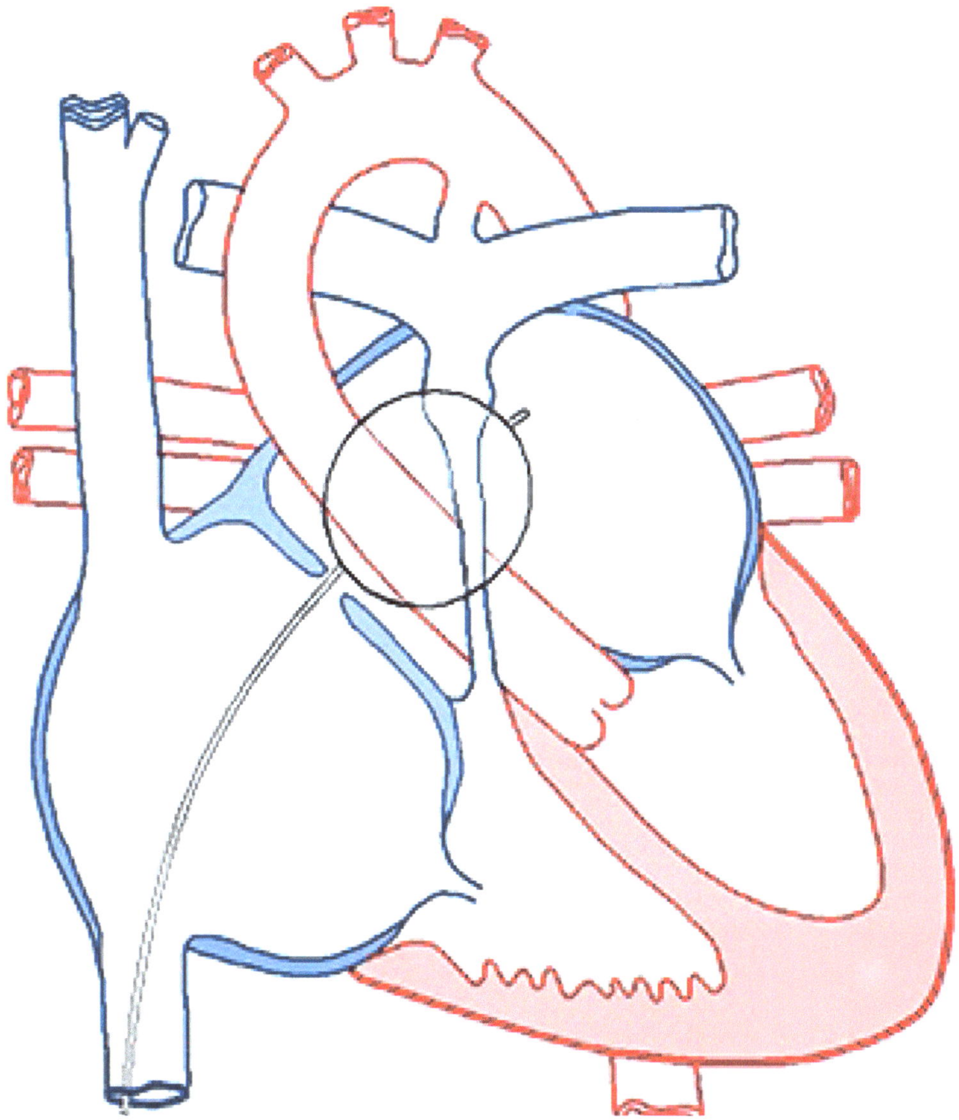

Figure 2: Balloon atrial septostomy in patient with pulmonary atresia

*Corresponding author Oran B: Medicana International Hospital, Department of Pediatric Cardiology, İzmir, Turkey
E-mail:boran@medicana.com.tr and bulentoran@hotmail.com

Blade Atrial Septostomy

Blade atrial septostomy is an interventional procedure in which a hole is created between the left and right atria. Access occurs via the femoral vein. Typical femoral vein puncture is performed and a blade septostomy catheter is advanced into the right atrium. The foramen ovale is crossed and the catheter is positioned in the left atrium.

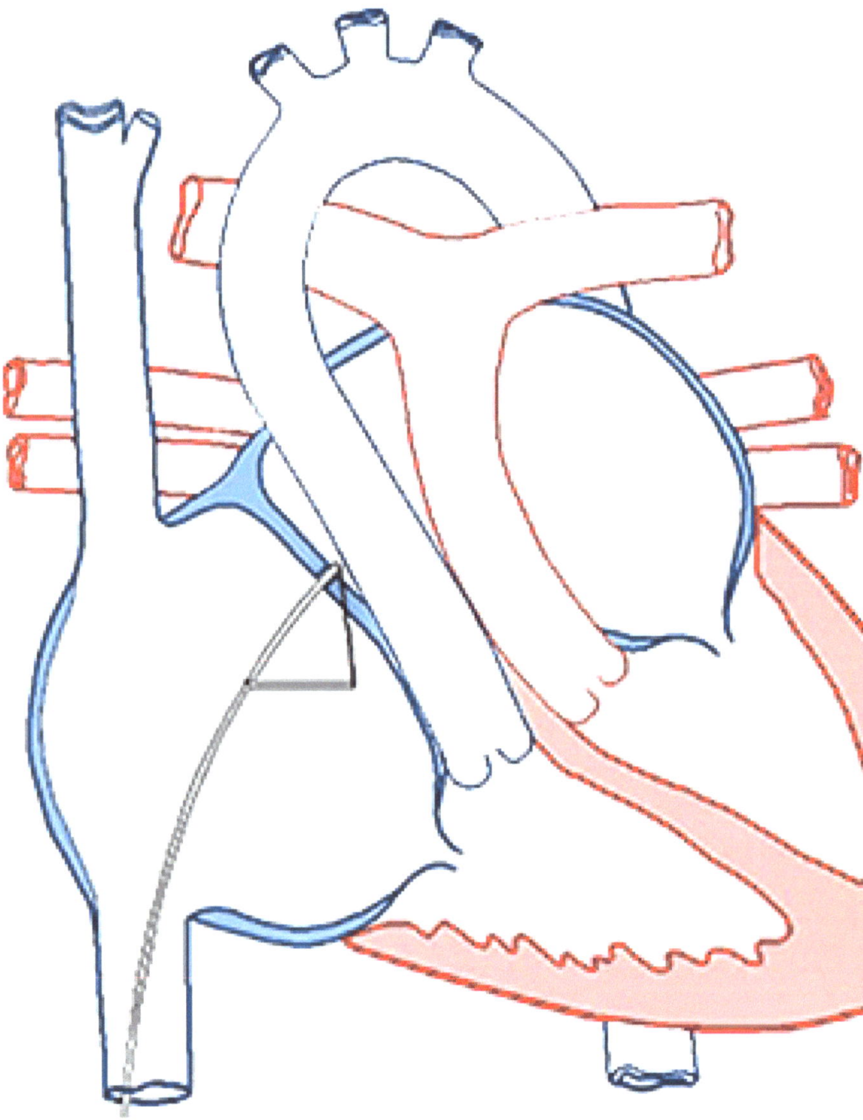

Figure 3: Blade atrial septostomy, transposition of the great arteries

*Corresponding author Oran B: Medicana International Hospital, Department of Pediatric Cardiology, İzmir, Turkey
E-mail:boran@medicana.com.tr and bulentoran@hotmail.com

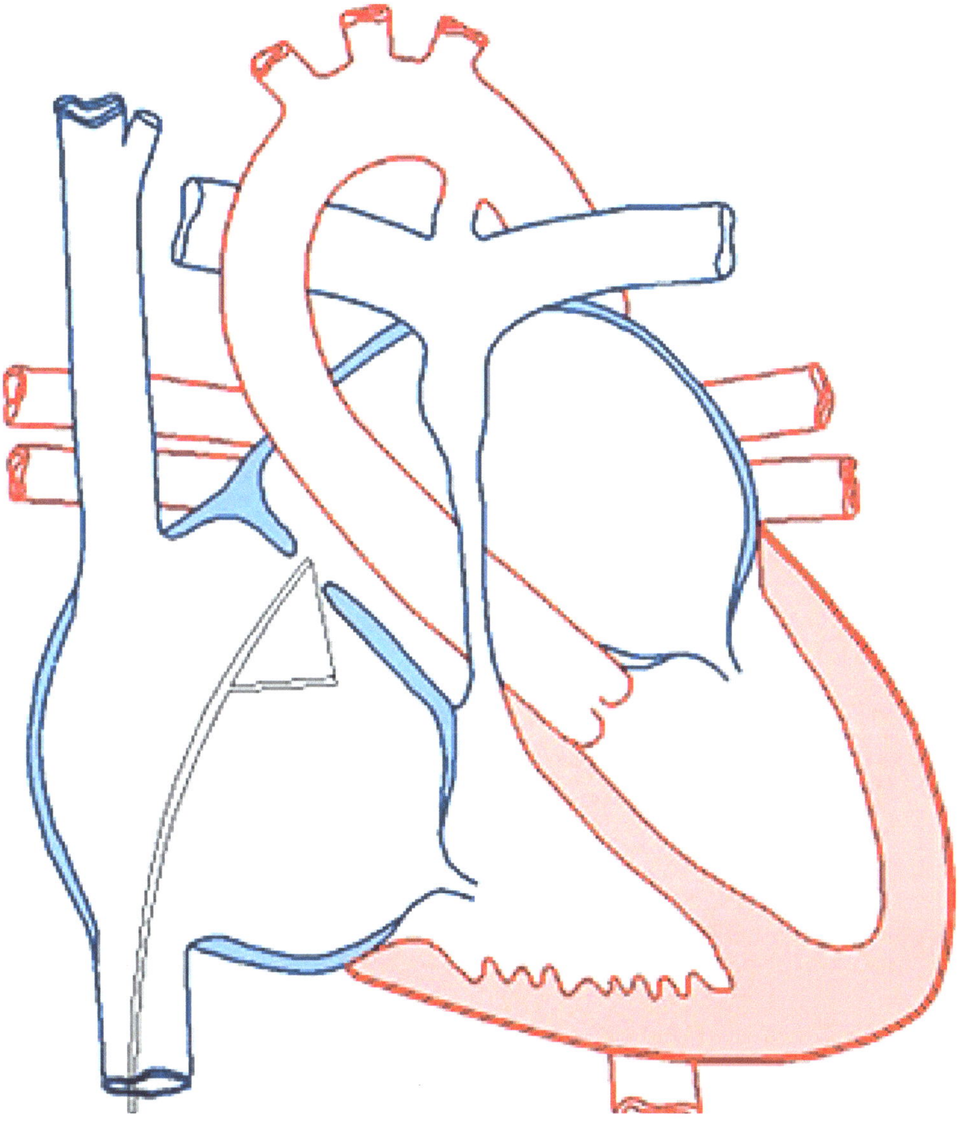

Figure 4: Blade atrial septostomy, pulmonary atresia

*Corresponding author Oran B: Medicana International Hospital, Department of Pediatric Cardiology, İzmir, Turkey
E-mail:boran@medicana.com.tr and bulentoran@hotmail.com

Pulmonary Balloon Valvuloplasty

Percutaneous pulmonary balloon valvuloplasty is the preferred procedure for treatment of uncomplicated severe valvar pulmonary stenosis. The right femoral vein serves as the entry point of the catheter, which is placed distal to the stenotic pulmonary valve.

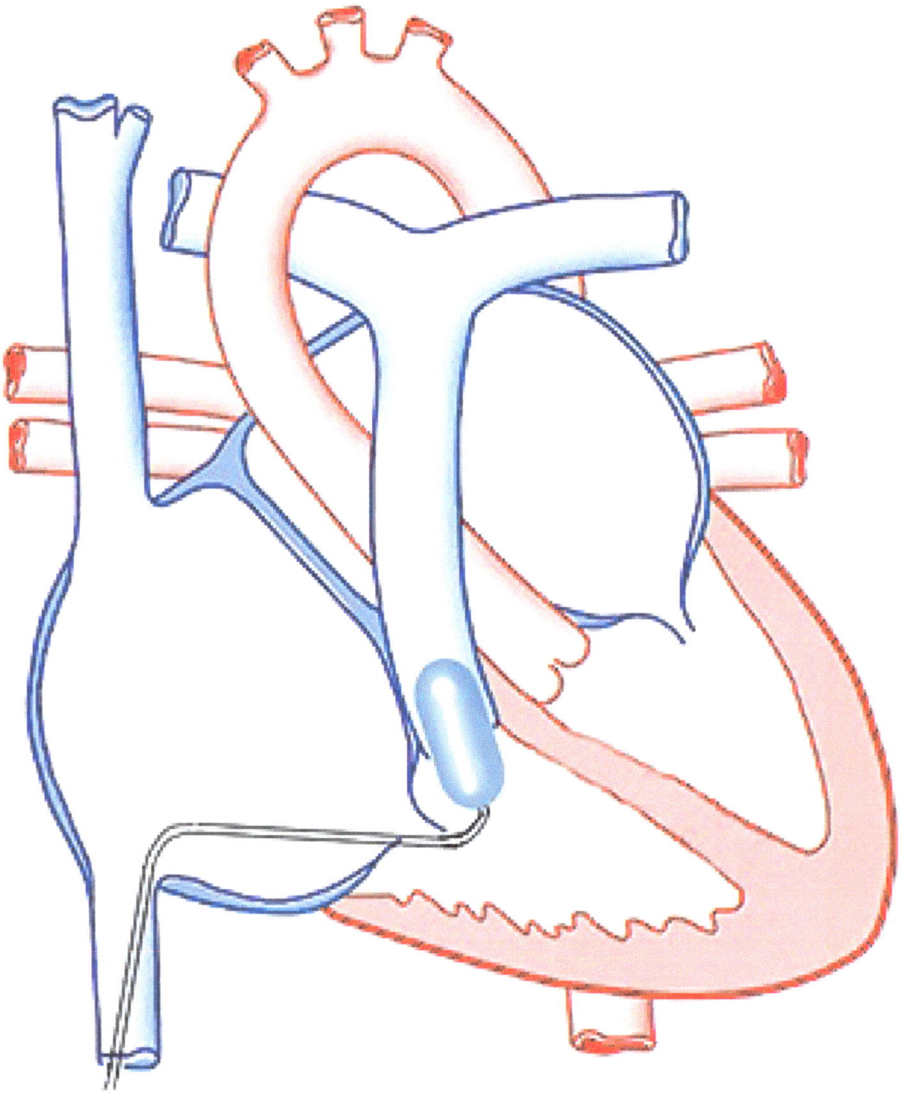

Figure 5: Pulmonary balloon valvuloplasty.

*Corresponding author Oran B: Medicana International Hospital, Department of Pediatric Cardiology, İzmir, Turkey
E-mail:boran@medicana.com.tr and bulentoran@hotmail.com

Aortic Baloon Valvuloplasty

Percutaneous aortic balloon valvuloplasty is the preferred procedure for treatment of uncomplicated severe valvar aortic stenosis. The right femoral artery serves as the entry point of the catheter, which is placed in the left ventricle via the aorta.

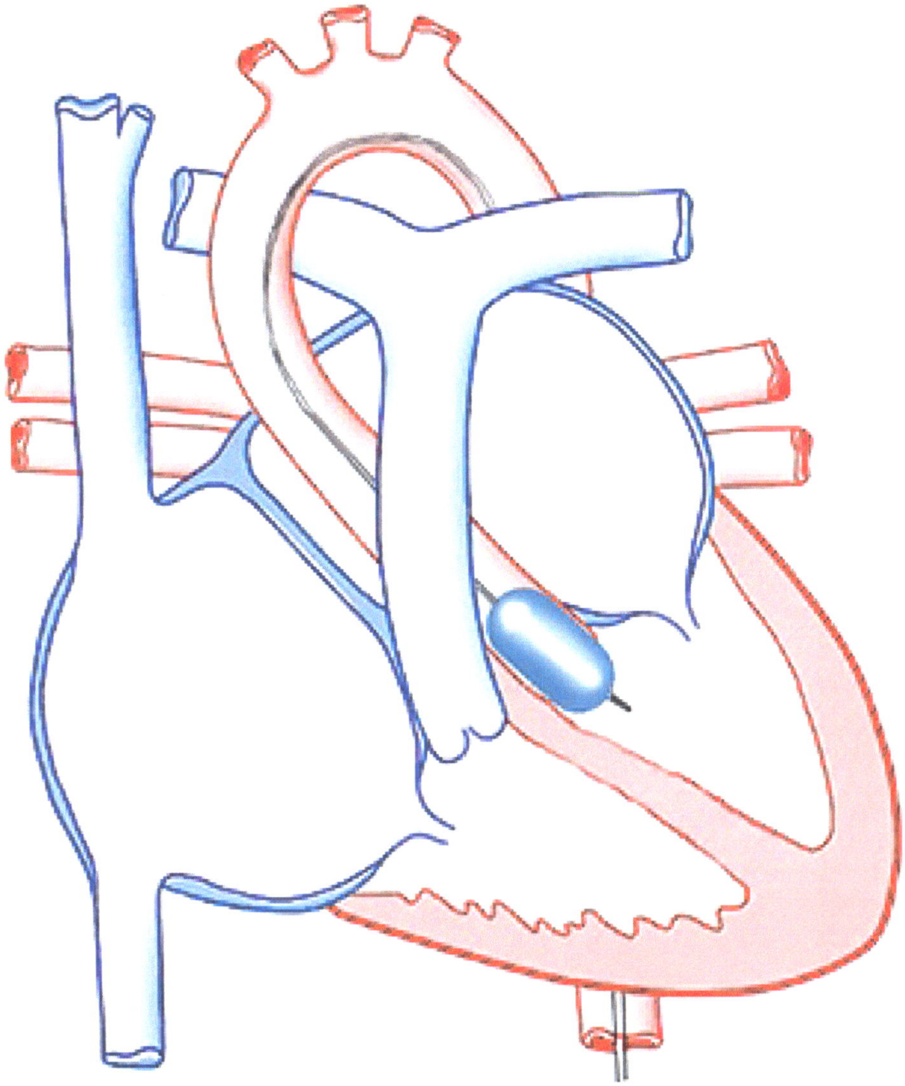

Figure 6: Aortic baloon valvuloplasty

*Corresponding author Oran B: Medicana International Hospital, Department of Pediatric Cardiology, İzmir, Turkey
E-mail:boran@medicana.com.tr and bulentoran@hotmail.com

Aortic Coarctation Angioplasty

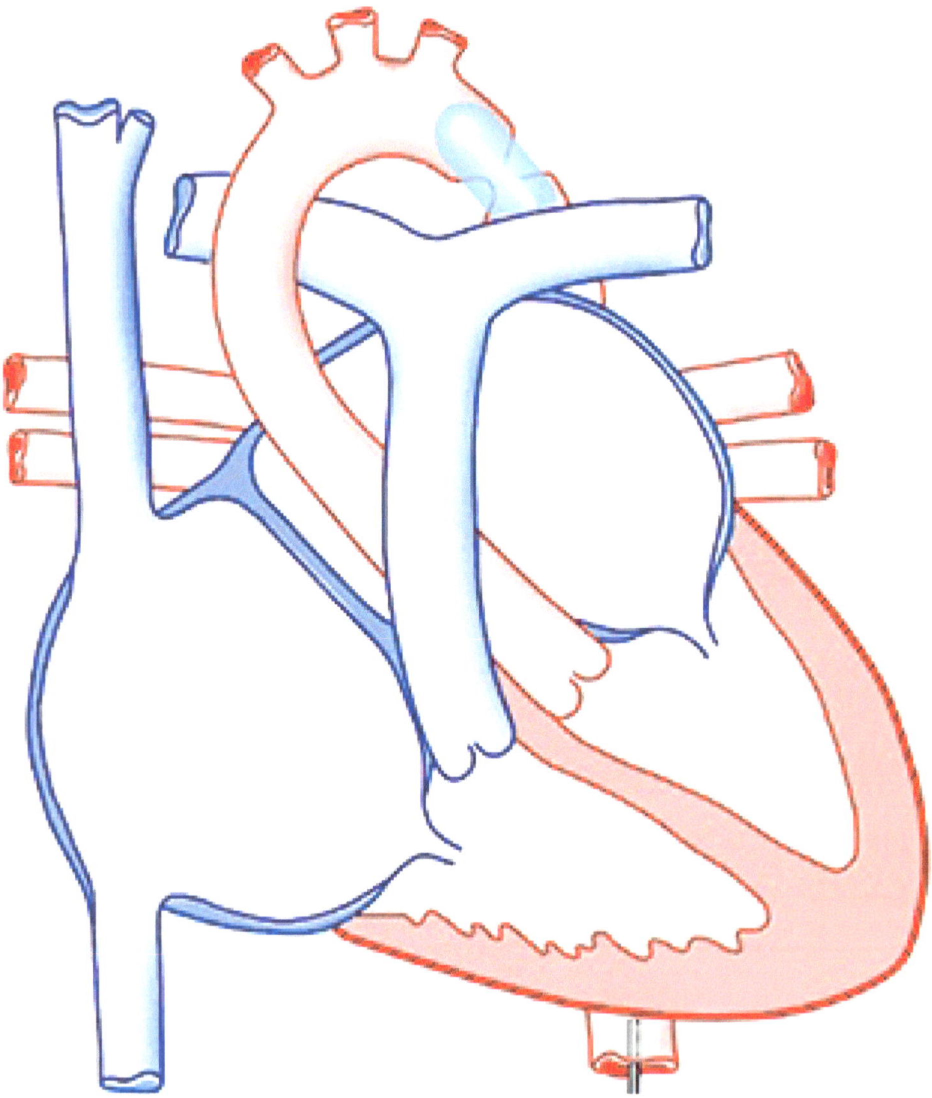

Figure 7: Balloon dilation of native aortic coarct / hypoplasia, (STS term: Balloon dilation)

*Corresponding author Oran B: Medicana International Hospital, Department of Pediatric Cardiology, İzmir, Turkey
E-mail:boran@medicana.com.tr and bulentoran@hotmail.com

Mitral Baloon Valvuloplasty

Mitral balloon valvuloplasty involves advancing a catheter over the wire across the interatrial septum after transseptal puncture, enlarging the opening and advancing an appropriately sized balloon across the mitral orifice, then inflating the balloon within the orifice.

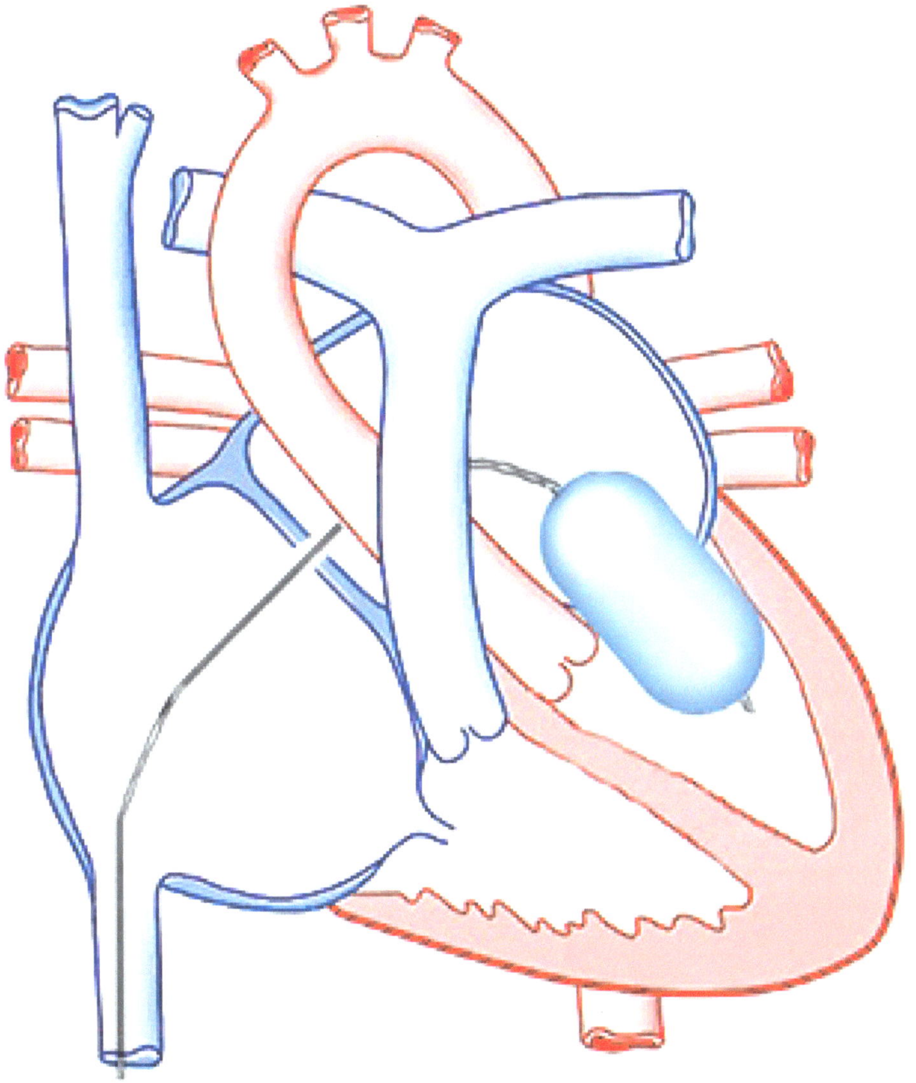

Figure 8: Mitral baloon valvuloplasty

*Corresponding author Oran B: Medicana International Hospital, Department of Pediatric Cardiology, İzmir, Turkey
E-mail:boran@medicana.com.tr and bulentoran@hotmail.com

Transcatheter Closure of Patent Ductus Arteriosus with an Occluder Devices

Several devices are currently available for percutaneous closure of PDA. The minimum diameter, aortic ampulla diameter, and duct length are measured. An endhole delivery catheter is passed through the duct from the pulmonary side into the descending aorta. The occluder is advanced through the catheter, then deployed in the appropriate position while the delivery catheter is withdrawn.

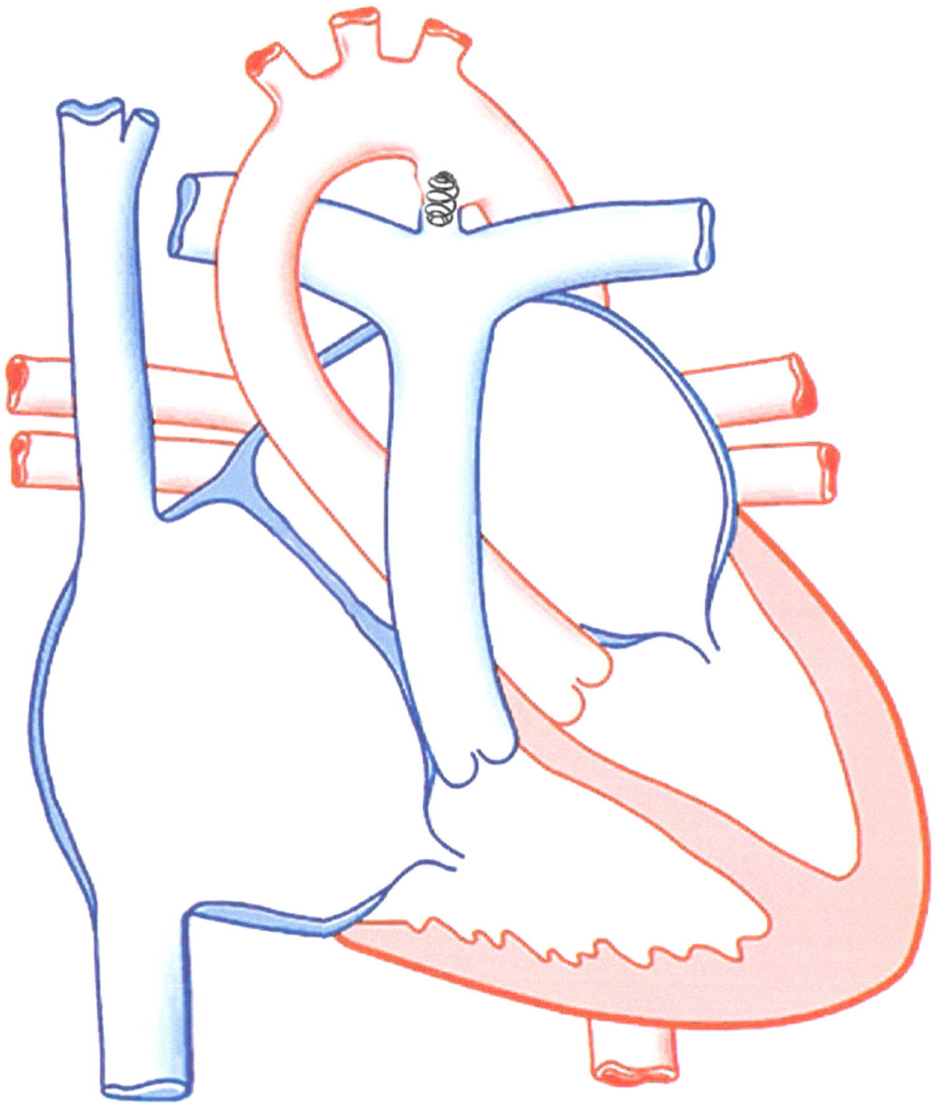

Figure 9: Transcatheter Closure of Patent Ductus Arteriosus with Devices.

*Corresponding author Oran B: Medicana International Hospital, Department of Pediatric Cardiology, İzmir, Turkey
E-mail:boran@medicana.com.tr and bulentoran@hotmail.com

Transcatheter Closure of the Atrial Septal Defect with an Occluder Devices

Transcatheter closure of secundum ASDs with an occluder device is an alternative to surgical repair. First, standard right heart catheterization is performed through the right femoral vein. The occluder device catheter is advanced into the right atrium after the balloon sizing procedure. The ASD is crossed and the delivery catheter is positioned in the left atrium. The occluder is advanced through the catheter, then deployed in the appropriate position while the delivery catheter is withdrawn.

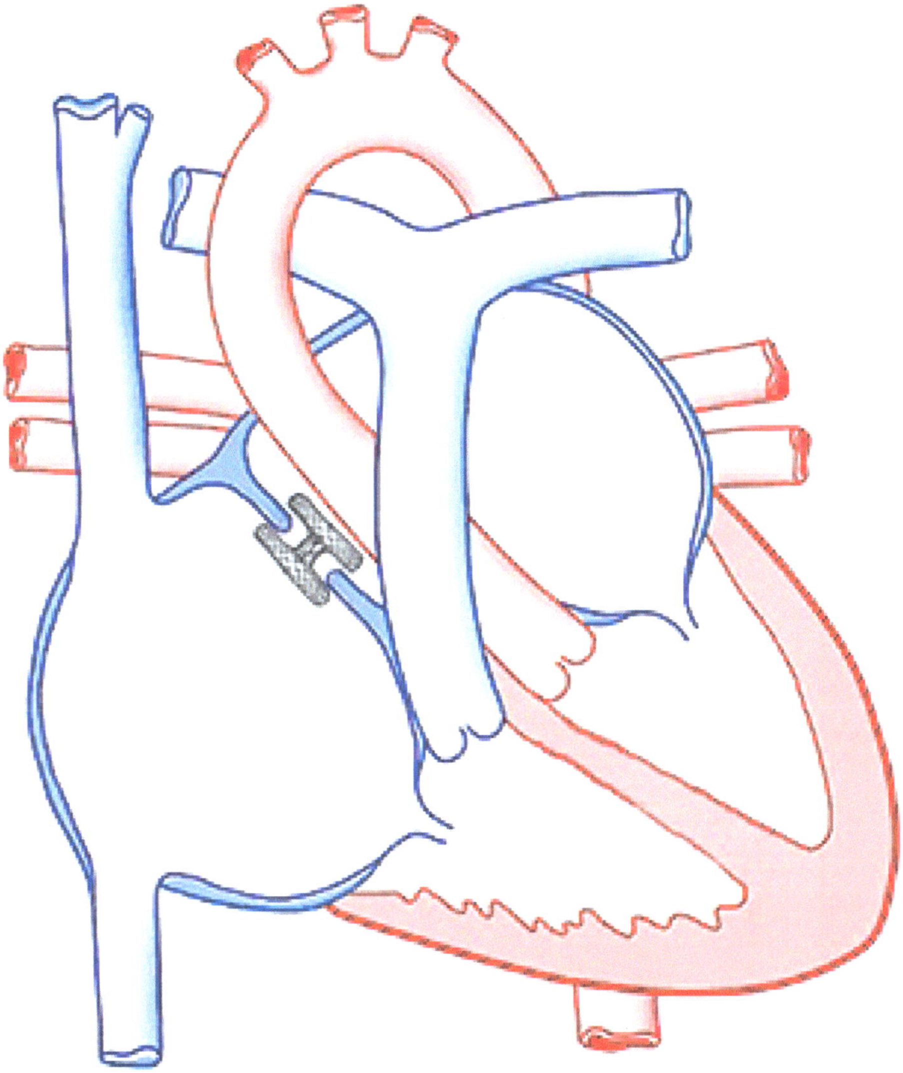

Figure 10: Transcatheter closure of the atrial septal defect with devices.

*Corresponding author Oran B: Medicana International Hospital, Department of Pediatric Cardiology, İzmir, Turkey
E-mail:boran@medicana.com.tr and bulentoran@hotmail.com

Transcatheter Closure of the Ventricular Septal Defect with an Occluder Devices

Transcatheter closure of VSDs with an occluder device is an alternative to surgical repair. First, standard right and left heart catheterization is performed through the right femoral vein and femoral artery. The delivery catheter is advanced into the right or left ventricle. Balloon sizing is not recommended due to associated risks. The VSD is crossed and the occluder device is positioned while the delivery catheter is withdrawn.

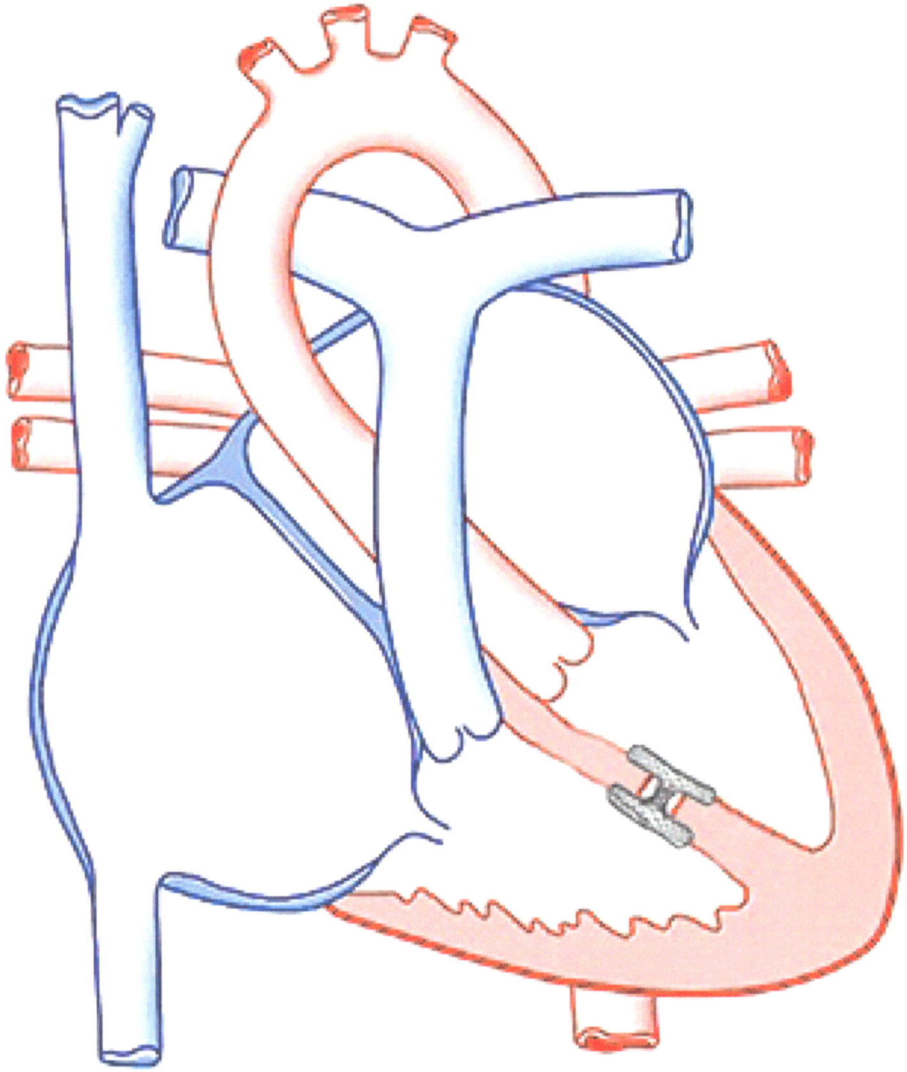

Figure 11: Transcatheter closure of the ventricular septal defect with devices.

*Corresponding author Oran B: Medicana International Hospital, Department of Pediatric Cardiology, İzmir, Turkey
E-mail:boran@medicana.com.tr and bulentoran@hotmail.com

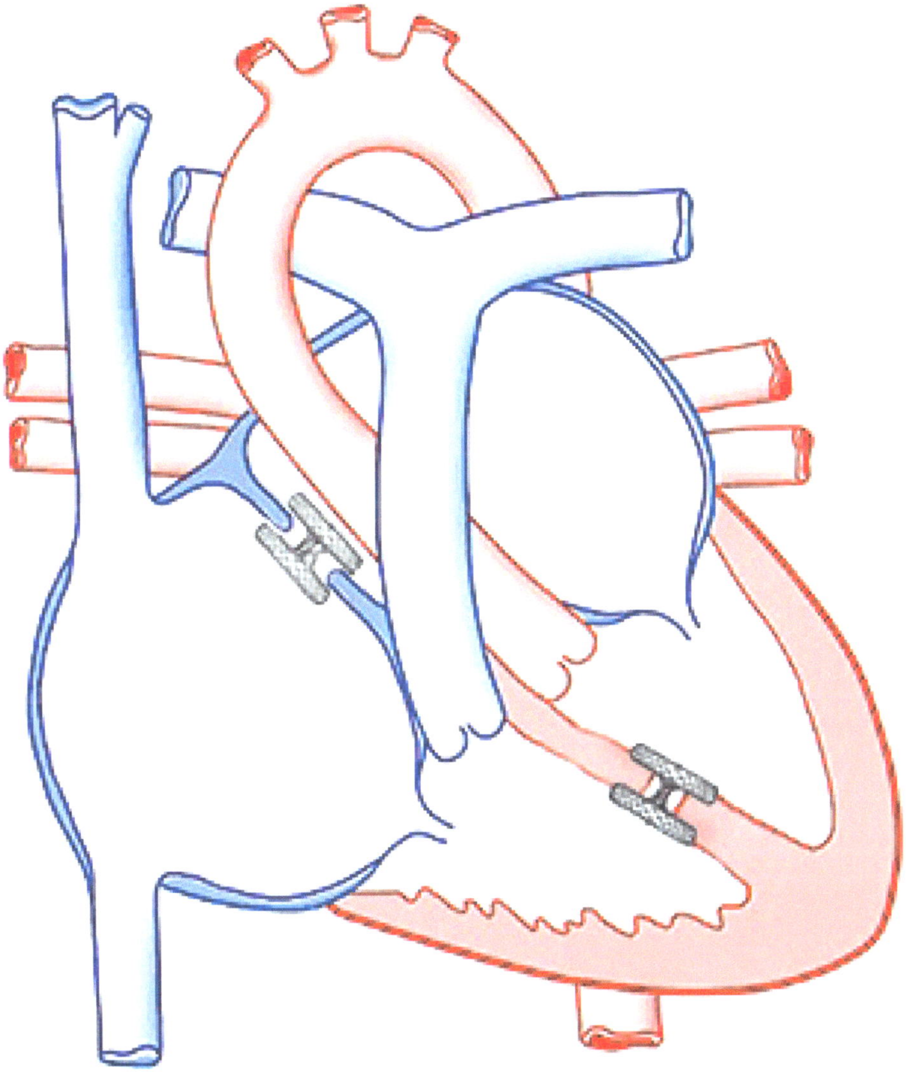

Figure 12: Transcatheter closure of ASD and VSD with devices.

*Corresponding author Oran B: Medicana International Hospital, Department of Pediatric Cardiology, İzmir, Turkey
E-mail:boran@medicana.com.tr and bulentoran@hotmail.com

Pulmonary Arterial Balloon Angioplasty/Stenting

Congenital or acquired peripheral pulmonary arterial stenosis may be related to genetic factors (e.g., Williams syndrome, Alagille syndrome, or congenital rubella syndrome) or result from surgical repair of congenital heart defects. (i.e., tetralogy of Fallot or a distally migrated pulmonary arterial band).

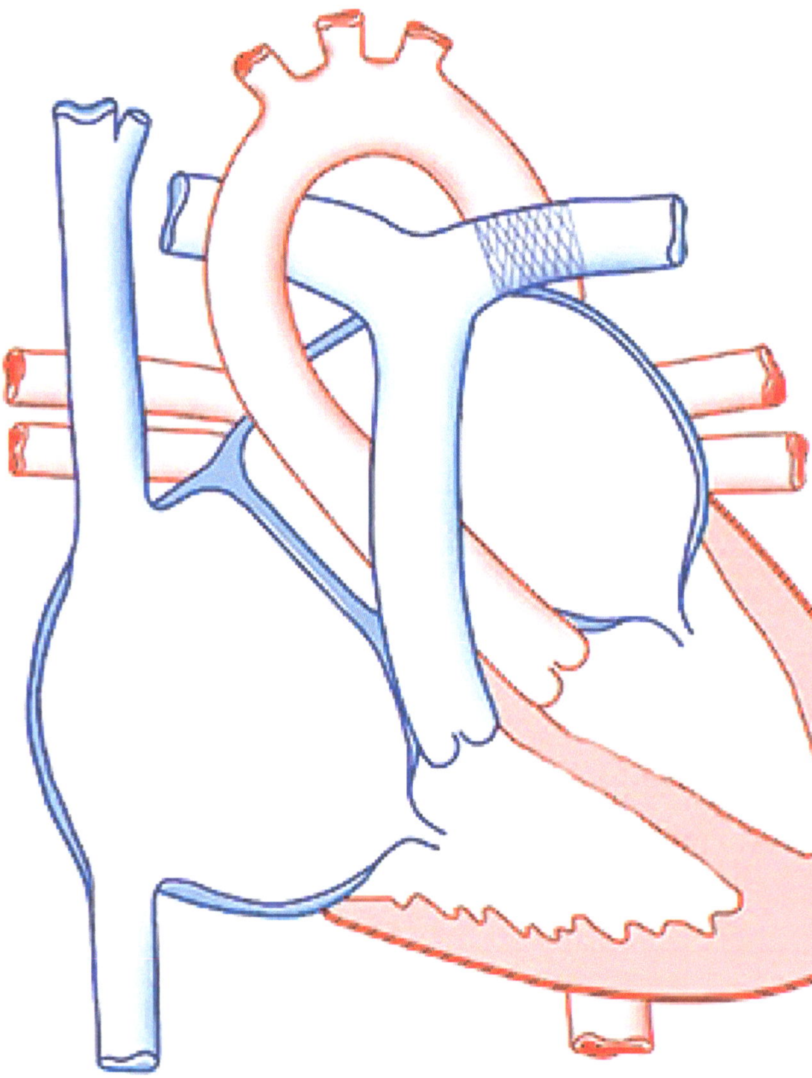

Figure 13: Balloon dilatation of left pulmonary artery stenosis with pulmonary arterial stenting.

*Corresponding author Oran B: Medicana International Hospital, Department of Pediatric Cardiology, İzmir, Turkey
E-mail:boran@medicana.com.tr and bulentoran@hotmail.com

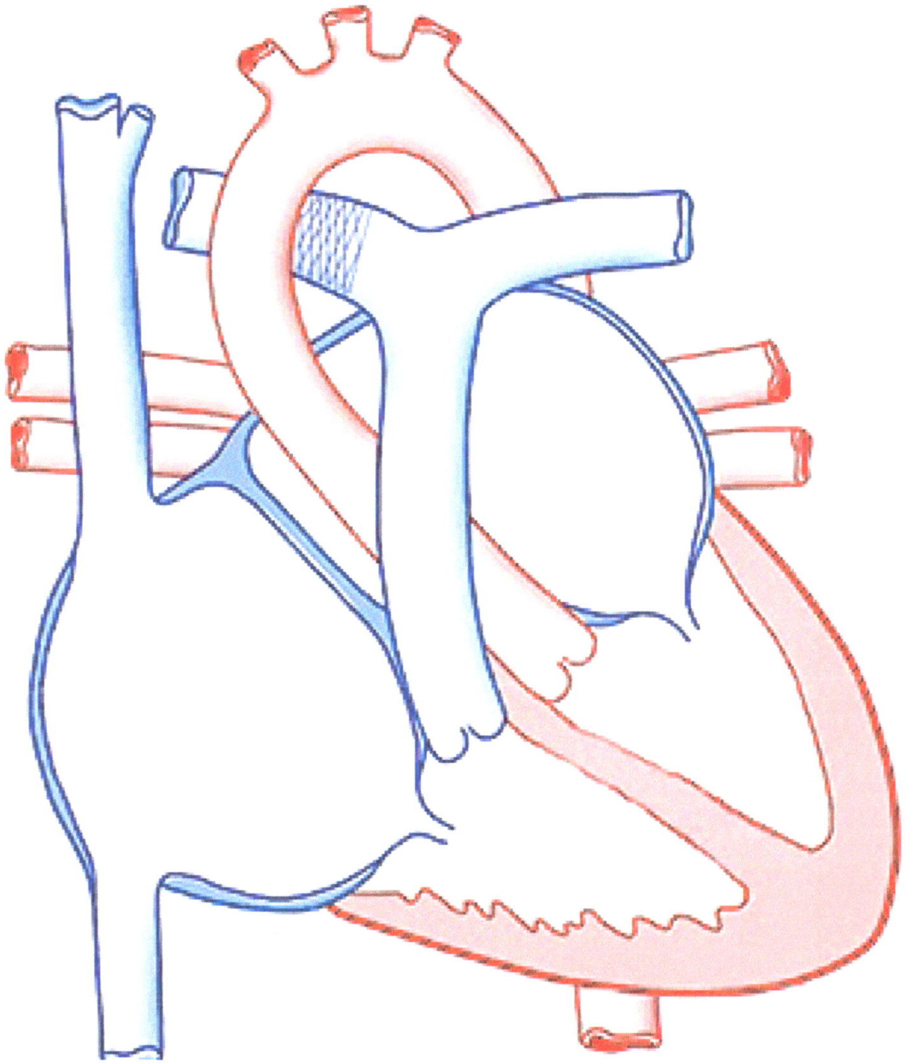

Figure 14: Balloon dilatation of right pulmonary artery stenosis with pulmonary arterial stenting.

*Corresponding author Oran B: Medicana International Hospital, Department of Pediatric Cardiology, İzmir, Turkey
E-mail:boran@medicana.com.tr and bulentoran@hotmail.com

Transcatheter Aortic Valve Implantation

Transcatheter aortic valve replacement (TAVR) or transcatheter aortic valve implantation (TAVI) is a minimally invasive procedure to replace a stenotic aortic valve that fails to open properly.

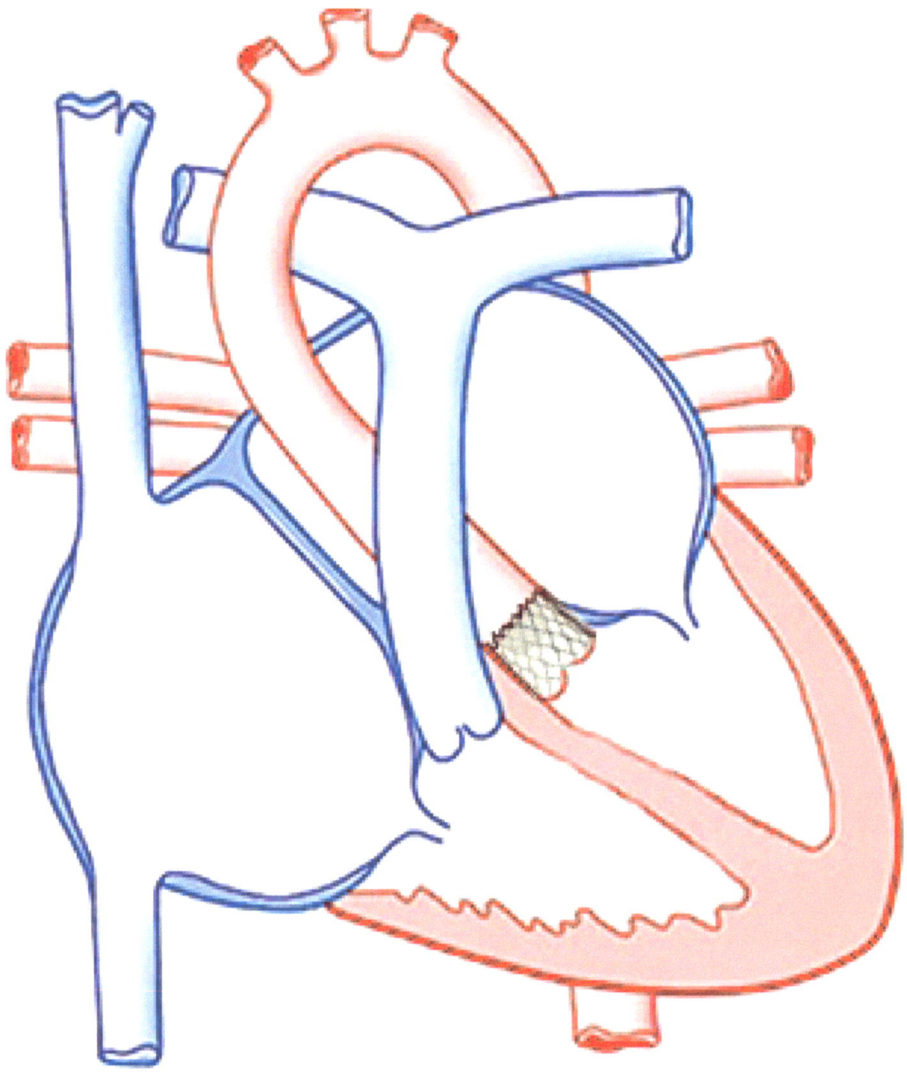

Figure 15: Transcatheter aortic valve replacement (TAVR) or transcatheter aortic valve implantation (TAVI).

*Corresponding author Oran B: Medicana International Hospital, Department of Pediatric Cardiology, İzmir, Turkey
E-mail:boran@medicana.com.tr and bulentoran@hotmail.com

Transcatheter Pulmonary Valve Replacement (TPVR) Procedure

Transcatheter pulmonary valve replacement (TPVR) has evolved into a viable alternative to surgical conduit or bioprosthetic valve replacement.

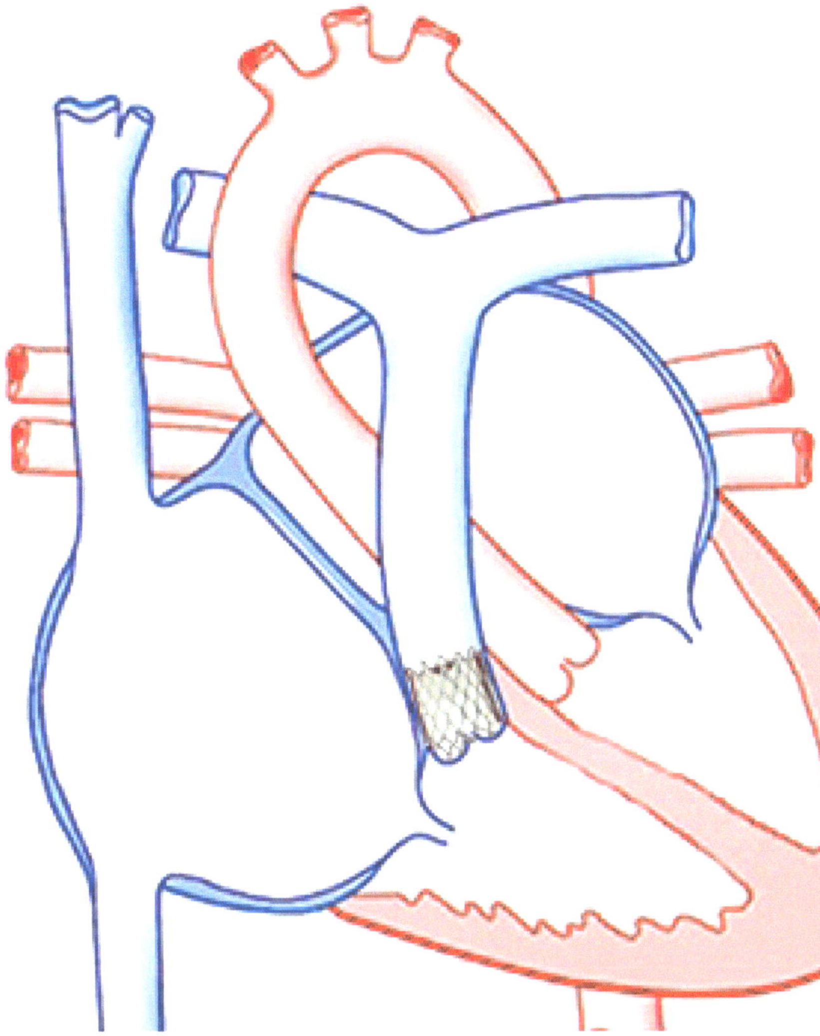

Figure 16: Transcatheter Pulmonary Valve Replacement (TPVR) Procedure.

*Corresponding author Oran B: Medicana International Hospital, Department of Pediatric Cardiology, İzmir, Turkey
E-mail:boran@medicana.com.tr and bulentoran@hotmail.com

*Corresponding author Oran B: Medicana International Hospital, Department of Pediatric Cardiology, İzmir, Turkey
E-mail:boran@medicana.com.tr and bulentoran@hotmail.com

CHAPTER 10

Surgical Procedures

Oran B.

Medicana International Hospital, Department of Pediatric Cardiology, İzmir, Turkey

*Corresponding author Oran B: Medicana International Hospital, Department of Pediatric Cardiology, İzmir, Turkey
E-mail:boran@medicana.com.tr and bulentoran@hotmail.com

*Corresponding author Oran B: Medicana International Hospital, Department of Pediatric Cardiology, İzmir, Turkey
E-mail:boran@medicana.com.tr and bulentoran@hotmail.com

Atrial Septal Defect and/or Ventricular Septal Defect Repair

Closure of large ASDs and/or VSDs by open-heart surgery is typically performed during infancy or childhood to prevent later complications. There is evidence that surgical repair before 25 years of age effectively mitigates later complications.

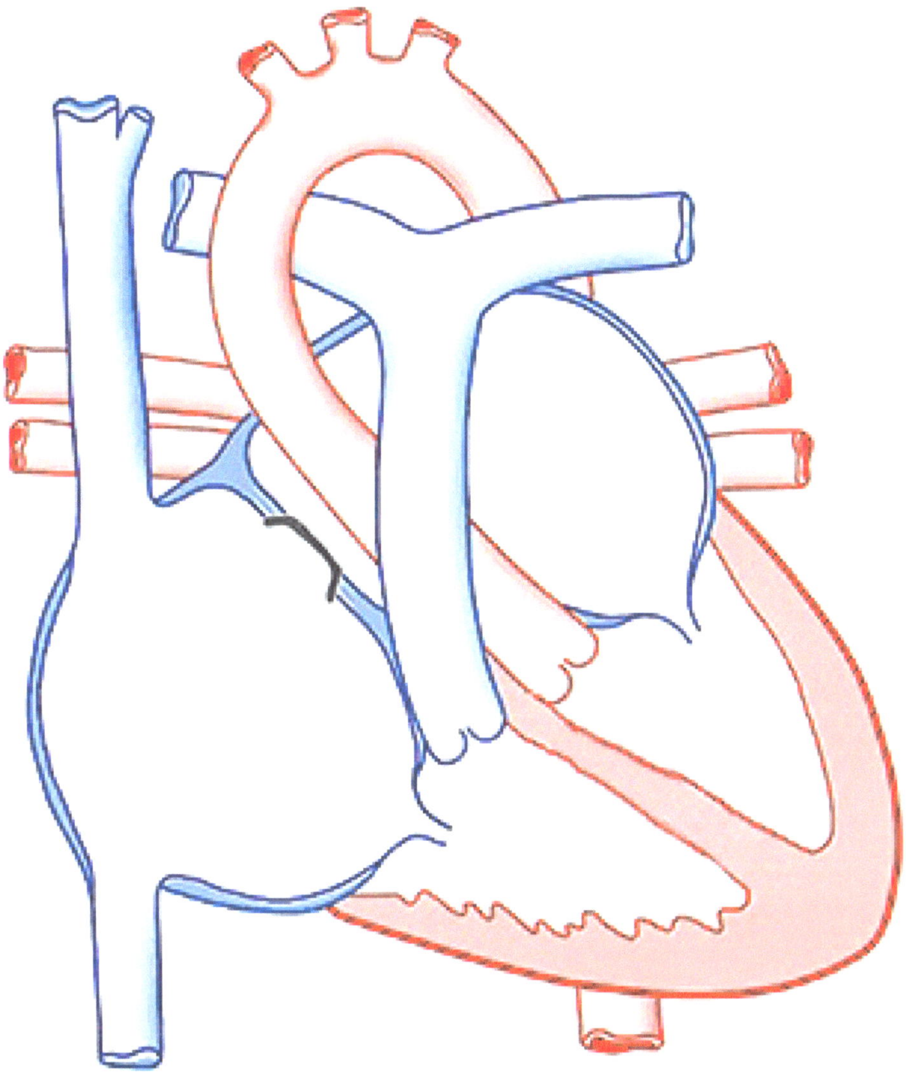

Figure 1: ASD closure.

*Corresponding author Oran B: Medicana International Hospital, Department of Pediatric Cardiology, İzmir, Turkey
E-mail:boran@medicana.com.tr and bulentoran@hotmail.com

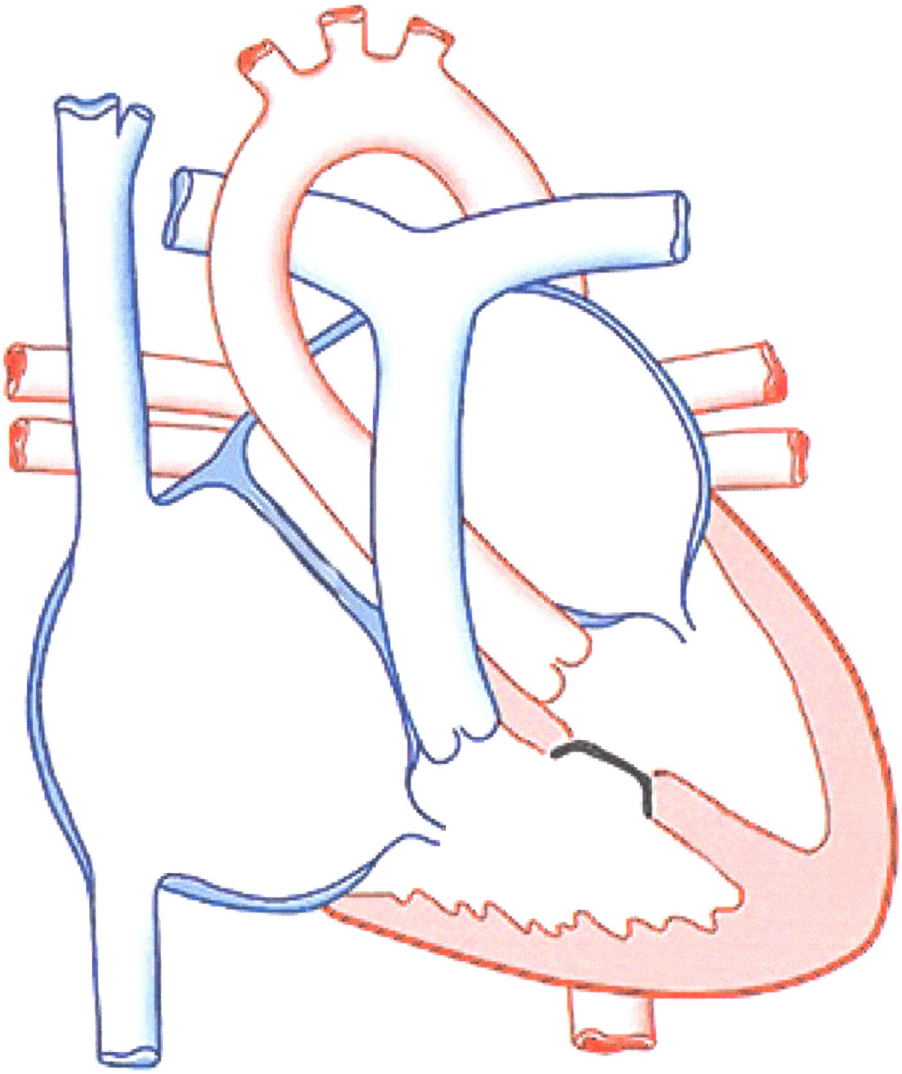

Figure 2: VSD closure.

*Corresponding author Oran B: Medicana International Hospital, Department of Pediatric Cardiology, İzmir, Turkey
E-mail:boran@medicana.com.tr and bulentoran@hotmail.com

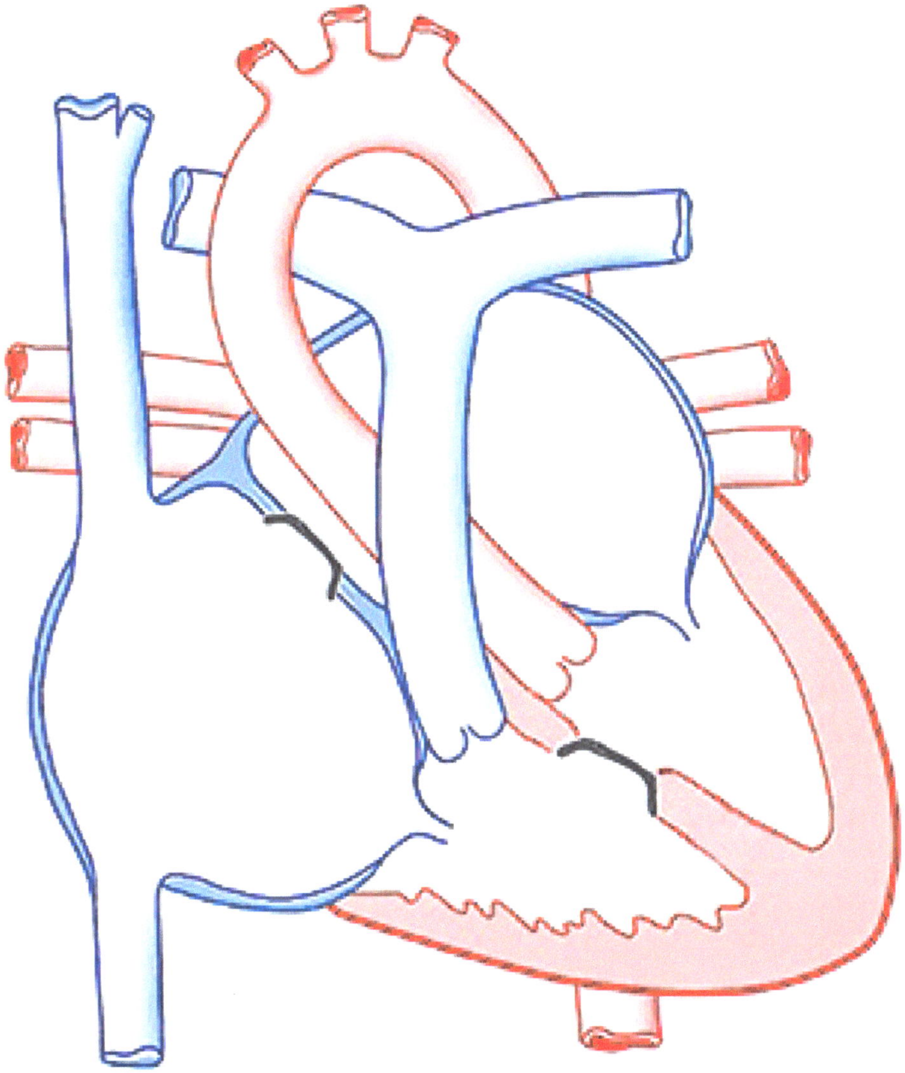

Figure 3: ASD and VSD closure.

*Corresponding author Oran B: Medicana International Hospital, Department of Pediatric Cardiology, İzmir, Turkey
E-mail:boran@medicana.com.tr and bulentoran@hotmail.com

Pulmonary Artery Banding

Pulmonary artery banding is a simple palliative surgical procedure for patients with both left-to-right shunt and pulmonary overcirculation. This staged approach for surgical correction of congenital heart defects is commonly used for infants with pulmonary overcirculation.

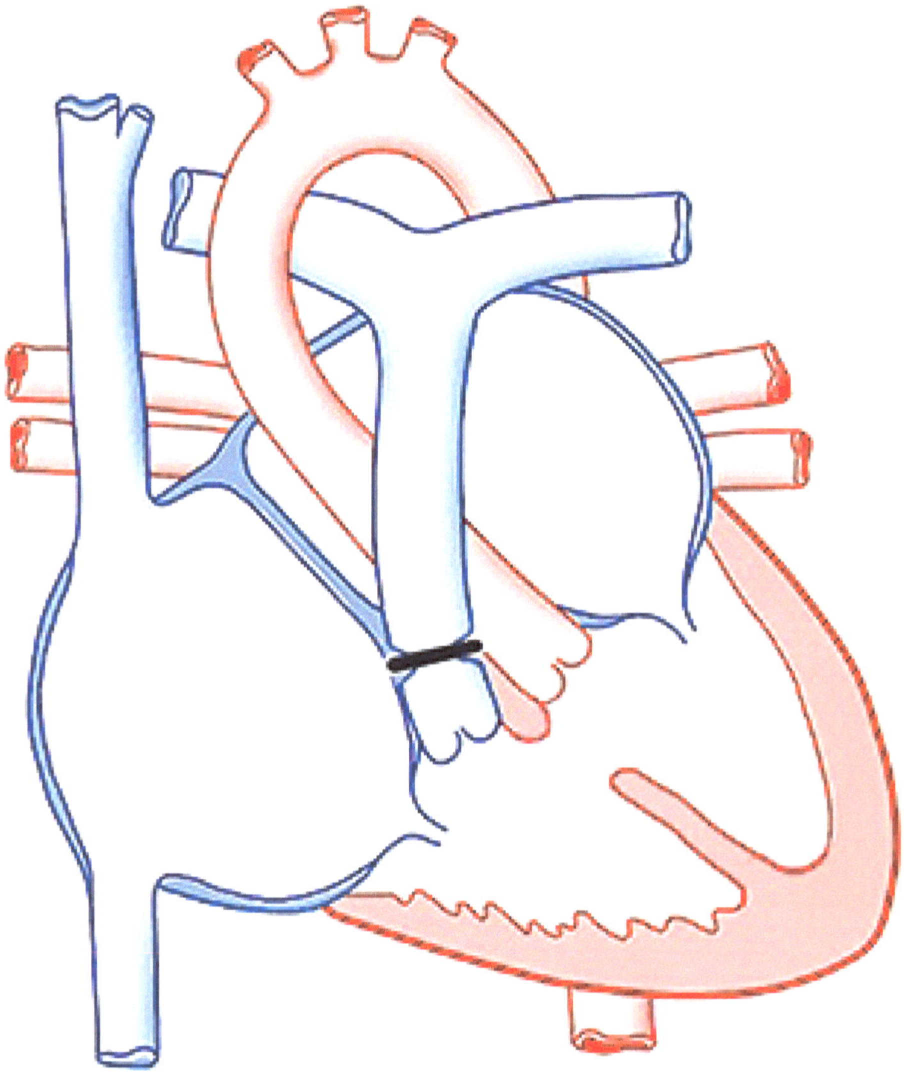

Figure 4: Pulmonary trunk band, VSD.

*Corresponding author Oran B: Medicana International Hospital, Department of Pediatric Cardiology, İzmir, Turkey
E-mail:boran@medicana.com.tr and bulentoran@hotmail.com

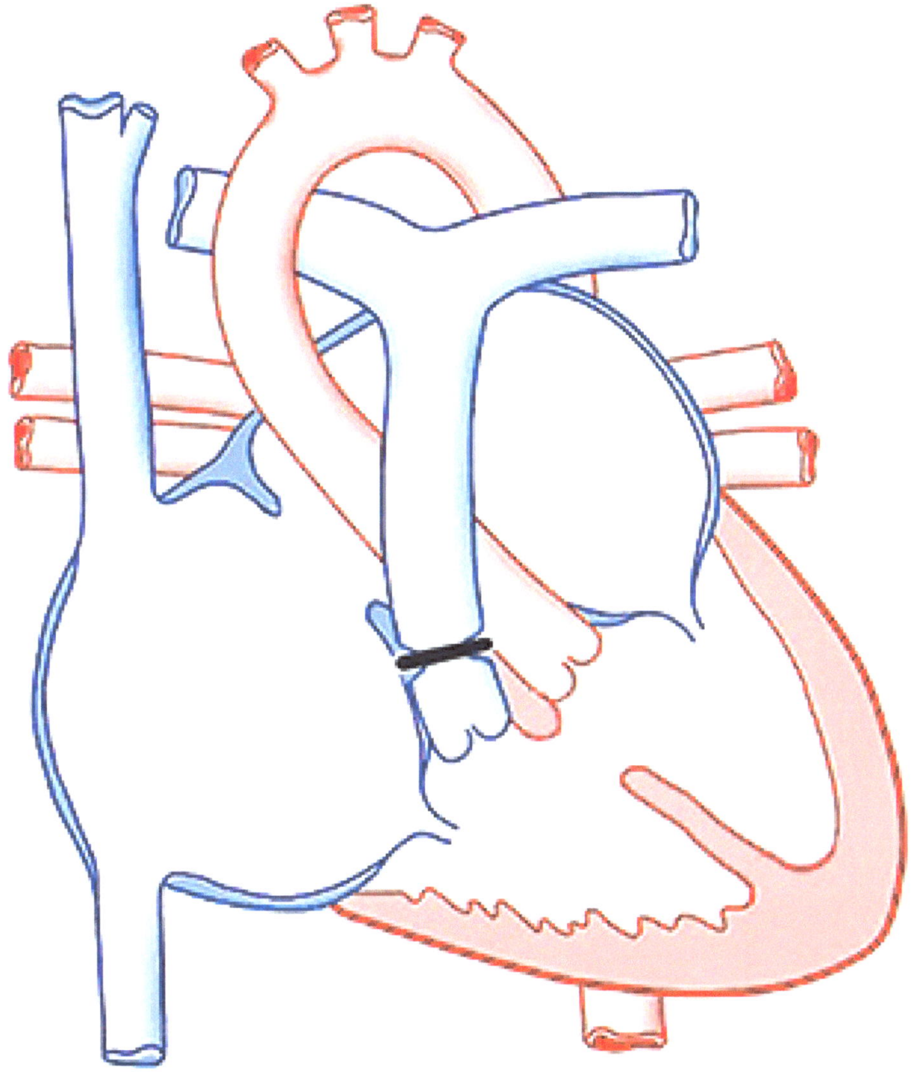

Figure 5: Pulmonary trunk band, ASD and VSD.

*Corresponding author Oran B: Medicana International Hospital, Department of Pediatric Cardiology, İzmir, Turkey
E-mail:boran@medicana.com.tr and bulentoran@hotmail.com

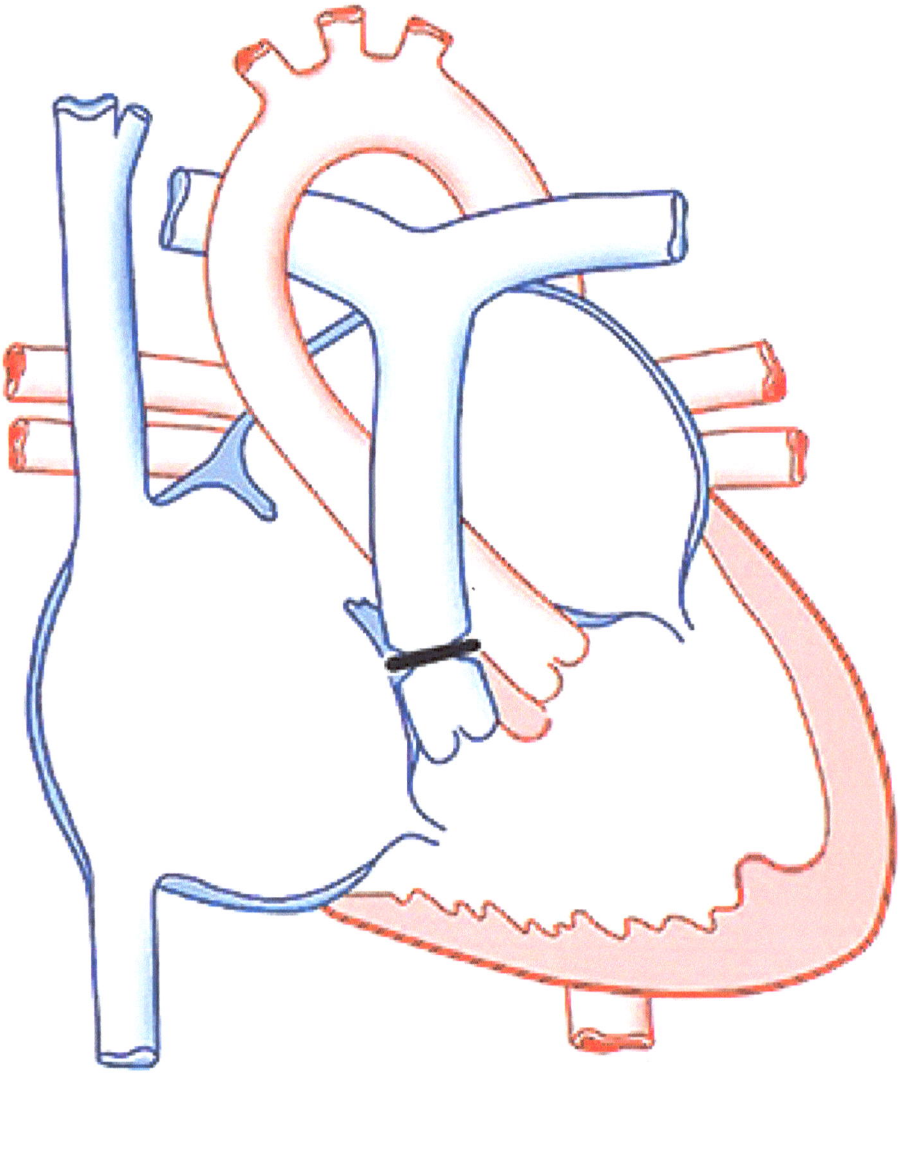

Figure 6: Pulmonary trunk band, solitary ventricle of indeterminate morphology, ASD.

*Corresponding author Oran B: Medicana International Hospital, Department of Pediatric Cardiology, İzmir, Turkey
E-mail:boran@medicana.com.tr and bulentoran@hotmail.com

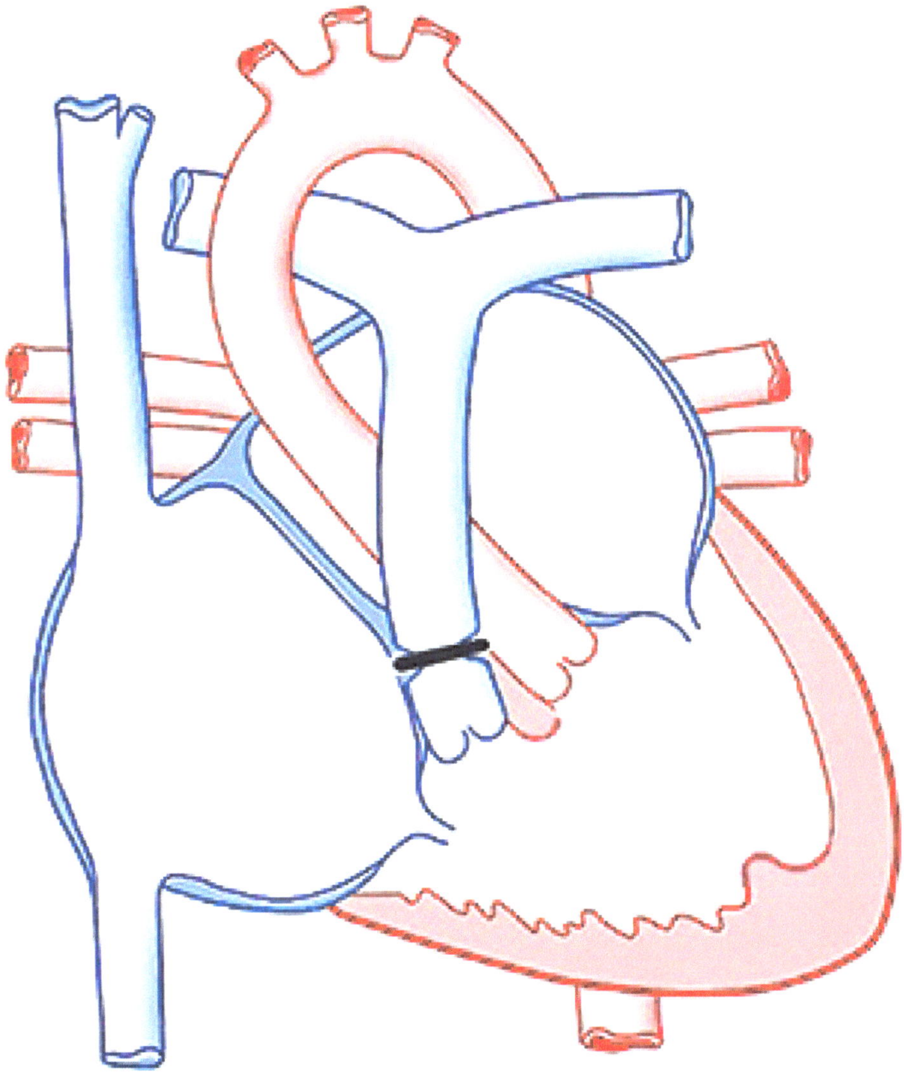

Figure 7: Pulmonary trunk band, solitary ventricle of indeterminate morphology.

*Corresponding author Oran B: Medicana International Hospital, Department of Pediatric Cardiology, İzmir, Turkey
E-mail:boran@medicana.com.tr and bulentoran@hotmail.com

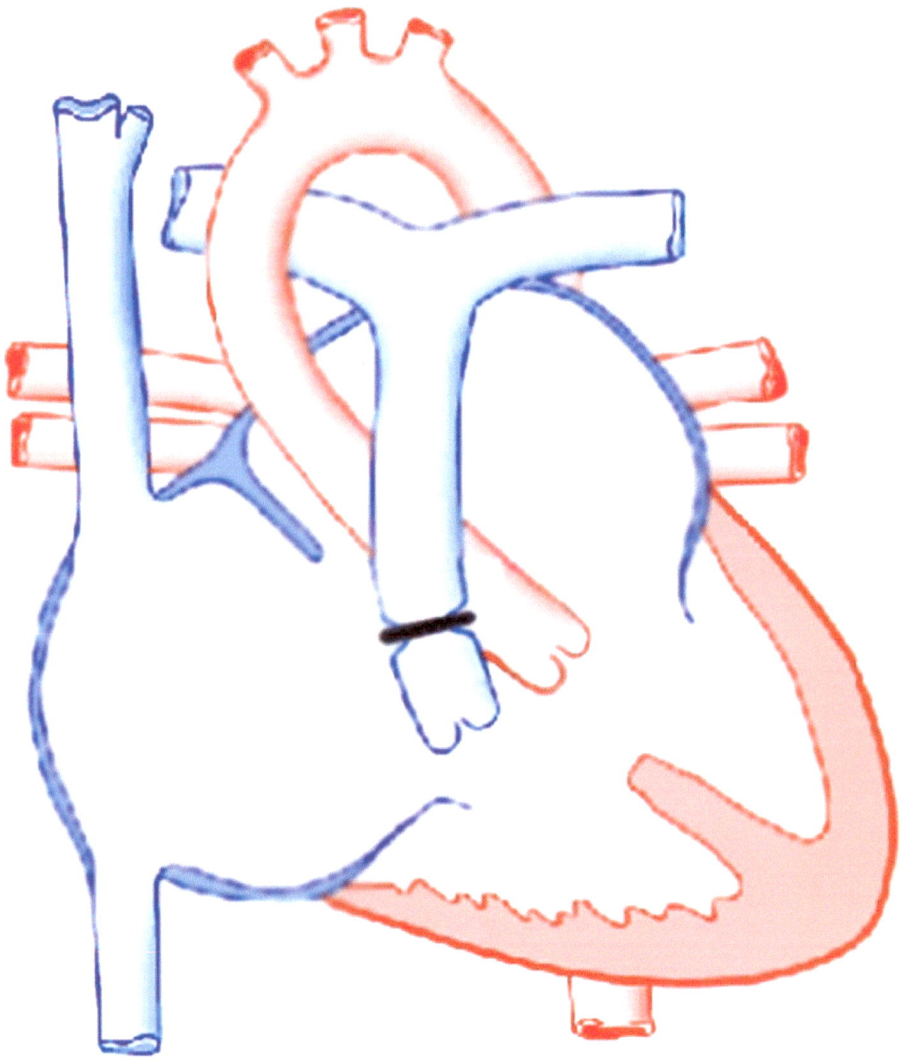

Figure 8: Pulmonary trunk band, complet AVSD.

*Corresponding author Oran B: Medicana International Hospital, Department of Pediatric Cardiology, İzmir, Turkey
E-mail:boran@medicana.com.tr and bulentoran@hotmail.com

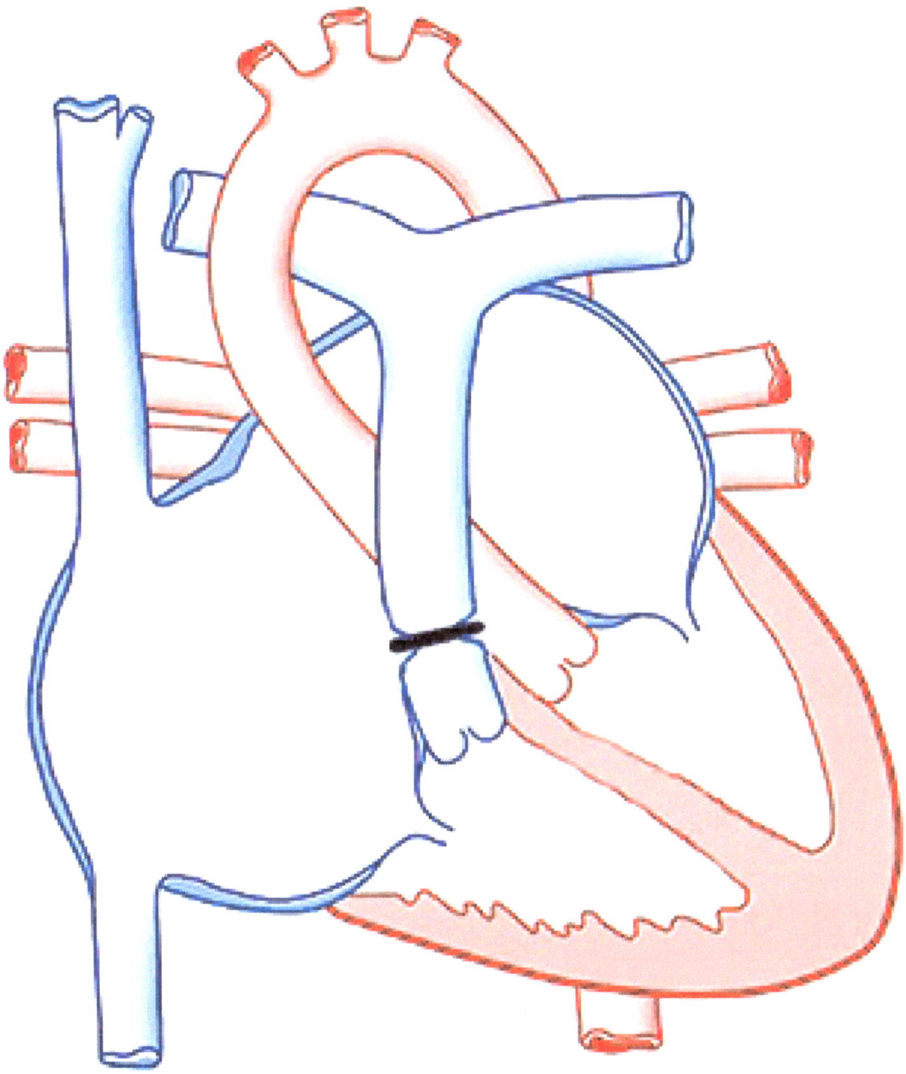

Figure 9: Pulmonary trunk band, common atrium.

*Corresponding author Oran B: Medicana International Hospital, Department of Pediatric Cardiology, İzmir, Turkey
E-mail:boran@medicana.com.tr and bulentoran@hotmail.com

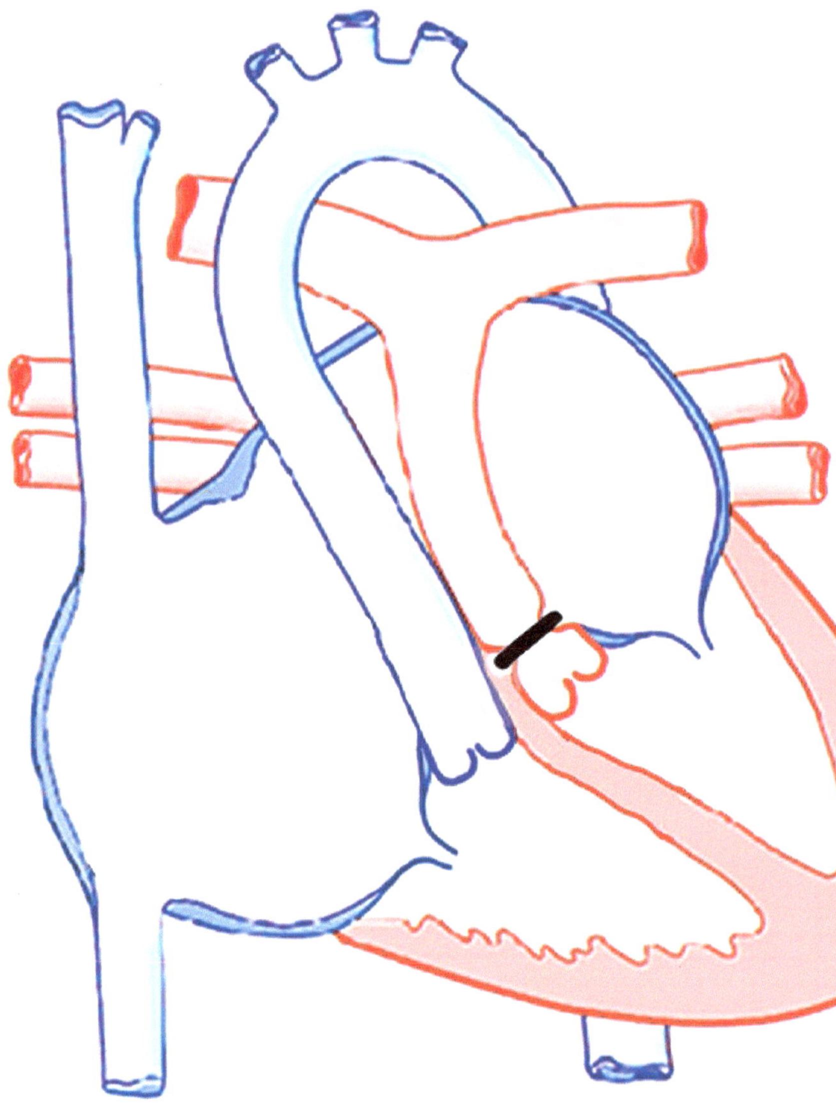

Figure 10: Pulmonary trunk band, Transposition of the great arteries, common atrium.

*Corresponding author Oran B: Medicana International Hospital, Department of Pediatric Cardiology, İzmir, Turkey
E-mail:boran@medicana.com.tr and bulentoran@hotmail.com

Pulmonary Artery Debanding

Debanding procedures are regularly performed several months after palliative surgery in combination with cardiac malformation repair. Accurate surgical timing is required for successful implementation of debanding procedures.

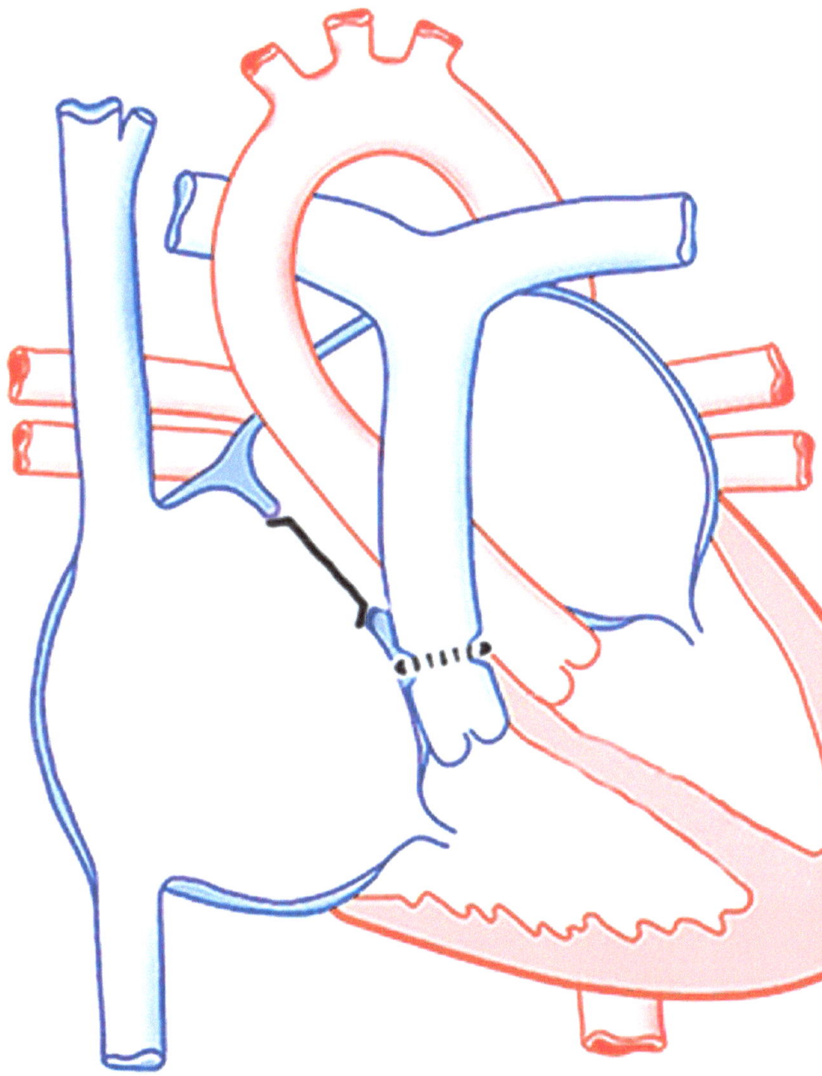

Figure 11: Pulmonary trunk band removal (de-band), ASD closure.

*Corresponding author Oran B: Medicana International Hospital, Department of Pediatric Cardiology, İzmir, Turkey
E-mail:boran@medicana.com.tr and bulentoran@hotmail.com

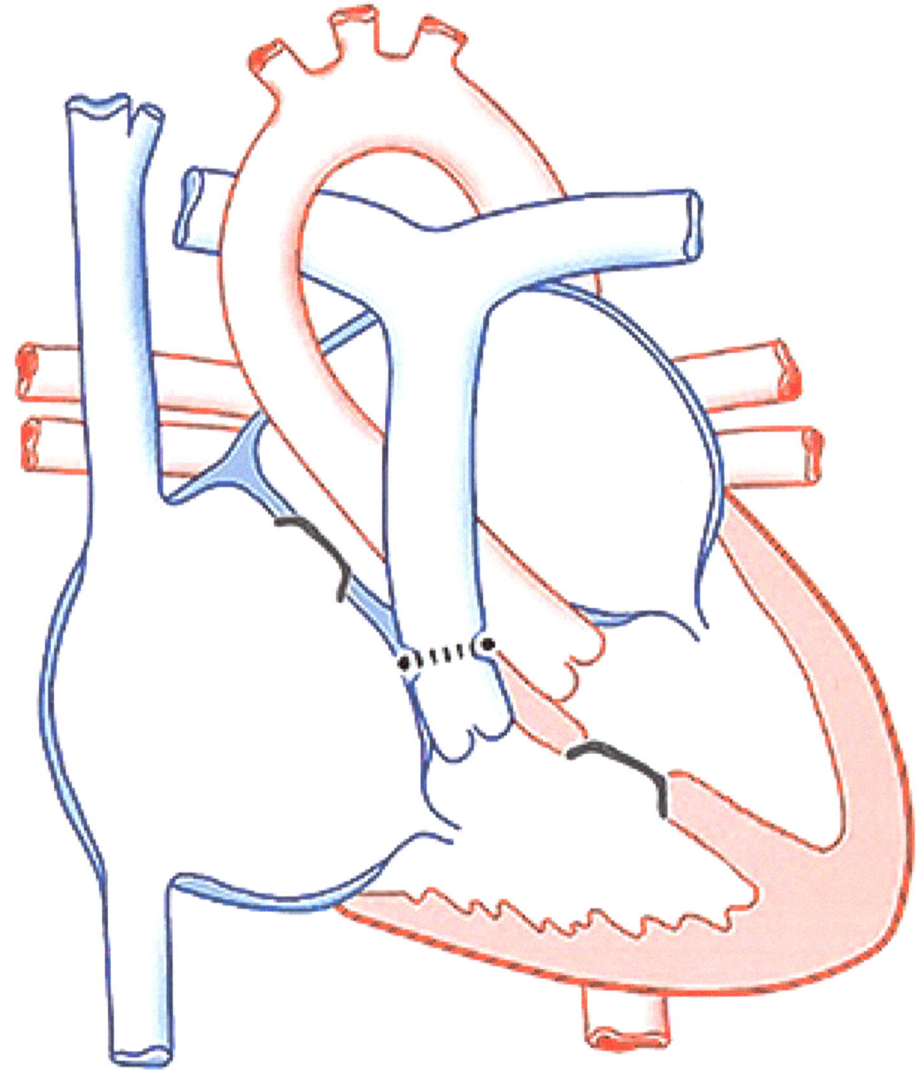

Figure 12: Pulmonary trunk band removal (de-band), ASD and VSD closure.

*Corresponding author Oran B: Medicana International Hospital, Department of Pediatric Cardiology, İzmir, Turkey
E-mail:boran@medicana.com.tr and bulentoran@hotmail.com

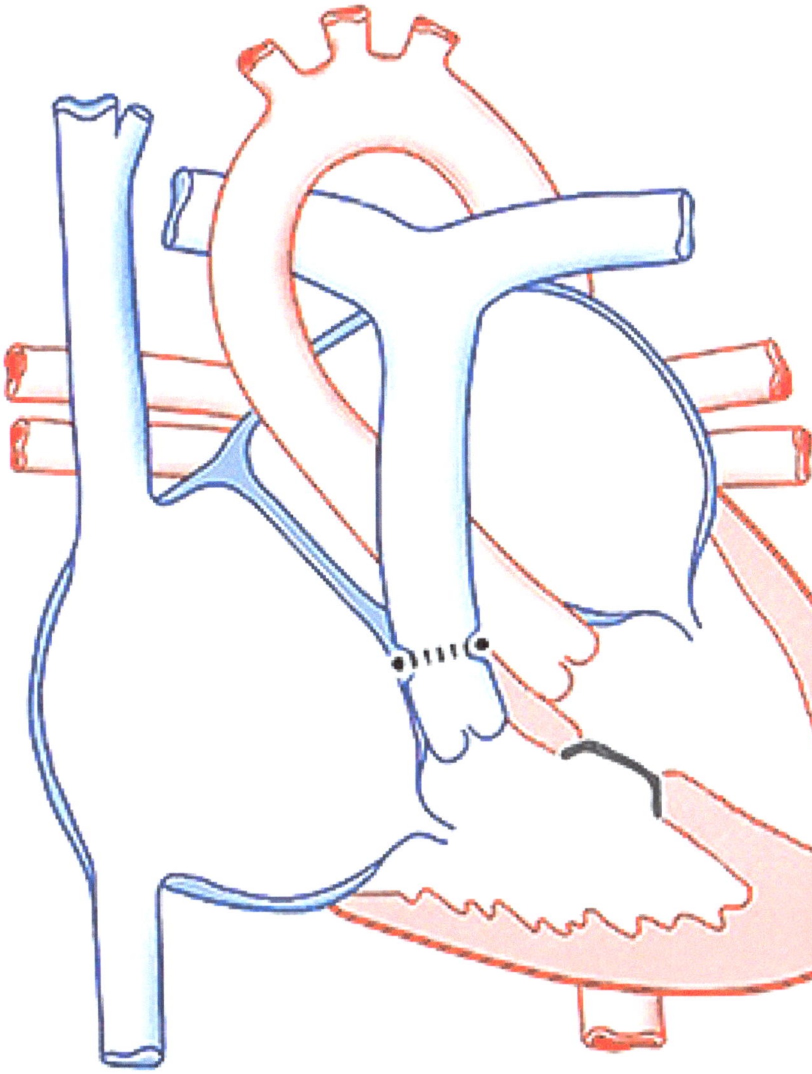

Figure 13: Pulmonary trunk band removal (de-band), VSD closure.

*Corresponding author Oran B: Medicana International Hospital, Department of Pediatric Cardiology, İzmir, Turkey
E-mail:boran@medicana.com.tr and bulentoran@hotmail.com

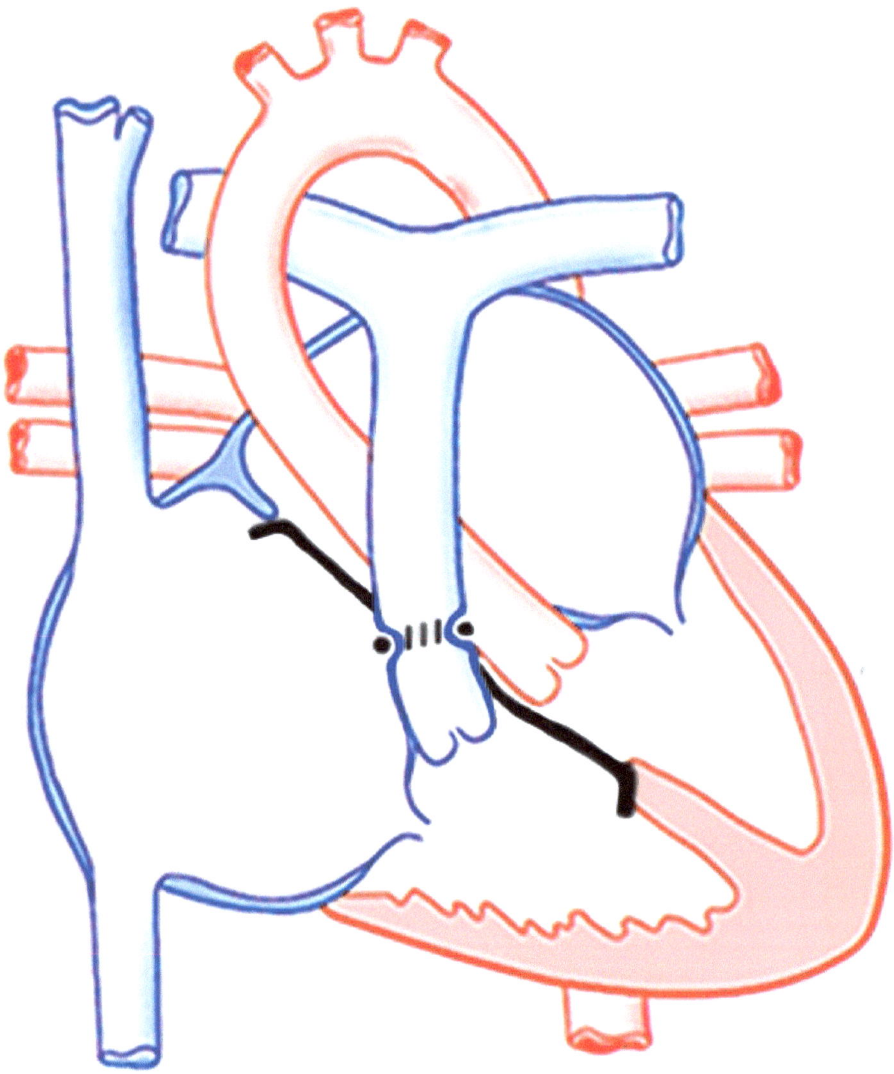

Figure 14: Pulmonary trunk band removal (de-band), AVSD closure.

*Corresponding author Oran B: Medicana International Hospital, Department of Pediatric Cardiology, İzmir, Turkey
E-mail:boran@medicana.com.tr and bulentoran@hotmail.com

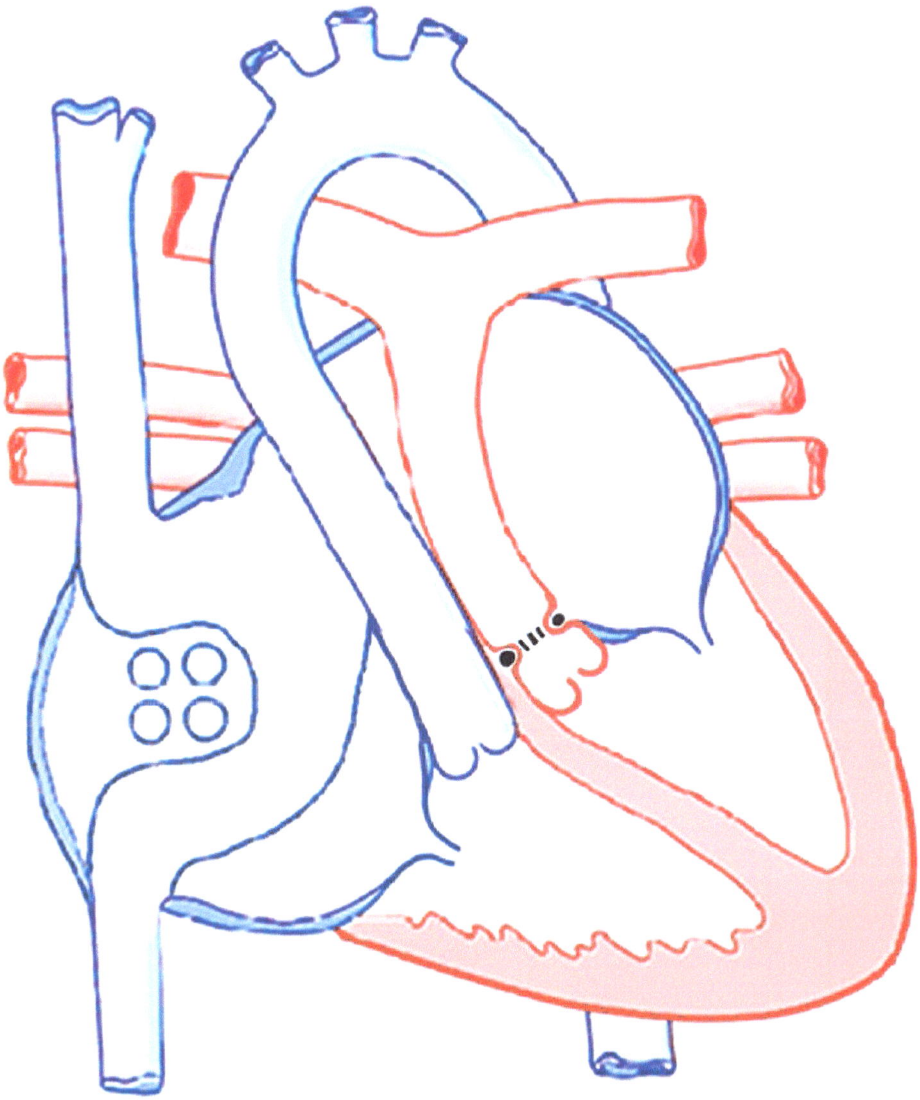

Figure 15: Mustard procedure (atrial inversion), pulmonary trunk band removal (de-band).

*Corresponding author Oran B: Medicana International Hospital, Department of Pediatric Cardiology, İzmir, Turkey
E-mail:boran@medicana.com.tr and bulentoran@hotmail.com

Aortopulmonary Window Closure

Surgical closure is recommended for all patients with an aortopulmonary window. This procedure should be performed near the time of diagnosis to prevent irreversible pulmonary vascular disease and Eisenmenger syndrome.

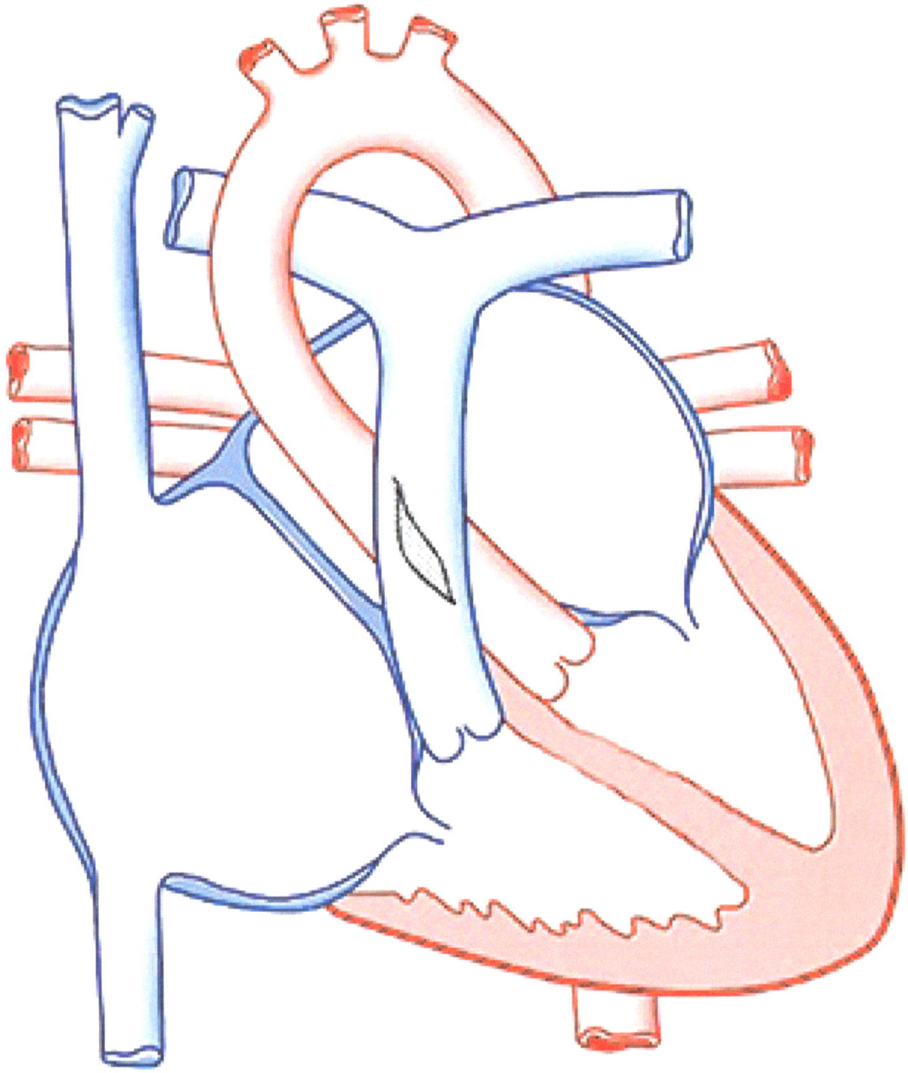

Figure 16: Aortopulmonary window closure.

*Corresponding author Oran B: Medicana International Hospital, Department of Pediatric Cardiology, İzmir, Turkey
E-mail:boran@medicana.com.tr and bulentoran@hotmail.com

Pulmonary Artery Origin from Ascending Aorta (hemitruncus) repair

Hemitruncus is a congenital deformity that results in early infant mortality. The repair of hemitruncus during early life is crucial for prevention of vascular obstructive disease and Eisenmenger syndrome.

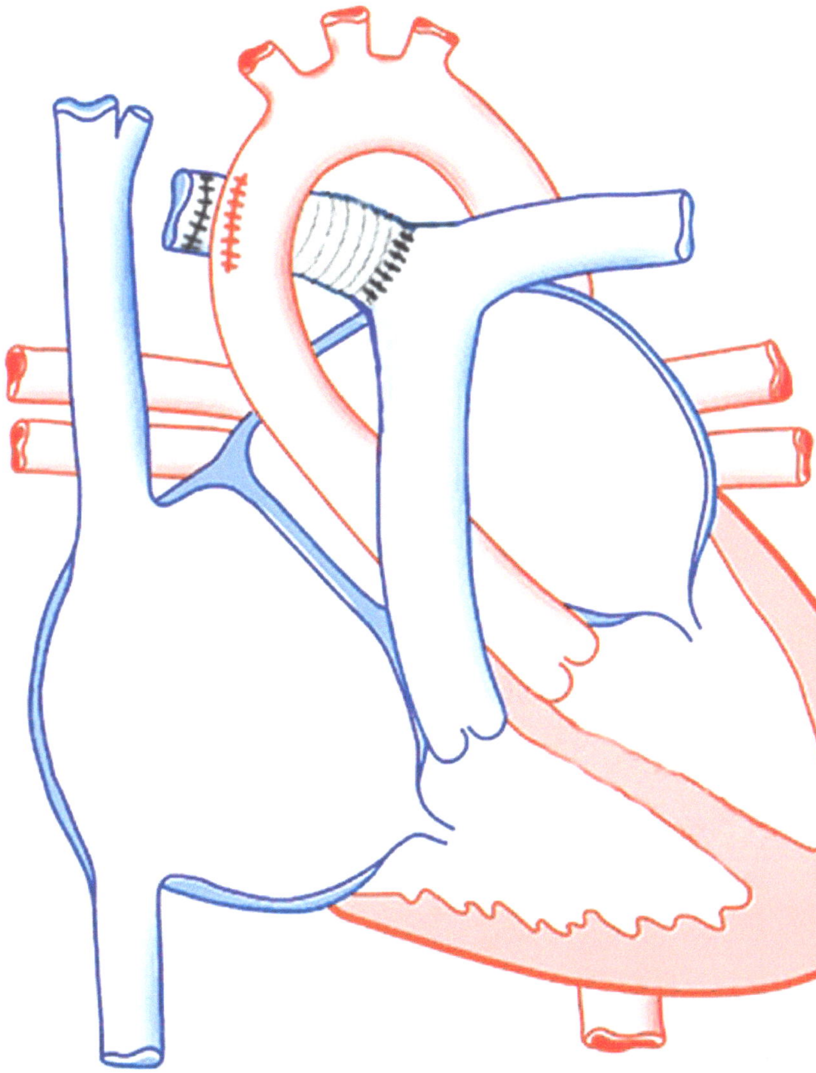

Figure 17: Pulmonary artery origin from ascending aorta (hemitruncus) repair.

*Corresponding author Oran B: Medicana International Hospital, Department of Pediatric Cardiology, İzmir, Turkey
E-mail:boran@medicana.com.tr and bulentoran@hotmail.com

Tetralogy of Fallot Repair

Surgical correction is required for tetralogy of Fallot defects. Total corrective repair includes closure of the VSD, removal of right ventricular outflow obstruction, and patch graft enlargement of the main pulmonary artery.

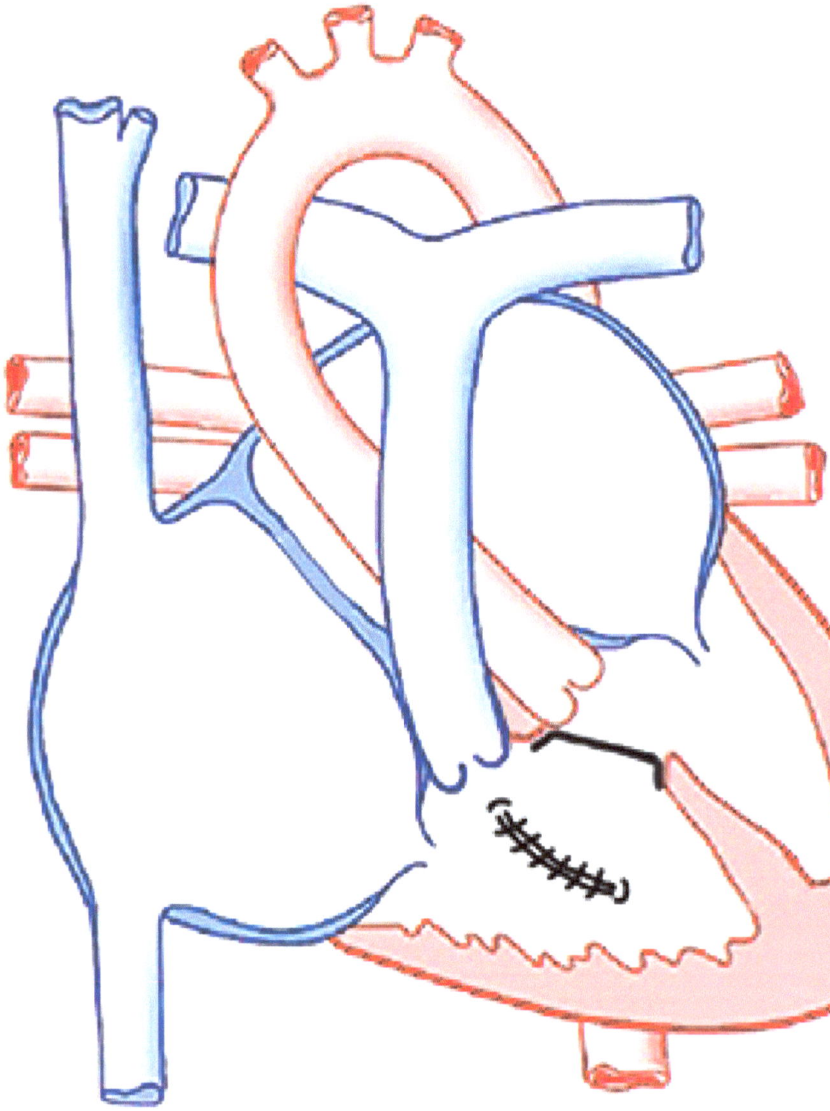

Figure 18: Tetralogy of Fallot repair without transannular patch, trans-RV approach.

*Corresponding author Oran B: Medicana International Hospital, Department of Pediatric Cardiology, İzmir, Turkey
E-mail:boran@medicana.com.tr and bulentoran@hotmail.com

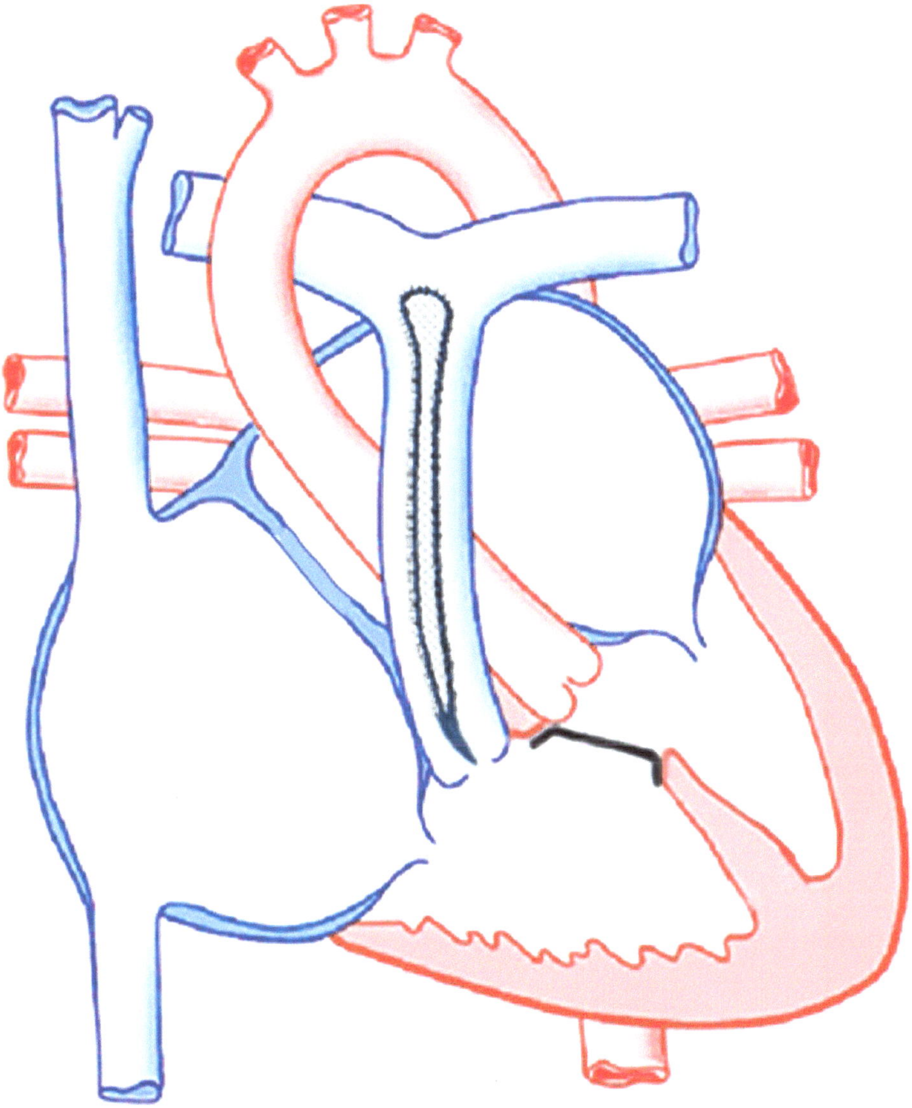

Figure 19: Tetralogy of Fallot repair with transannular patch, trans-RV approach.

*Corresponding author Oran B: Medicana International Hospital, Department of Pediatric Cardiology, İzmir, Turkey
E-mail:boran@medicana.com.tr and bulentoran@hotmail.com

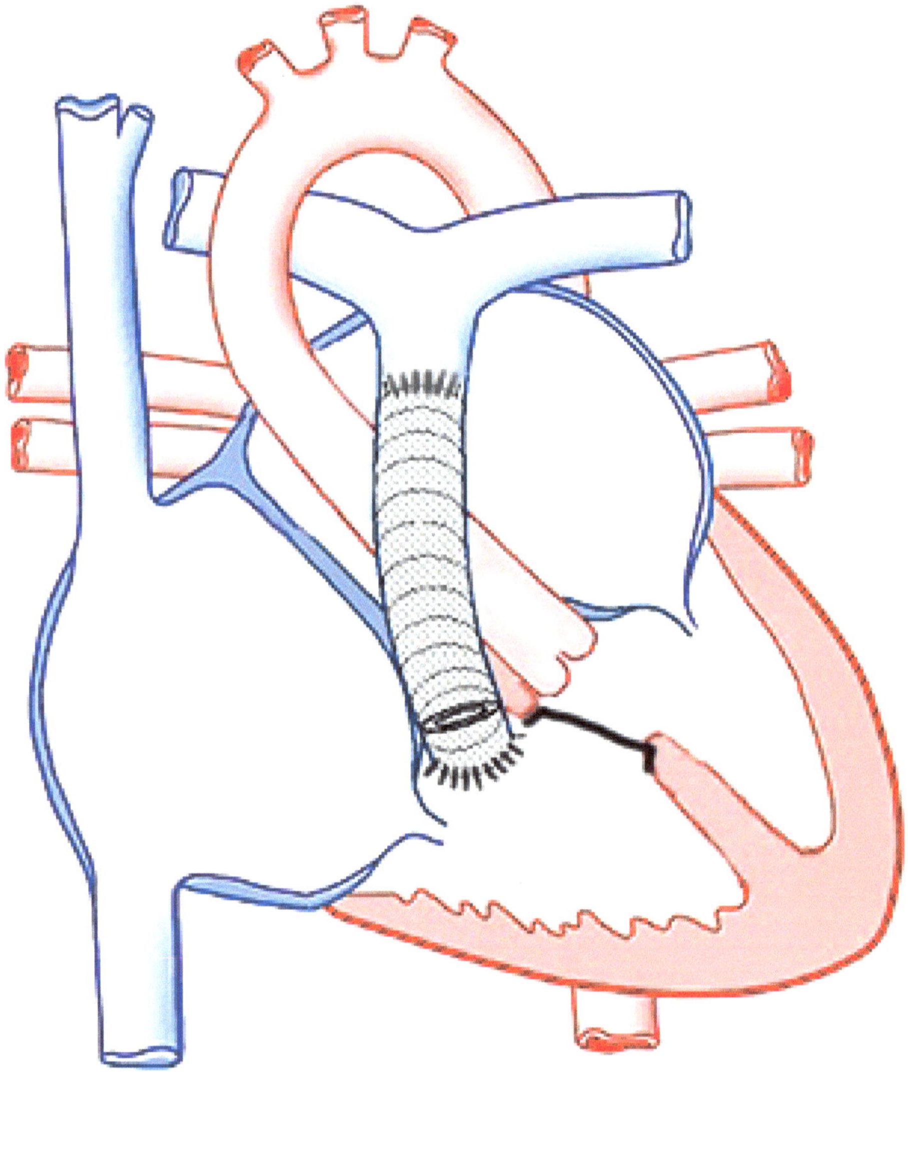

Figure 20: Fallot tetralogy repair, right ventricle to pulmonary artery conduit.

*Corresponding author Oran B: Medicana International Hospital, Department of Pediatric Cardiology, İzmir, Turkey
E-mail:boran@medicana.com.tr and bulentoran@hotmail.com

Reconstruction of the Pulmonary Artery

Branch pulmonary artery stenosis may be congenital or acquired. Treatment options include surgical patch arterioplasty and hybrid procedures with stents or conduit placement.

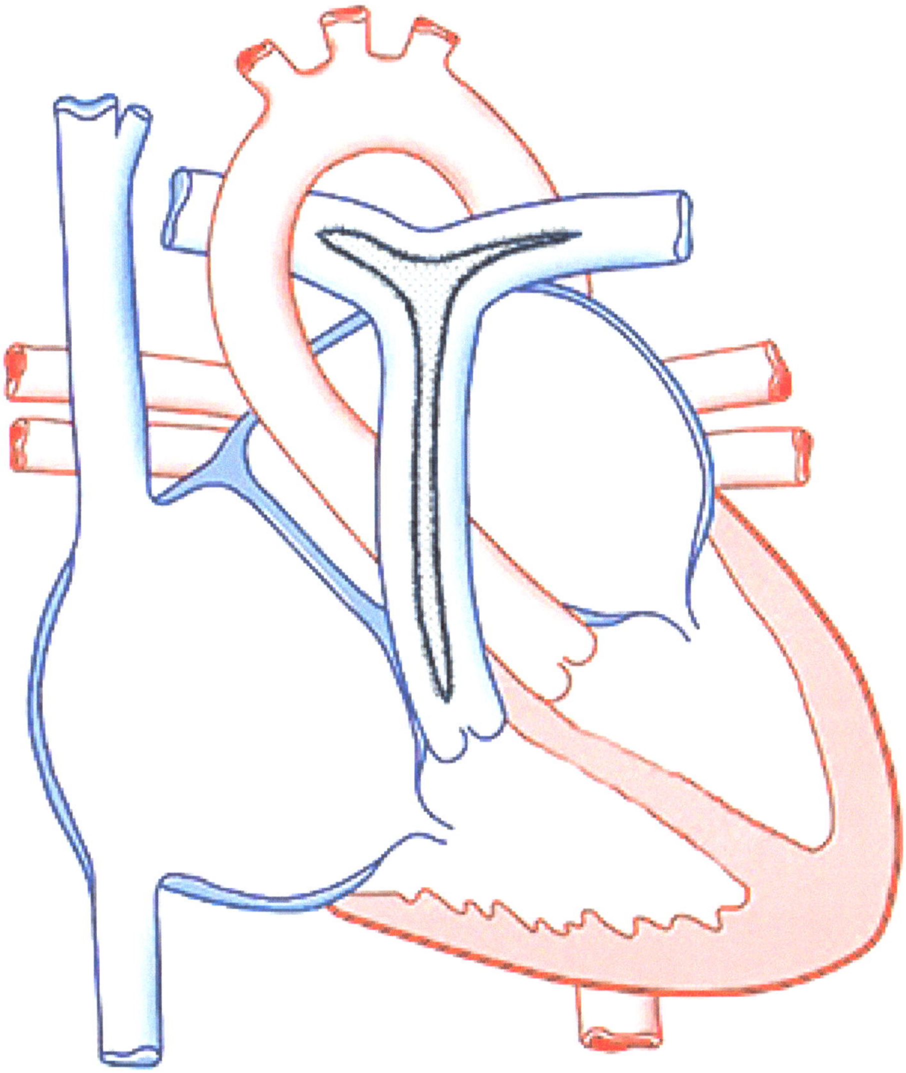

Figure 21: Pulmonary arterioplasty / reconstruction-peripheral (at/beyond hilar bifurcation).

*Corresponding author Oran B: Medicana International Hospital, Department of Pediatric Cardiology, İzmir, Turkey
E-mail:boran@medicana.com.tr and bulentoran@hotmail.com

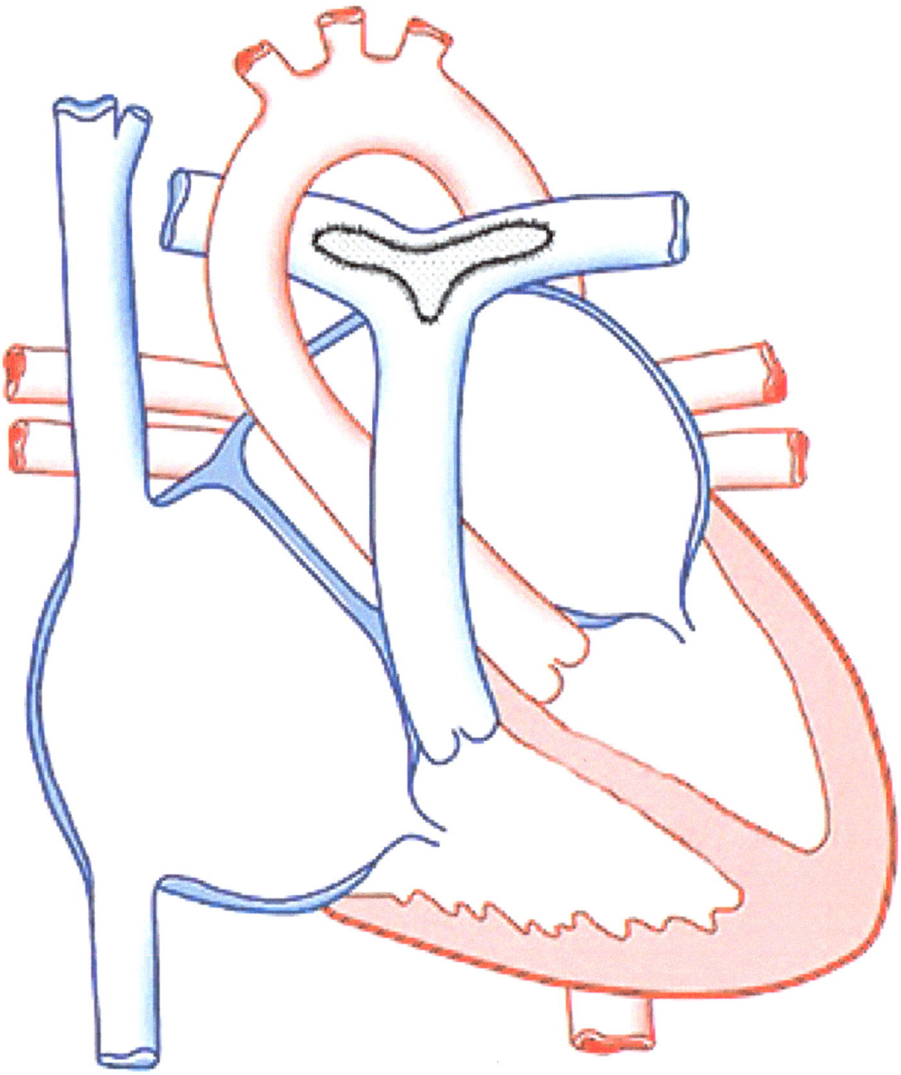

Figure 22: Pulmonary arterioplasty / reconstruction-peripheral.

*Corresponding author Oran B: Medicana International Hospital, Department of Pediatric Cardiology, İzmir, Turkey
E-mail:boran@medicana.com.tr and bulentoran@hotmail.com

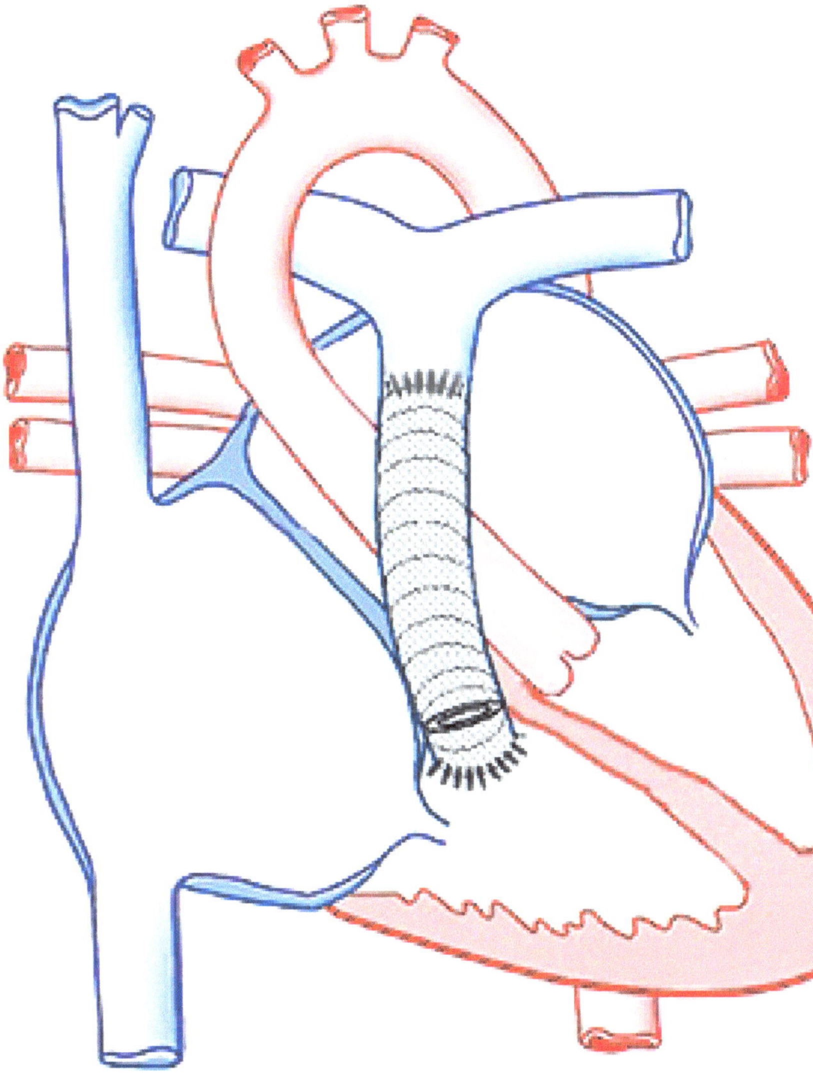

Figure 23: Right ventricle to pulmonary artery conduit construction.

*Corresponding author Oran B: Medicana International Hospital, Department of Pediatric Cardiology, İzmir, Turkey
E-mail:boran@medicana.com.tr and bulentoran@hotmail.com

Mitral and Aortic Valve Replacement

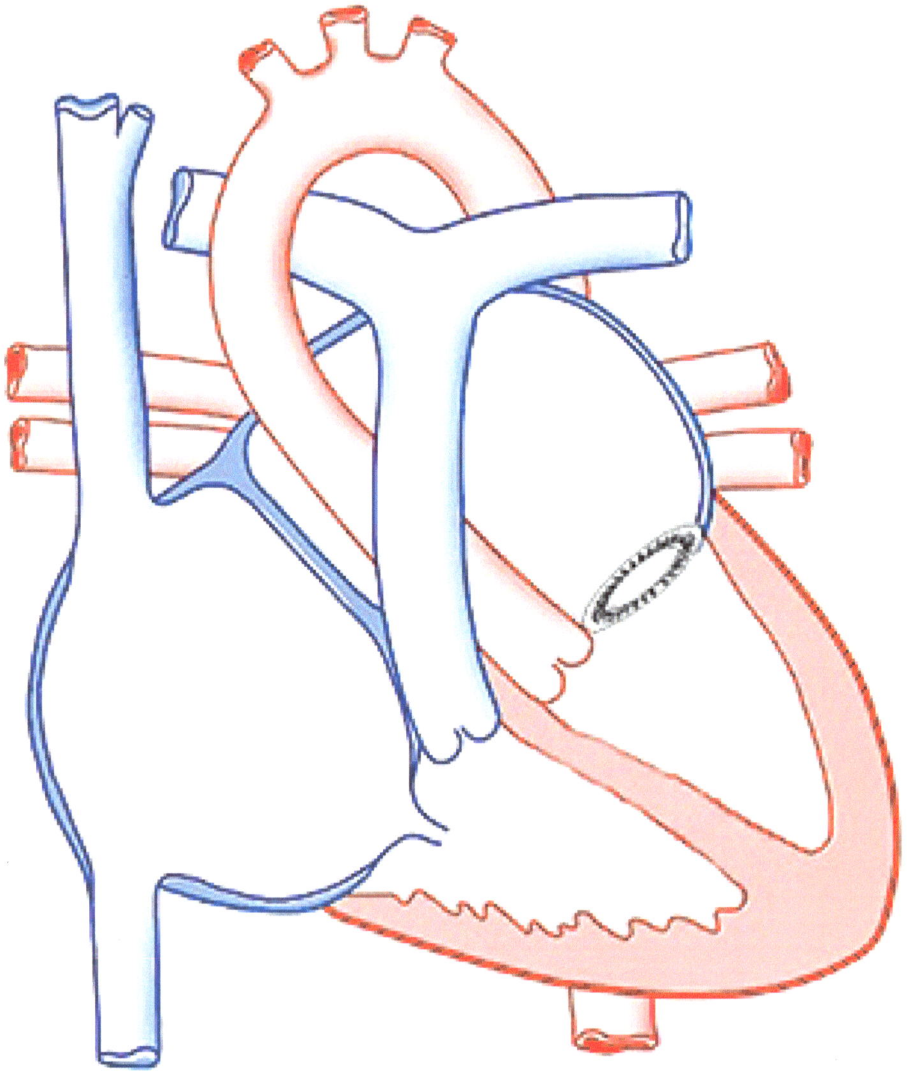

Figure 24: Mitral valvar replacement.

*Corresponding author Oran B: Medicana International Hospital, Department of Pediatric Cardiology, İzmir, Turkey
E-mail:boran@medicana.com.tr and bulentoran@hotmail.com

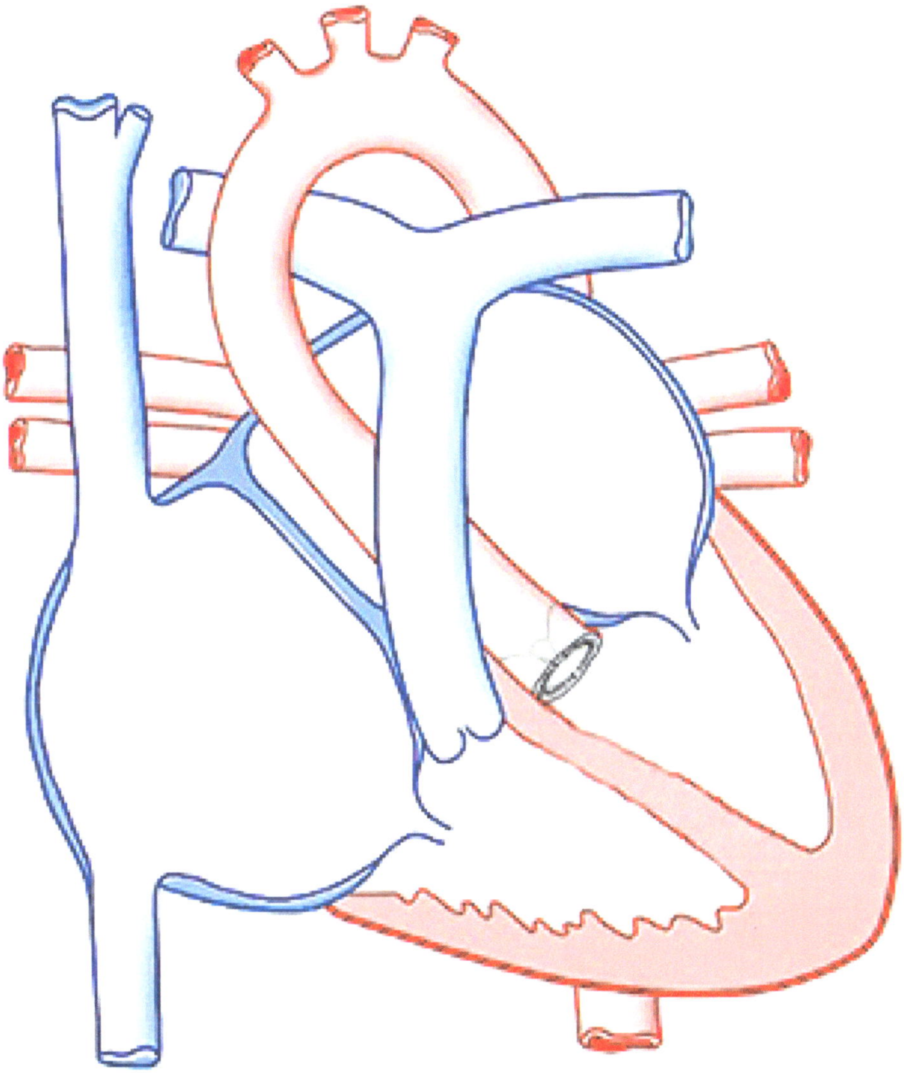

Figure 25: Aortic valve replacement.

*Corresponding author Oran B: Medicana International Hospital, Department of Pediatric Cardiology, İzmir, Turkey
E-mail:boran@medicana.com.tr and bulentoran@hotmail.com

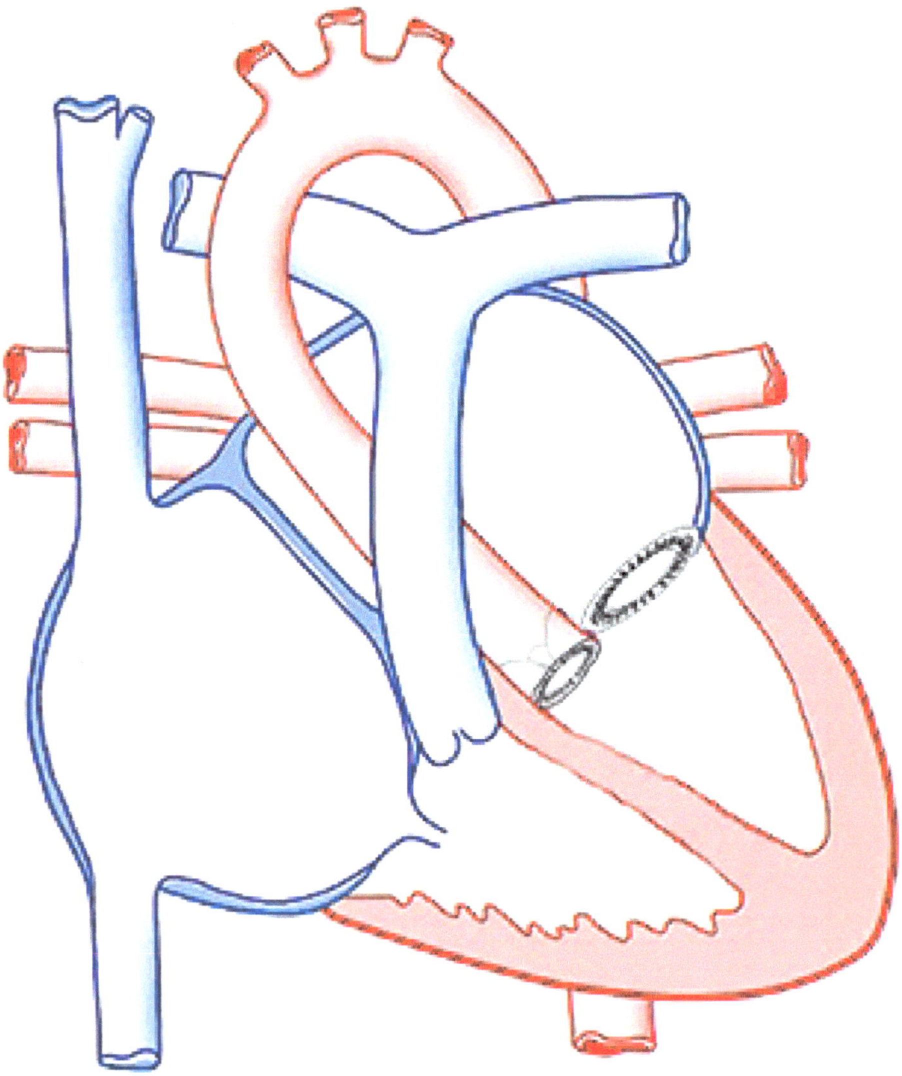

Figure 26: Mitral valve replacement and Aortic valve replacement.

*Corresponding author Oran B: Medicana International Hospital, Department of Pediatric Cardiology, İzmir, Turkey
E-mail:boran@medicana.com.tr and bulentoran@hotmail.com

Surgical Closure of the Patent Ductus Arteriosus

Standard surgical treatments for large PDA during infancy are surgical ligation or surgical ligation and division.

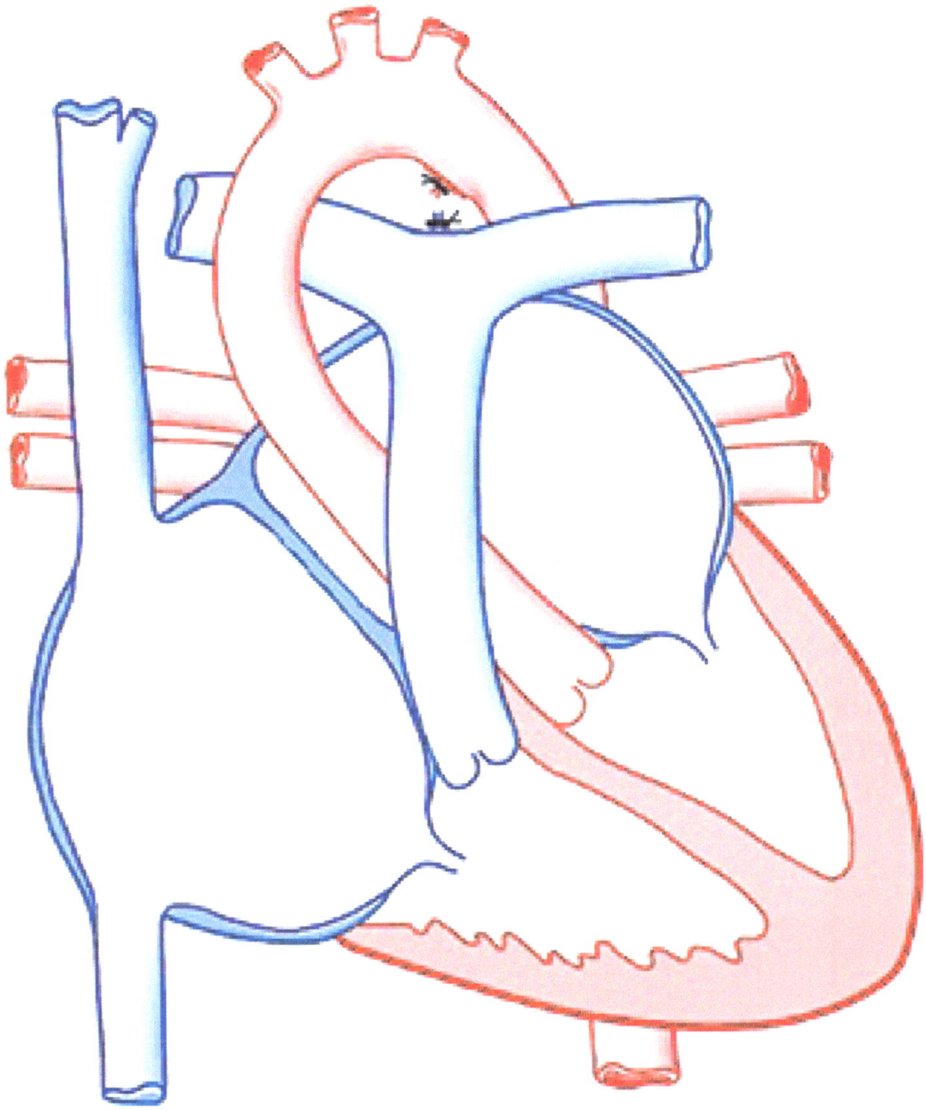

Figure 27: Patent arterial duct closure – surgical.

*Corresponding author Oran B: Medicana International Hospital, Department of Pediatric Cardiology, İzmir, Turkey
E-mail:boran@medicana.com.tr and bulentoran@hotmail.com

Norwood Procedure

Infants with hypoplastic left heart syndrome will not survive without a series of surgical procedures to rebuild the heart. The surgical goal is to rebuild portions of the heart and redirect blood flow. Norwood procedures are open-heart surgical procedures for newborn infants. Collectively, the Norword procedures build a new aorta, cause the right ventricle to pump through the new aorta, and produce a new path to the pulmonary artery.

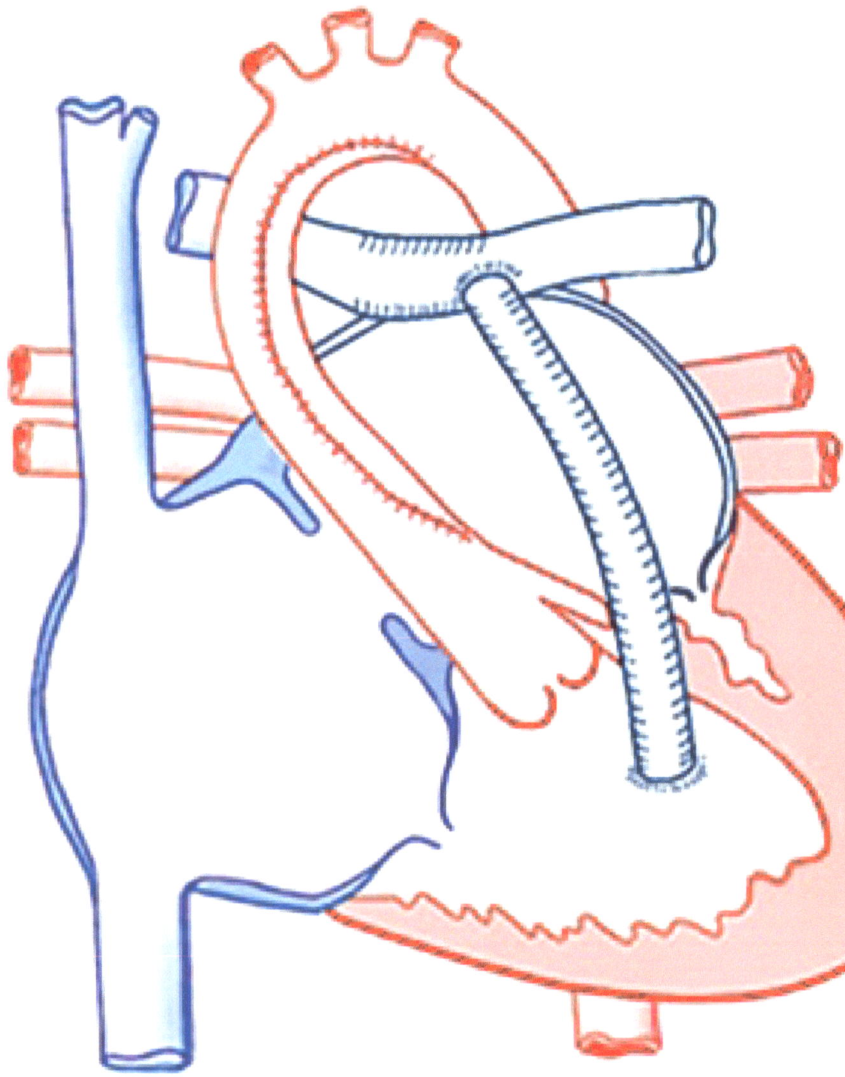

Figure 28: Norwood type procedure.

*Corresponding author Oran B: Medicana International Hospital, Department of Pediatric Cardiology, İzmir, Turkey
E-mail:boran@medicana.com.tr and bulentoran@hotmail.com

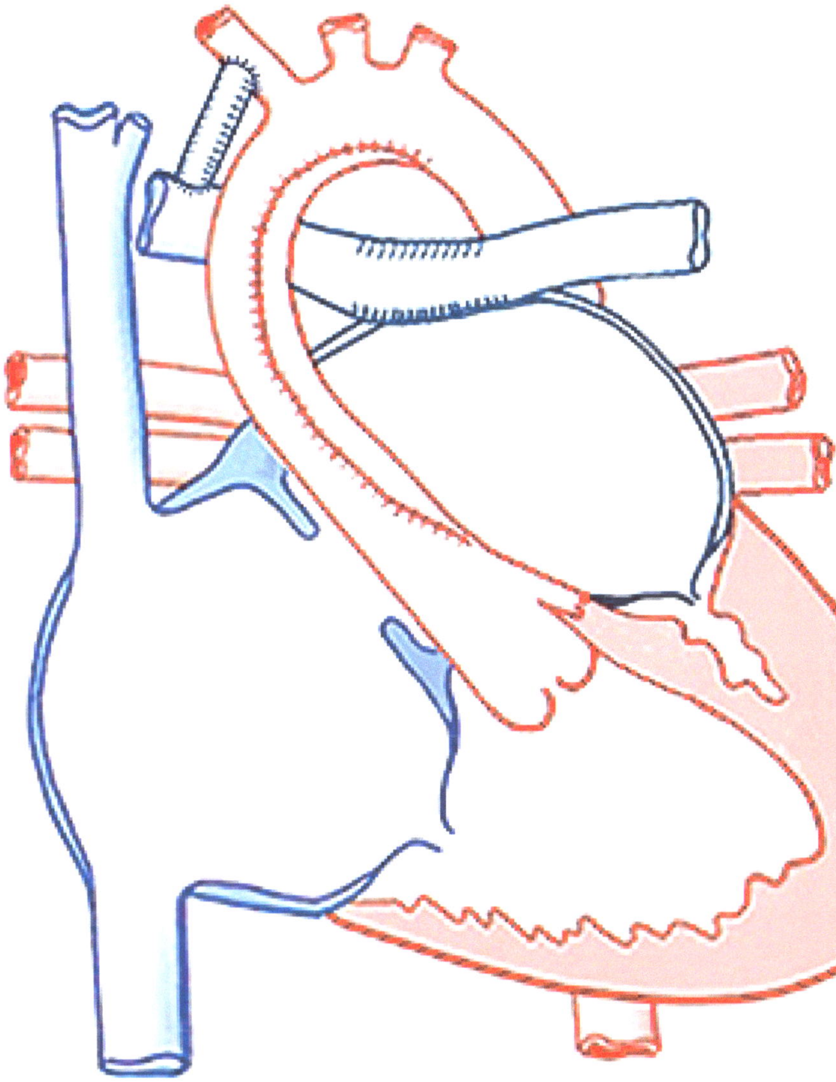

Figure 29: Norwood type procedure.

*Corresponding author Oran B: Medicana International Hospital, Department of Pediatric Cardiology, İzmir, Turkey
E-mail:boran@medicana.com.tr and bulentoran@hotmail.com

Arterial Switch Procedure

The arterial switch is a surgical procedure for treatment of transposition of the great arteries. Large arteries with ventriculoarterial discordance are crossed and reanastomosed. Coronary arteries are reimplanted into the new aorta (neo-aorta) and VSDs are closed.

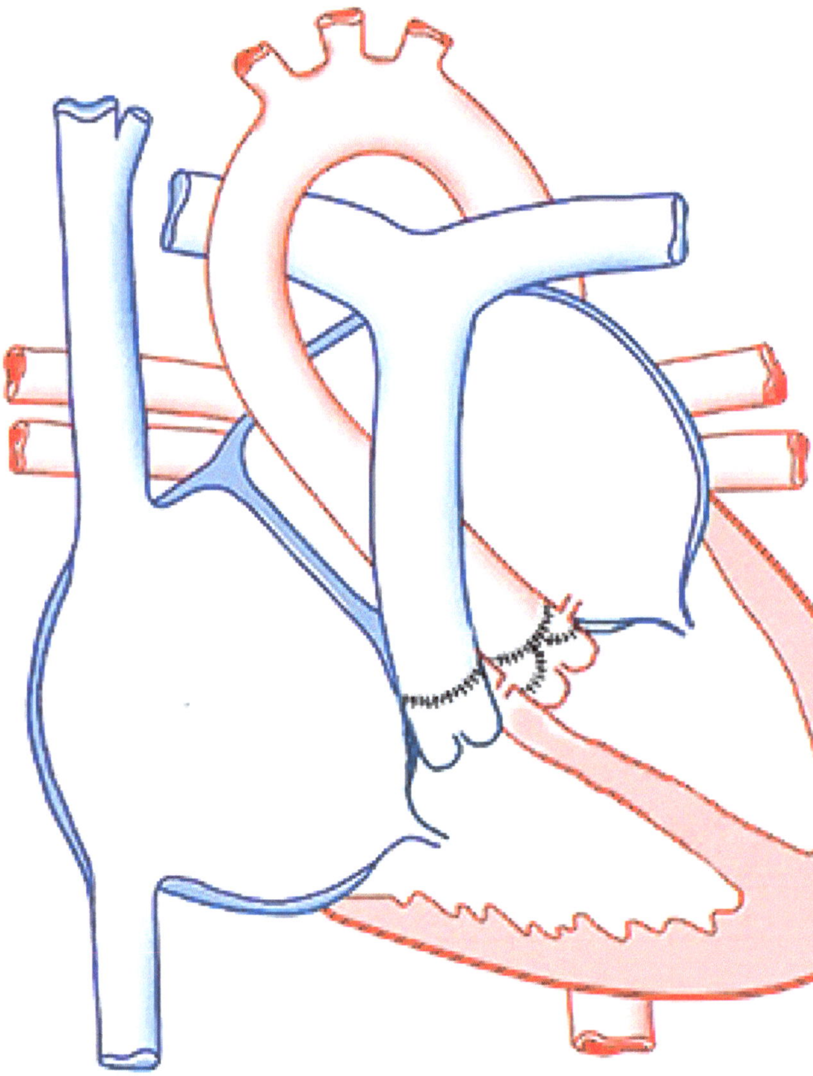

Figure 30: Arterial switch procedure.

*Corresponding author Oran B: Medicana International Hospital, Department of Pediatric Cardiology, İzmir, Turkey
E-mail:boran@medicana.com.tr and bulentoran@hotmail.com

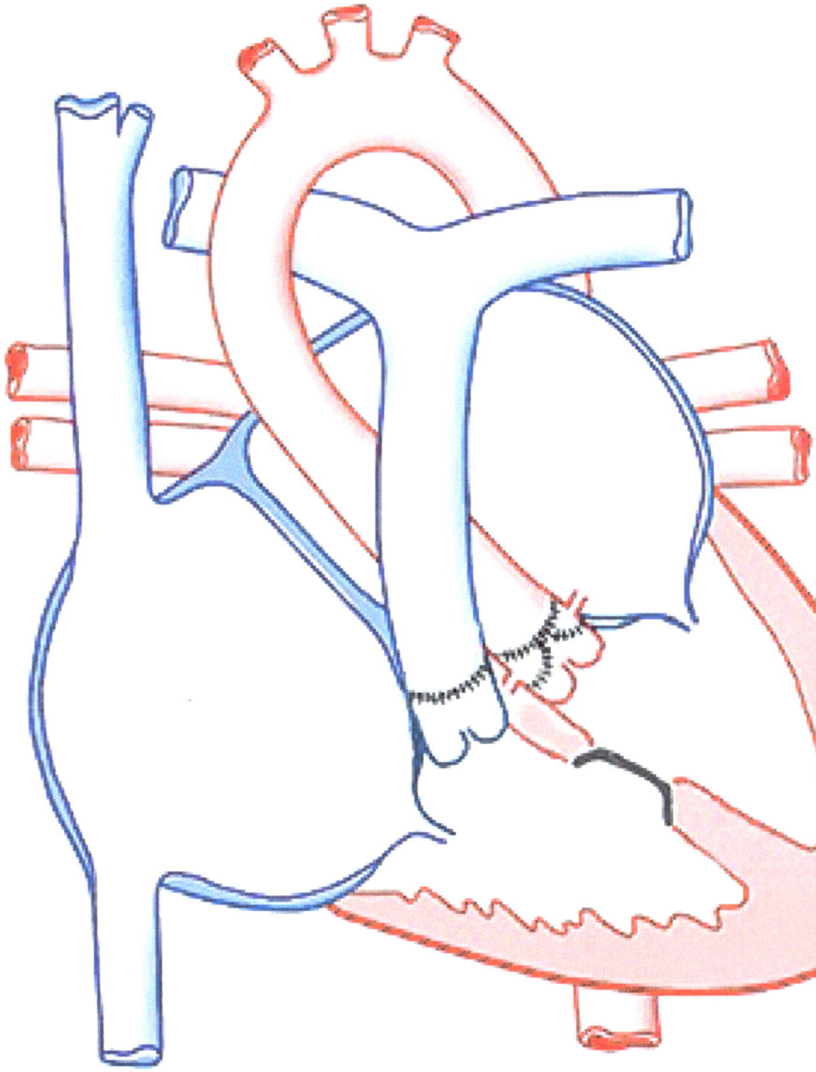

Figure 31: Arterial switch procedure and VSD closure.

*Corresponding author Oran B: Medicana International Hospital, Department of Pediatric Cardiology, İzmir, Turkey
E-mail:boran@medicana.com.tr and bulentoran@hotmail.com

Mustard Procedure

Transposition of the great arteries is a birth defect characterized by reversal of the two great arteries. Surgical intervention can include correction of the blood flow at the atrial level using the Mustard procedure, a type of atrial switch procedure.

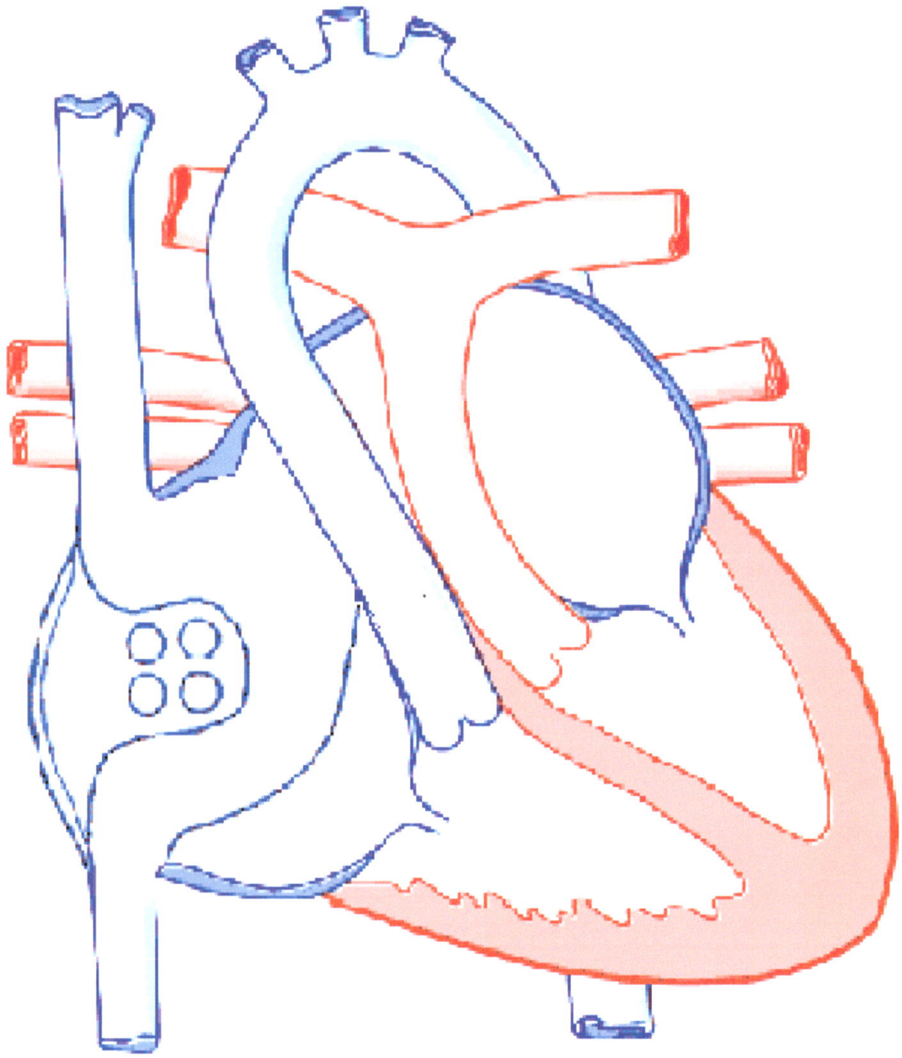

Figure 32: Mustard procedure (atrial inversion).

*Corresponding author Oran B: Medicana International Hospital, Department of Pediatric Cardiology, İzmir, Turkey
E-mail:boran@medicana.com.tr and bulentoran@hotmail.com

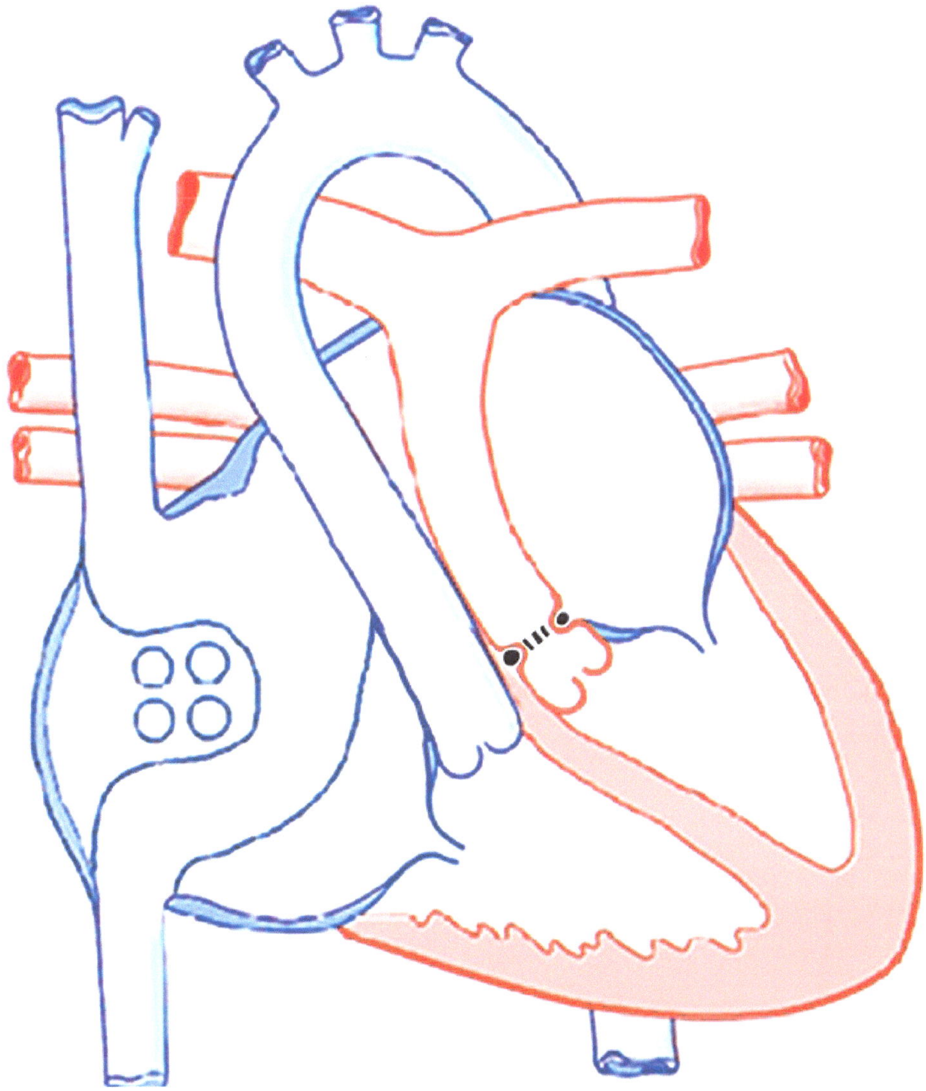

Figure 33: Mustard procedure (atrial inversion), pulmonary trunk band removal (de-band).

*Corresponding author Oran B: Medicana International Hospital, Department of Pediatric Cardiology, İzmir, Turkey
E-mail:boran@medicana.com.tr and bulentoran@hotmail.com

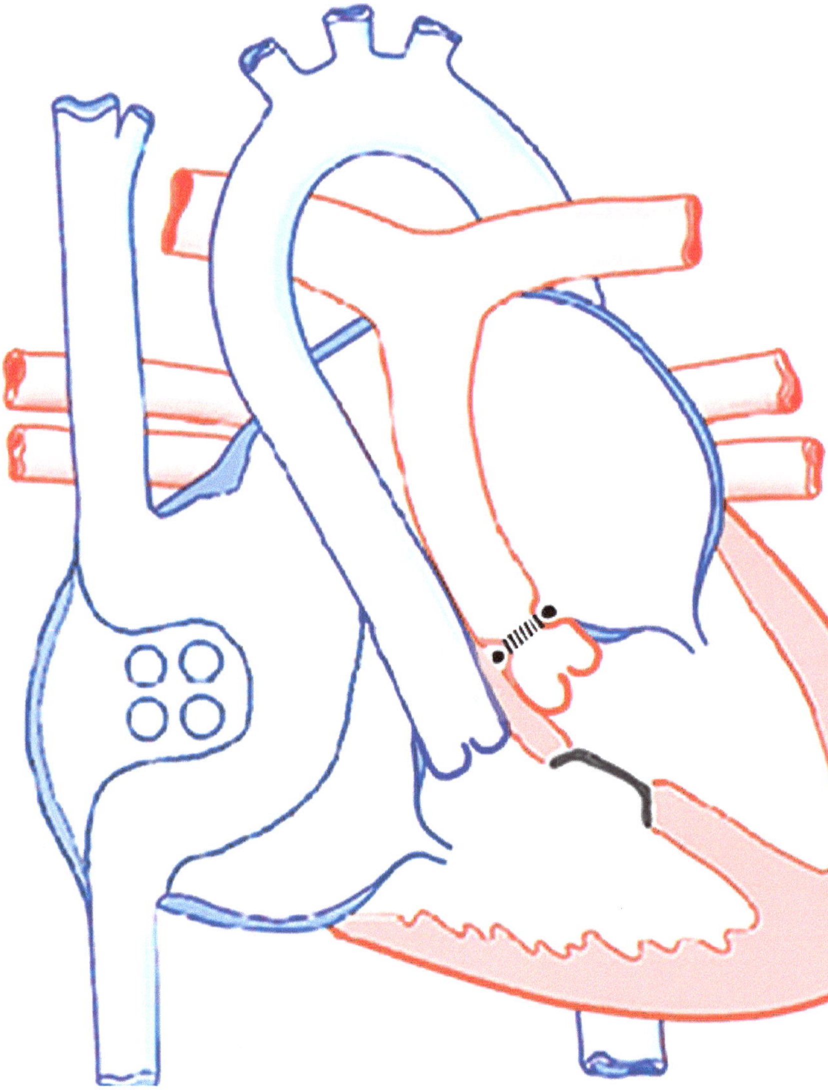

Figure 34: Mustard procedure (atrial inversion), pulmonary trunk band removal (de-band), VSD closure.

*Corresponding author Oran B: Medicana International Hospital, Department of Pediatric Cardiology, İzmir, Turkey
E-mail:boran@medicana.com.tr and bulentoran@hotmail.com

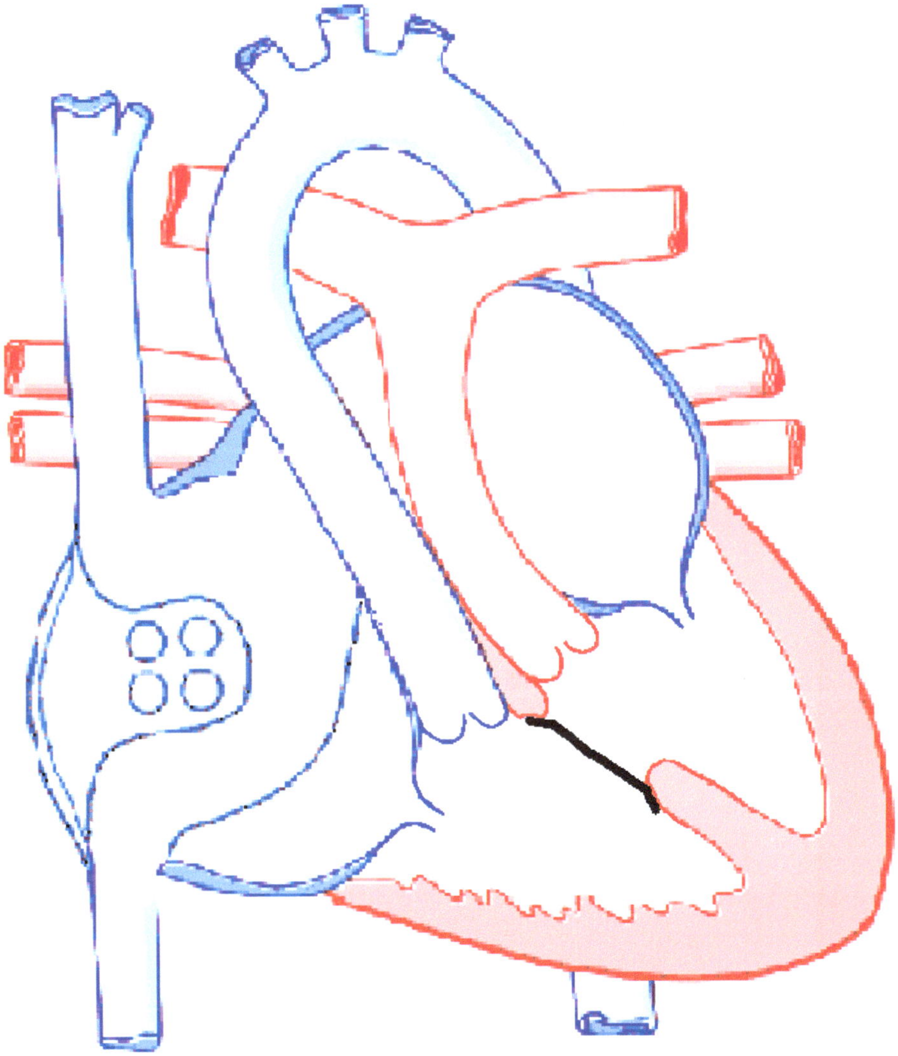

Figure 35: Mustard procedure (atrial inversion), VSD closure.

*Corresponding author Oran B: Medicana International Hospital, Department of Pediatric Cardiology, İzmir, Turkey
E-mail:boran@medicana.com.tr and bulentoran@hotmail.com

Rastelli Procedure

The Rastelli procedure is a corrective operation for patients with transposition of the great arteries, VSDs, and pulmonary stenosis. This procedure includes right ventriculotomy, VSD closure, and the creation of an intracardiac baffle from the left ventricle to the aorta. In addition, it includes production of an external valved conduit that connects the right ventricle to the pulmonary artery.

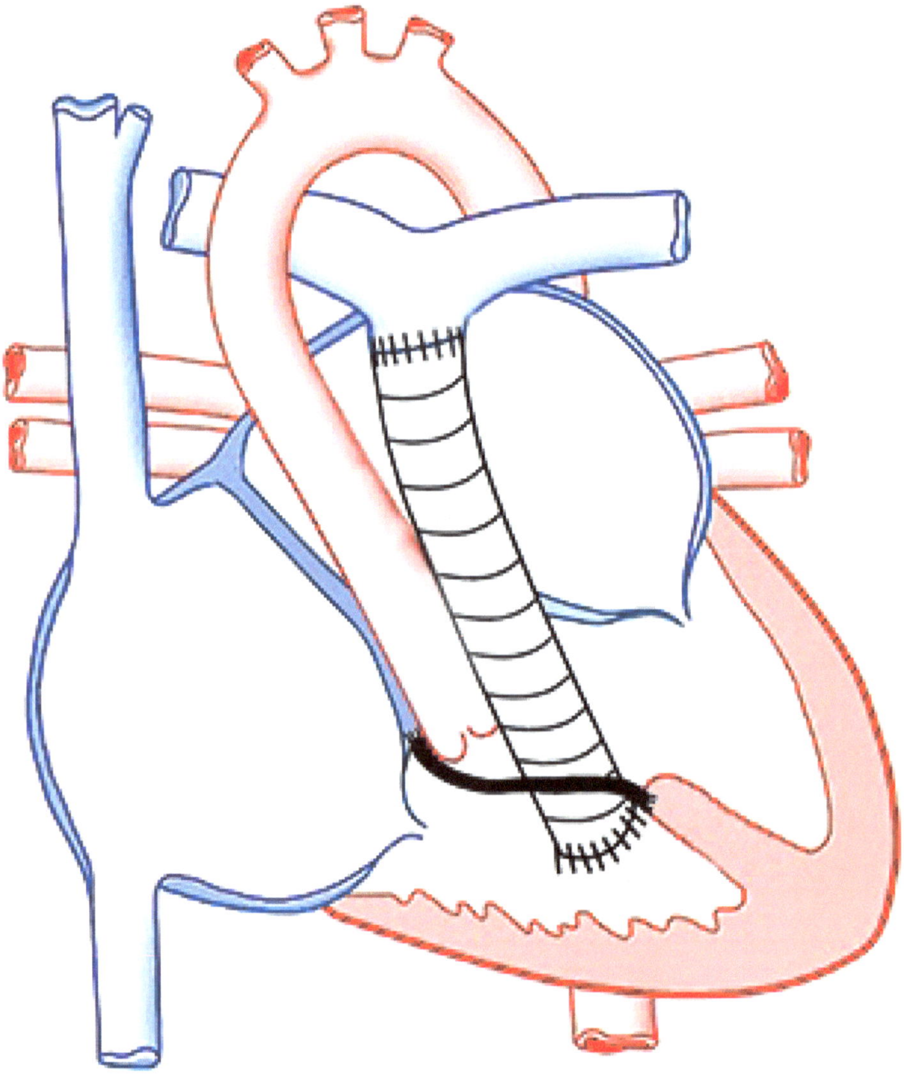

Figure 36: Rastelli procedure: LV to Ao via VSD & RV to pulm trunk conduit.

*Corresponding author Oran B: Medicana International Hospital, Department of Pediatric Cardiology, İzmir, Turkey
E-mail:boran@medicana.com.tr and bulentoran@hotmail.com

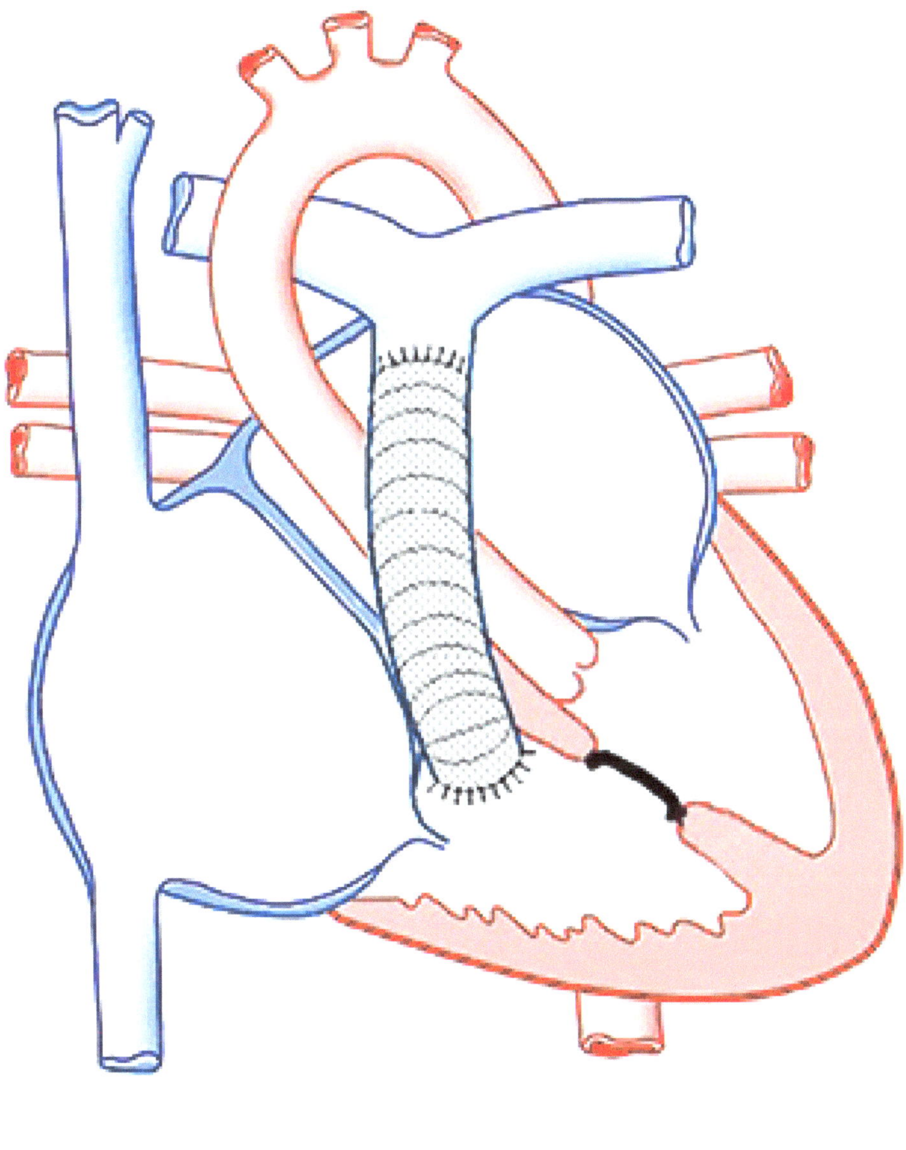

Figure 37: Rastelli procedure, ventricular septal defect closure.

*Corresponding author Oran B: Medicana International Hospital, Department of Pediatric Cardiology, İzmir, Turkey
E-mail:boran@medicana.com.tr and bulentoran@hotmail.com

Double Outlet Right Ventricular Repair

A decision between "single ventricle solution" or "double ventricle solution" should consider the locations, diameters, and number of VSDs, atrioventricular valve anomalies, and any other anomalies. If the locations, numbers, and relationship of VSDs to the large arteries and the size of both ventricles are appropriate, the "double ventricle solution" is indicated. If complete correction is not immediately possible, a modified Blalock-Taussig shunt should be applied. If ventricular size is not appropriate and atrioventricular valves exhibit anomalies, then the "single ventricle solution" or the "one and a half ventricle solution" (biventricular septation + bidirectional Glenn anastomosis) should be performed.

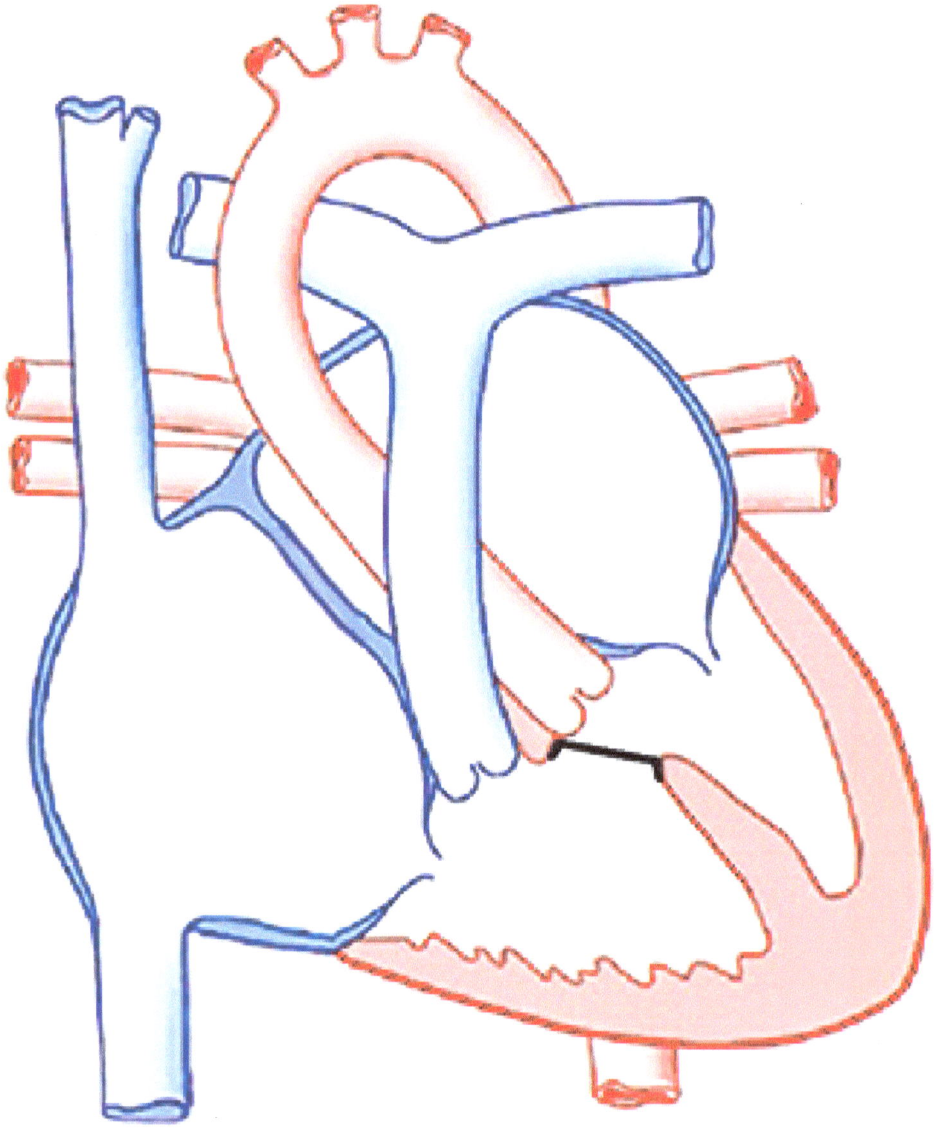

Figure 38: Double outlet right ventricular repair.

*Corresponding author Oran B: Medicana International Hospital, Department of Pediatric Cardiology, İzmir, Turkey
E-mail:boran@medicana.com.tr and bulentoran@hotmail.com

Double Outlet Left Ventricular Repair

A double outlet left ventricle with two well-developed ventricles is surgically treated by closure of VSDs, closure of the native left ventricle-pulmonary outflow, and placement of a right ventricle-pulmonary artery extracardiac conduit.

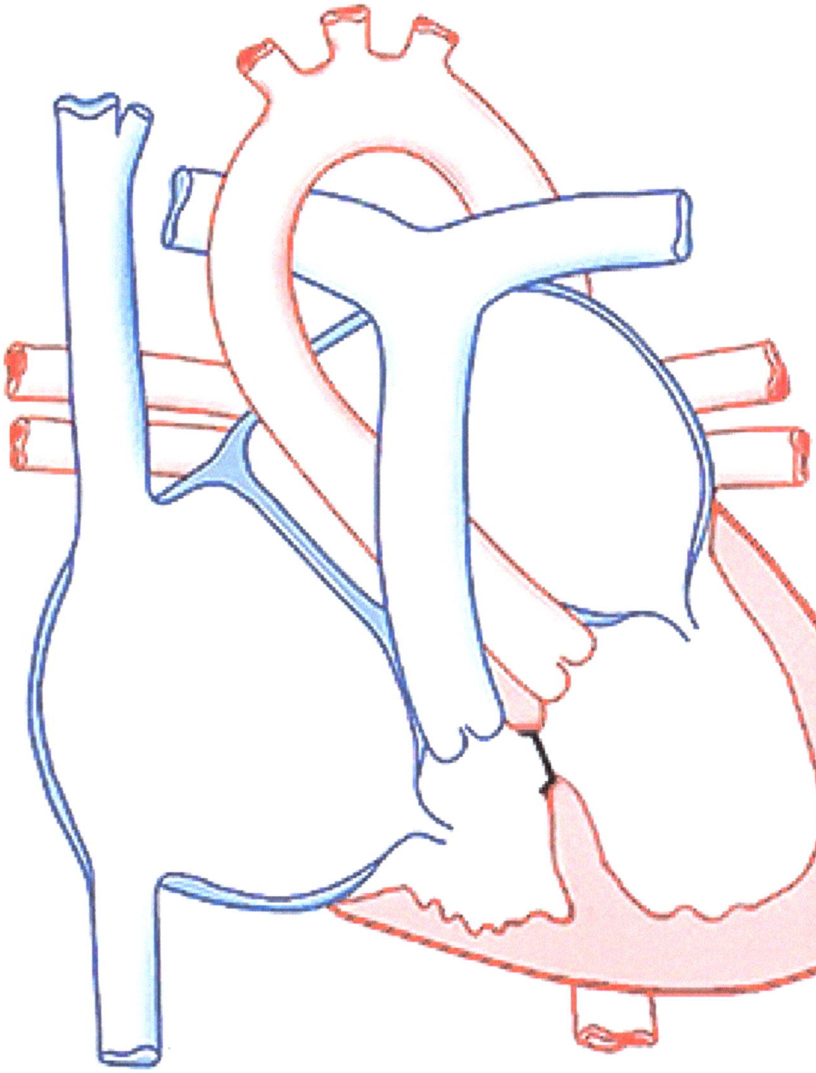

Figure 39: Double outlet left ventricular repair.

*Corresponding author Oran B: Medicana International Hospital, Department of Pediatric Cardiology, İzmir, Turkey
E-mail:boran@medicana.com.tr and bulentoran@hotmail.com

Repair of Coarctation of the Aorta

Open-heart surgery is not required to correct coarctation of the aorta. Surgical techniques include removal of the narrow aortic segment with end-to-end or end-to-side anastomosis or sutures to the hypoplastic segment with a patch, using a portion of the subclavian artery or a synthetic graft.

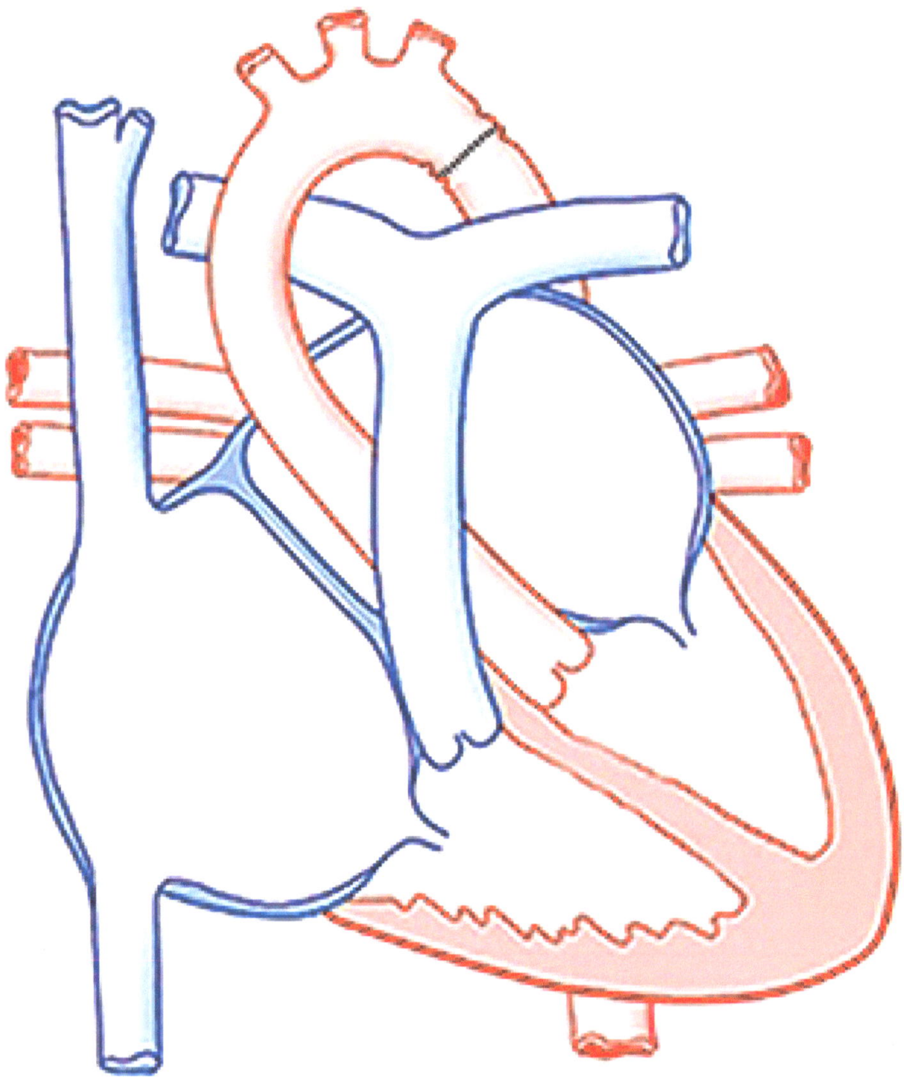

Figure 40: Aortic coarct/hypoplasia repair: resection & end/end anast.

*Corresponding author Oran B: Medicana International Hospital, Department of Pediatric Cardiology, İzmir, Turkey
E-mail:boran@medicana.com.tr and bulentoran@hotmail.com

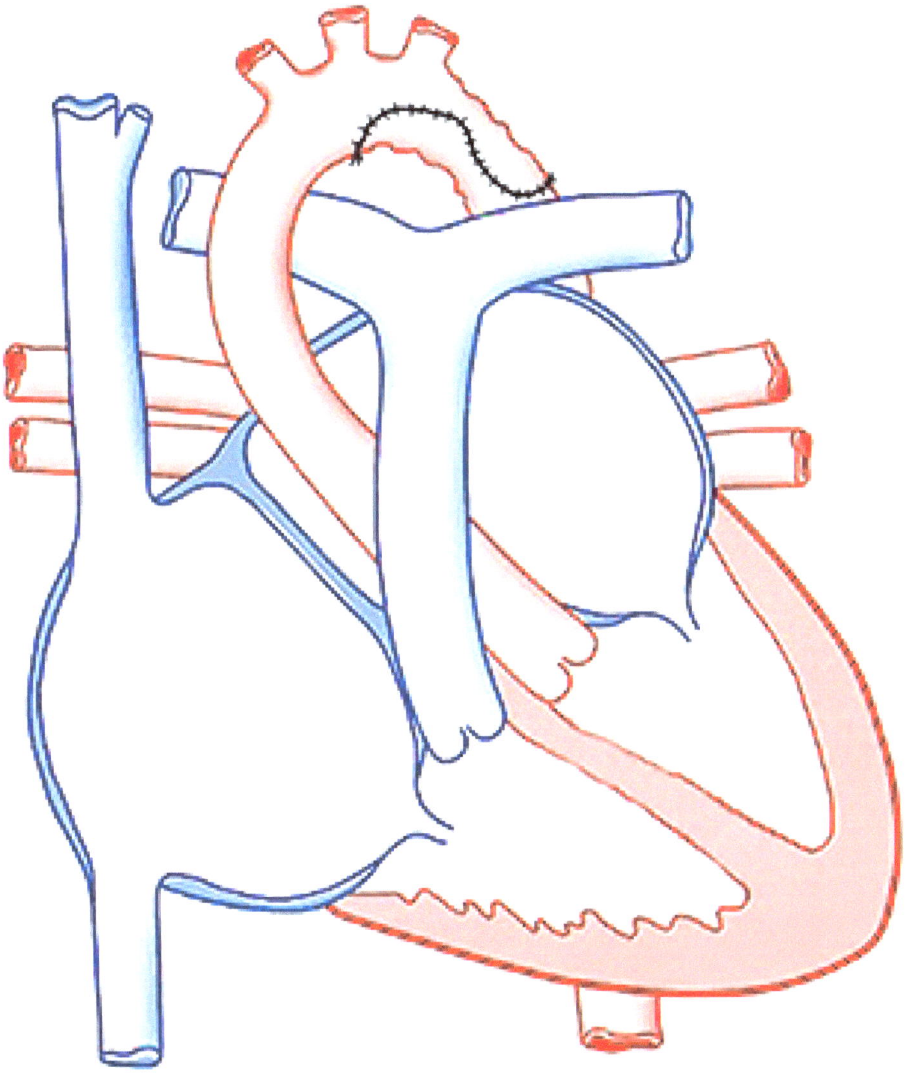

Figure 41: Aortic coarct/hypoplasia repair: extended resection & end/end anast.

*Corresponding author Oran B: Medicana International Hospital, Department of Pediatric Cardiology, İzmir, Turkey
E-mail:boran@medicana.com.tr and bulentoran@hotmail.com

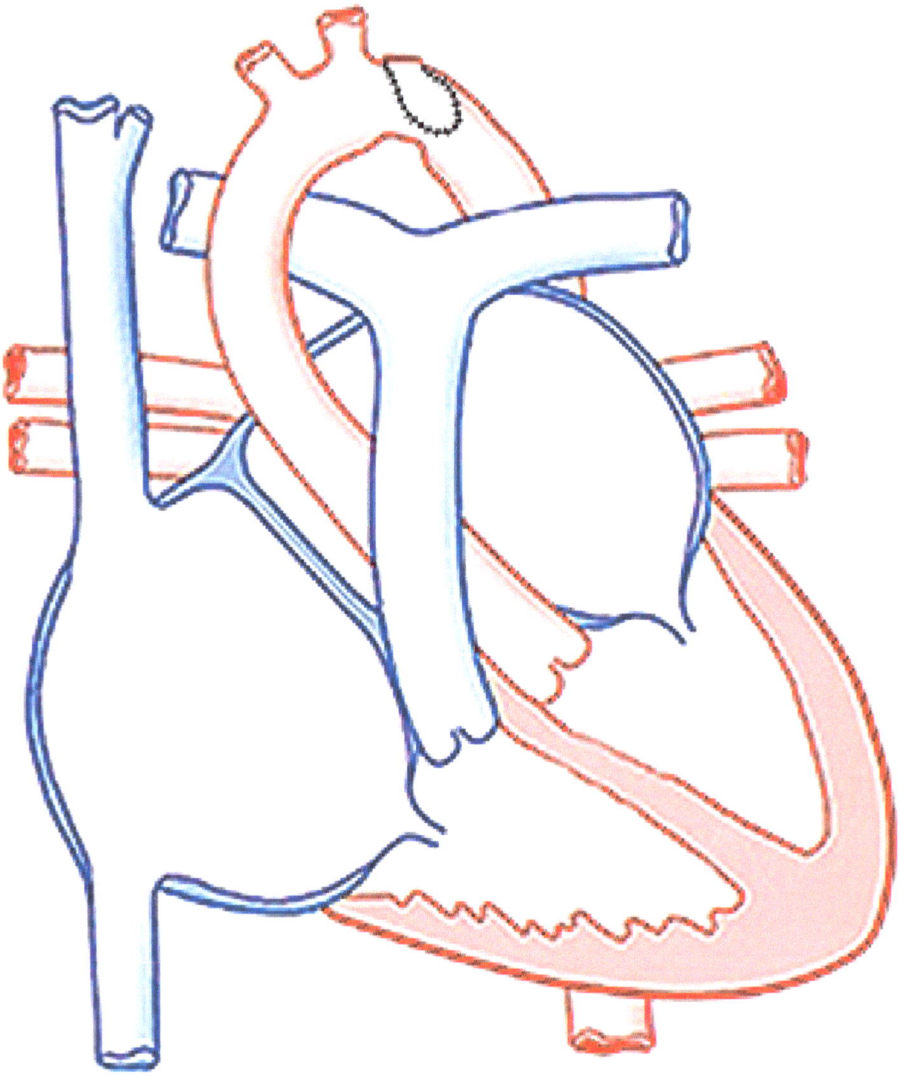

Figure 42: Aortic coarct/hypoplasia repair: subclavian flap aortoplasty.

*Corresponding author Oran B: Medicana International Hospital, Department of Pediatric Cardiology, İzmir, Turkey
E-mail:boran@medicana.com.tr and bulentoran@hotmail.com

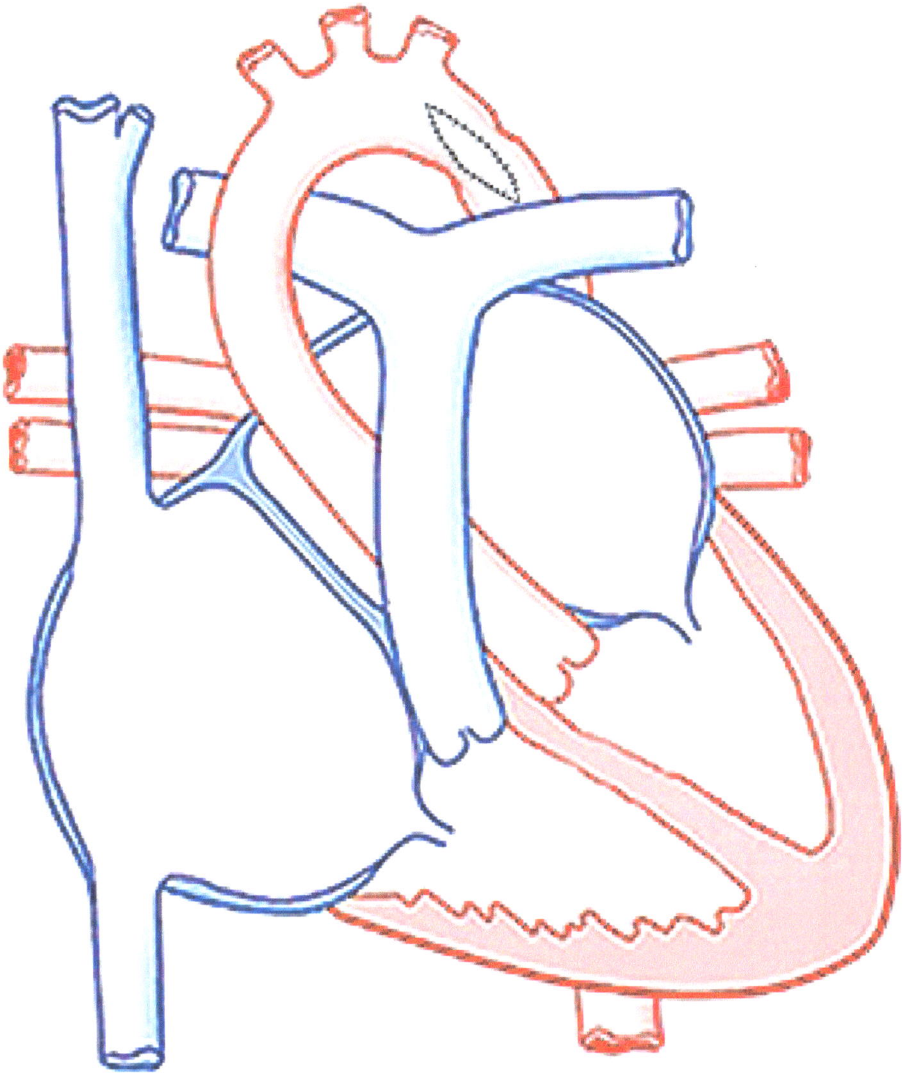

Figure 43: Aortic coarct/hypoplasia repair: patch aortoplasty.

*Corresponding author Oran B: Medicana International Hospital, Department of Pediatric Cardiology, İzmir, Turkey
E-mail:boran@medicana.com.tr and bulentoran@hotmail.com

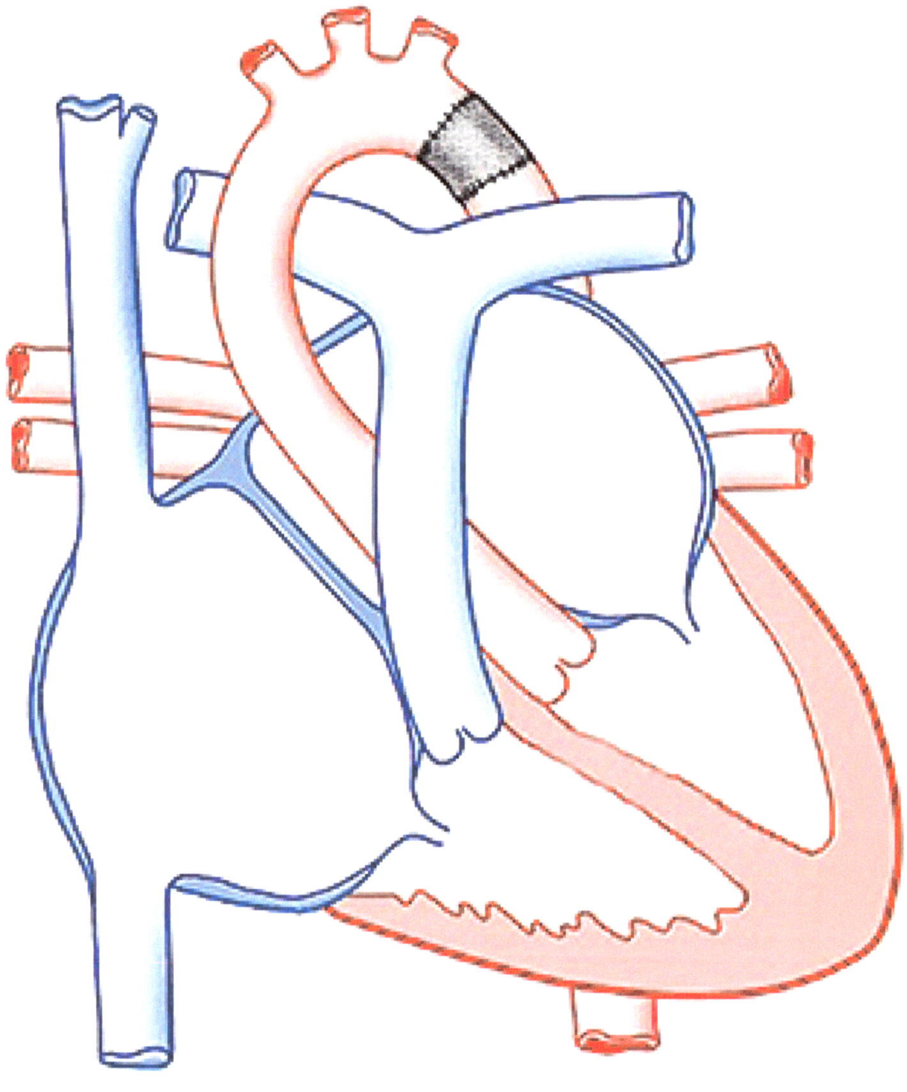

Figure 44: Aortic coarct/hypoplasia repair: resection + insertion tube graft.

*Corresponding author Oran B: Medicana International Hospital, Department of Pediatric Cardiology, İzmir, Turkey
E-mail:boran@medicana.com.tr and bulentoran@hotmail.com

Interrupted Aortic Arch Repair

Surgical intervention is required for survival in patients with an interrupted aortic arch. The procedure involves end-to-end or end-to-side anastomosis and/or application of a patch using graft tissue. The postoperative survival rate is high.

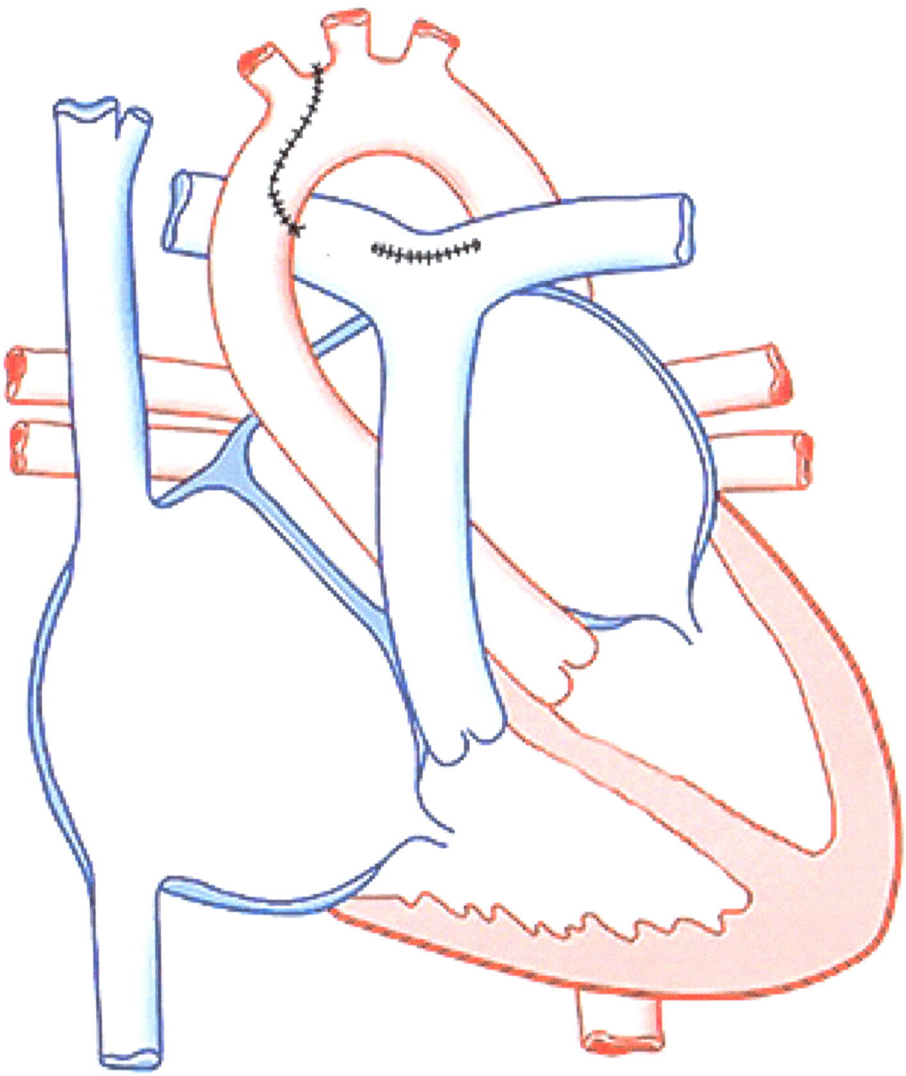

Figure 45: Interrupted aortic arch repair type-I.

*Corresponding author Oran B: Medicana International Hospital, Department of Pediatric Cardiology, İzmir, Turkey
E-mail:boran@medicana.com.tr and bulentoran@hotmail.com

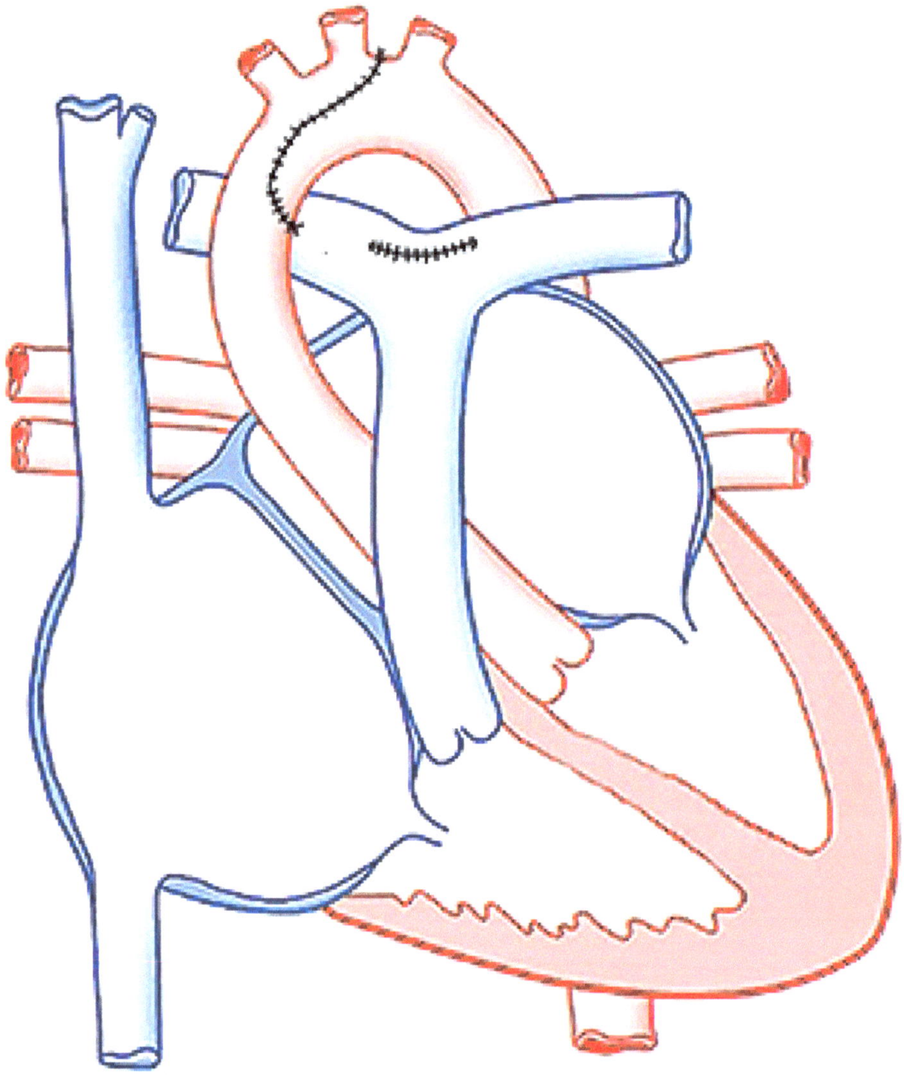

Figure 46: Interrupted aortic arch repair type-ll.

*Corresponding author Oran B: Medicana International Hospital, Department of Pediatric Cardiology, İzmir, Turkey
E-mail:boran@medicana.com.tr and bulentoran@hotmail.com

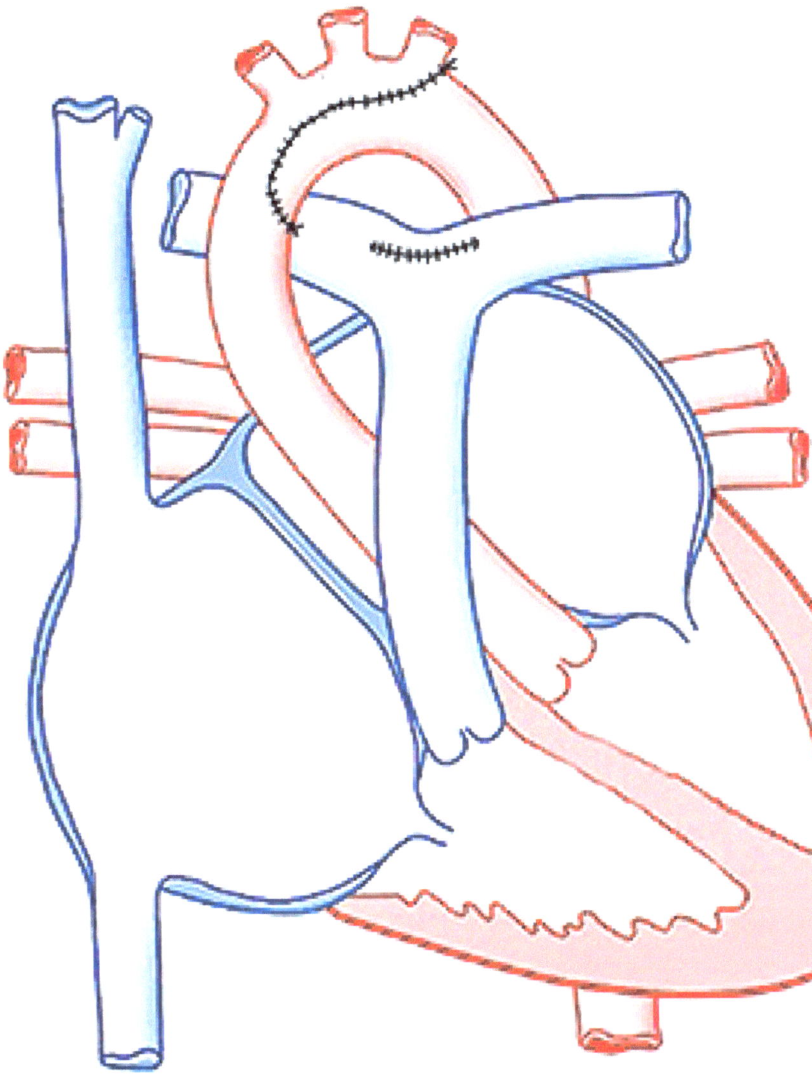

Figure 47: Interrupted aortic arch repair type-lll.

*Corresponding author Oran B: Medicana International Hospital, Department of Pediatric Cardiology, İzmir, Turkey
E-mail:boran@medicana.com.tr and bulentoran@hotmail.com

Konno Procedure

The Konno surgical procedure corrects tunnel-type subvalvar aortic stenosis. The right ventriculotomy and left ventricular outflow tract are enlarged with a patch; aortic valve replacement may also be required. Often, the "Ross procedure" and the "Ross-Konno procedure" are performed together.

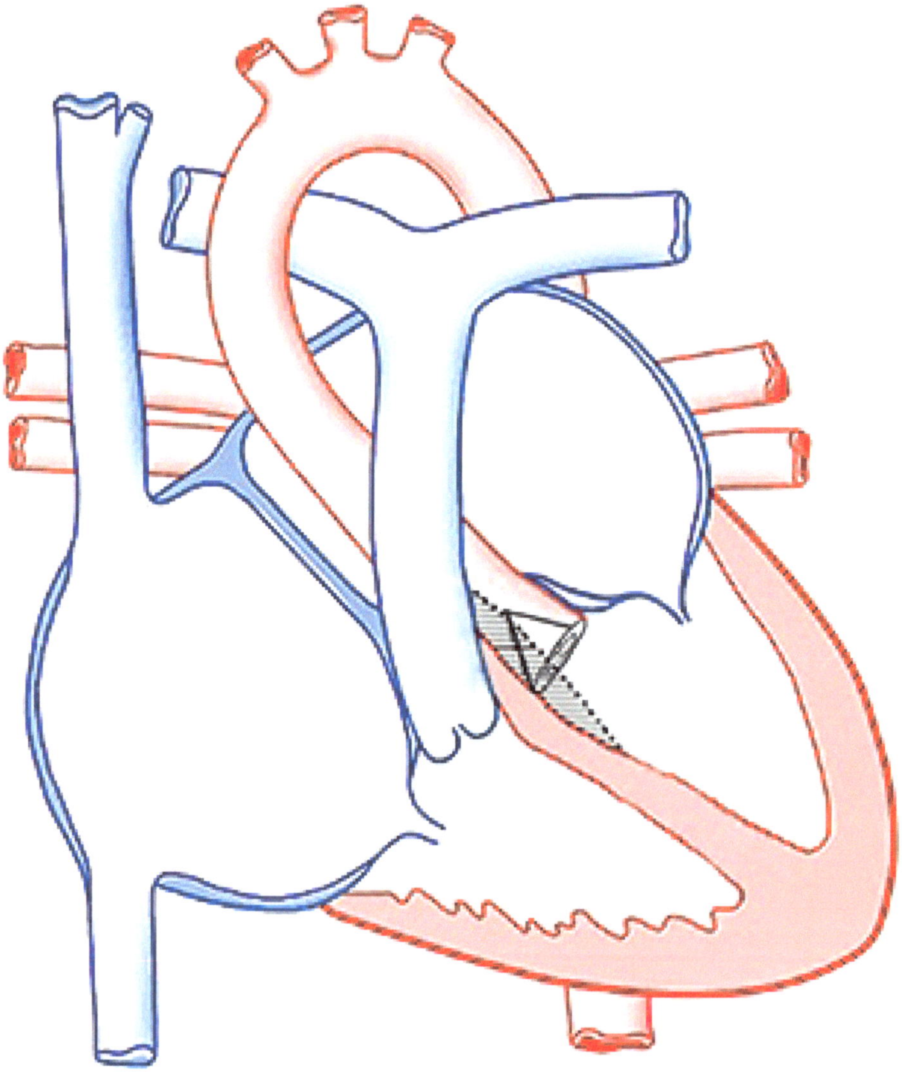

Figure 48: left ventricular outflow tract obstruction relief - complex (Konno etc).

*Corresponding author Oran B: Medicana International Hospital, Department of Pediatric Cardiology, İzmir, Turkey
E-mail:boran@medicana.com.tr and bulentoran@hotmail.com

Modified Blalock-Taussig Shunt with ASD and Pulmonary Atresia

The Blalock-Taussig shunt is a palliative shunt between the subclavian and pulmonary arteries. The modified Blalock-Taussig shunt procedure involves interposition of an expanded polytetrafluoroethylene vascular graft between the subclavian and pulmonary arteries.

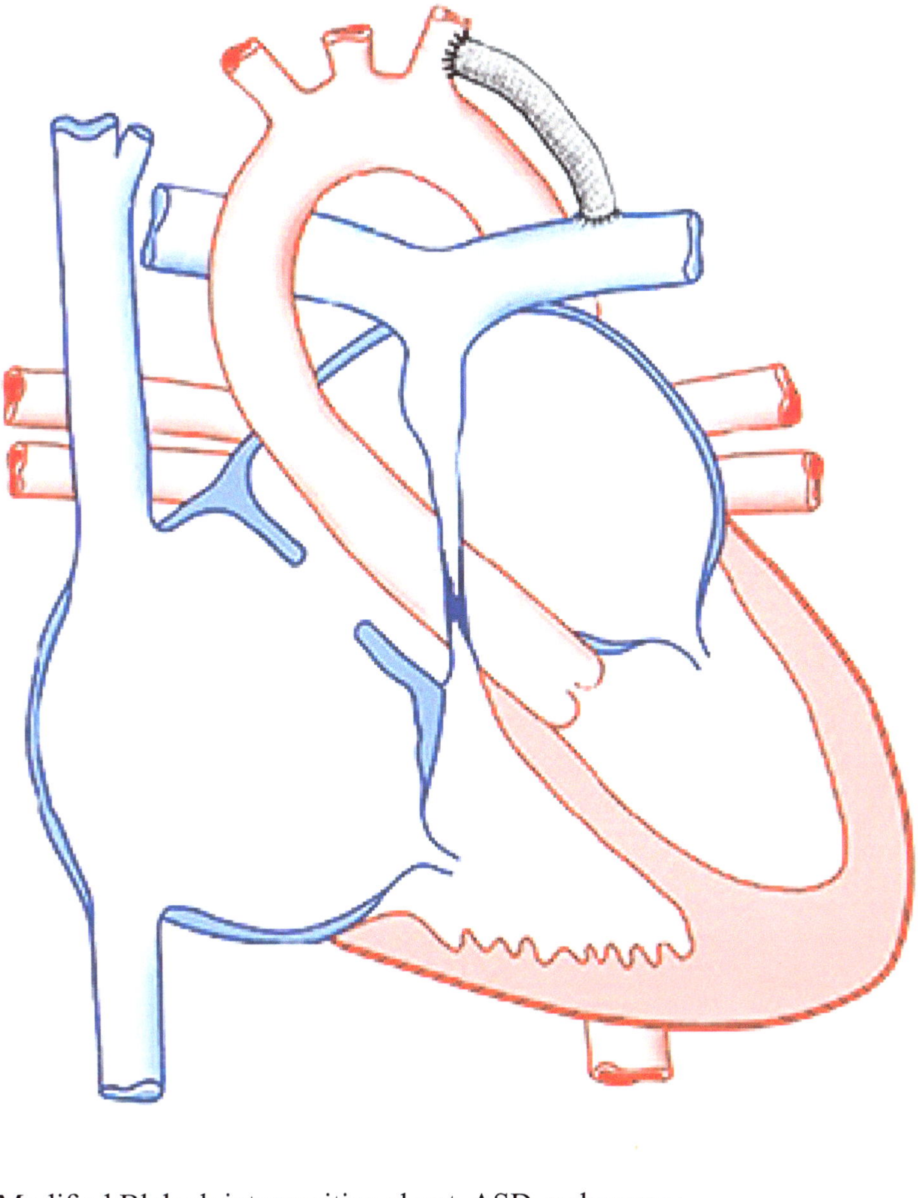

Figure 49: Modified Blalock interposition shunt, ASD, pulmonary.

*Corresponding author Oran B: Medicana International Hospital, Department of Pediatric Cardiology, İzmir, Turkey
E-mail:boran@medicana.com.tr and bulentoran@hotmail.com

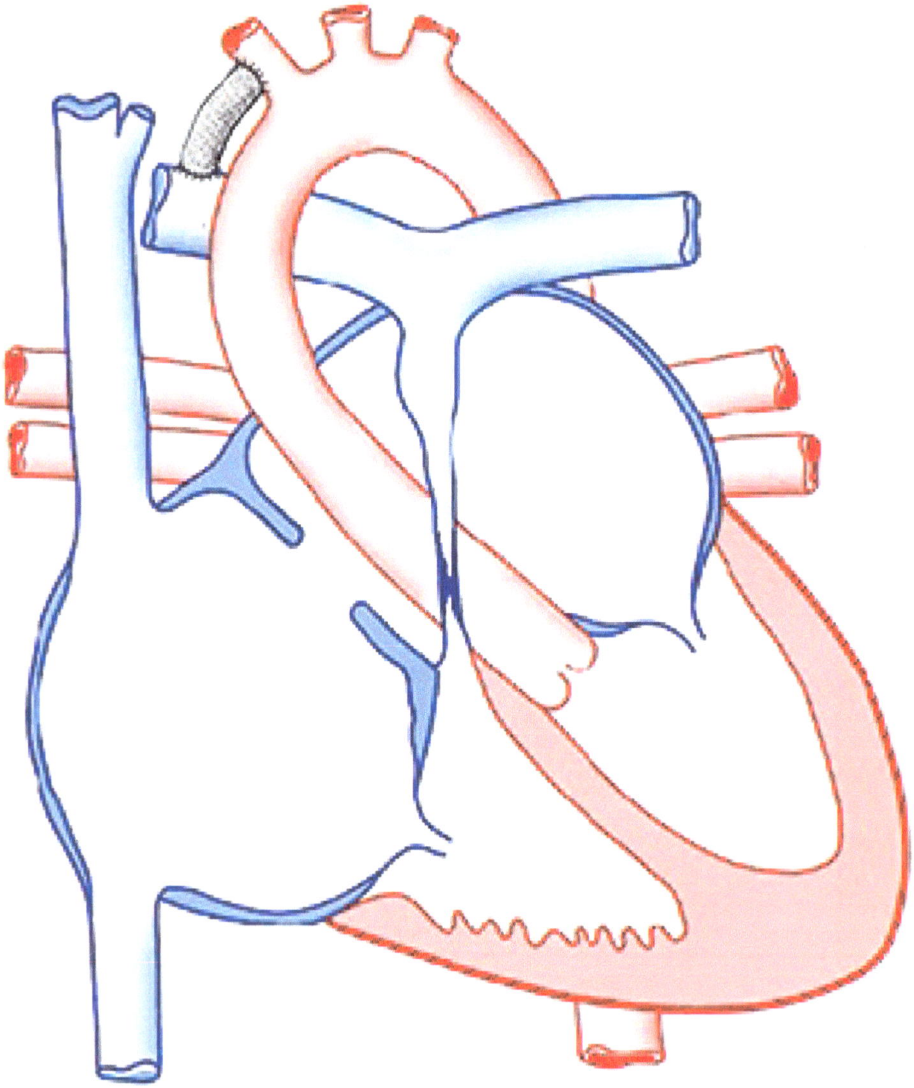

Figure 50: Modified Blalock interposition shunt, ASD, pulmonary.

*Corresponding author Oran B: Medicana International Hospital, Department of Pediatric Cardiology, İzmir, Turkey
E-mail:boran@medicana.com.tr and bulentoran@hotmail.com

One and a half Ventricle Repair

One and a half ventricle repair is useful for patients with limited right ventricular diameter and function. The right ventricular outflow tract stenosis is removed, the tricuspid valve is repaired, and the right atrial volume is reduced by plication. In addition, a bidirectional Glenn shunt is applied to increase pulmonary blood flow.

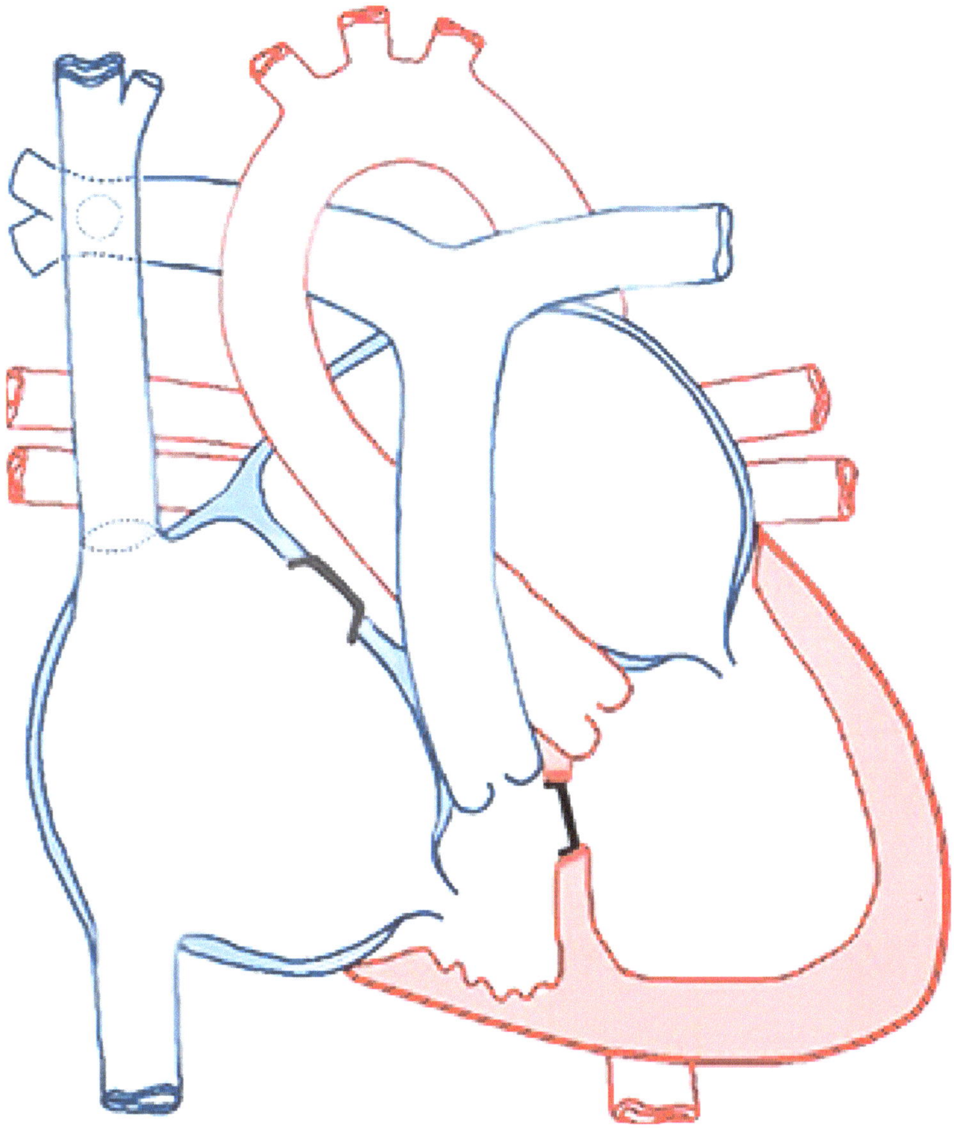

Figure 51: One and a half ventricle repair.

*Corresponding author Oran B: Medicana International Hospital, Department of Pediatric Cardiology, İzmir, Turkey
E-mail:boran@medicana.com.tr and bulentoran@hotmail.com

Bidirectional Glenn (cavo-pulmonary) Anastomosis

The Glenn shunt is performed to increase pulmonary blood flow in patients with pulmonary atresia or severe pulmonary stenosis. The bidirectional Glenn shunt procedure, in which end-to-side anastomosis is performed between the divided vena cava superior and the undivided pulmonary artery, is preferred over the Glenn shunt. This procedure ensures that both lungs receive blood.

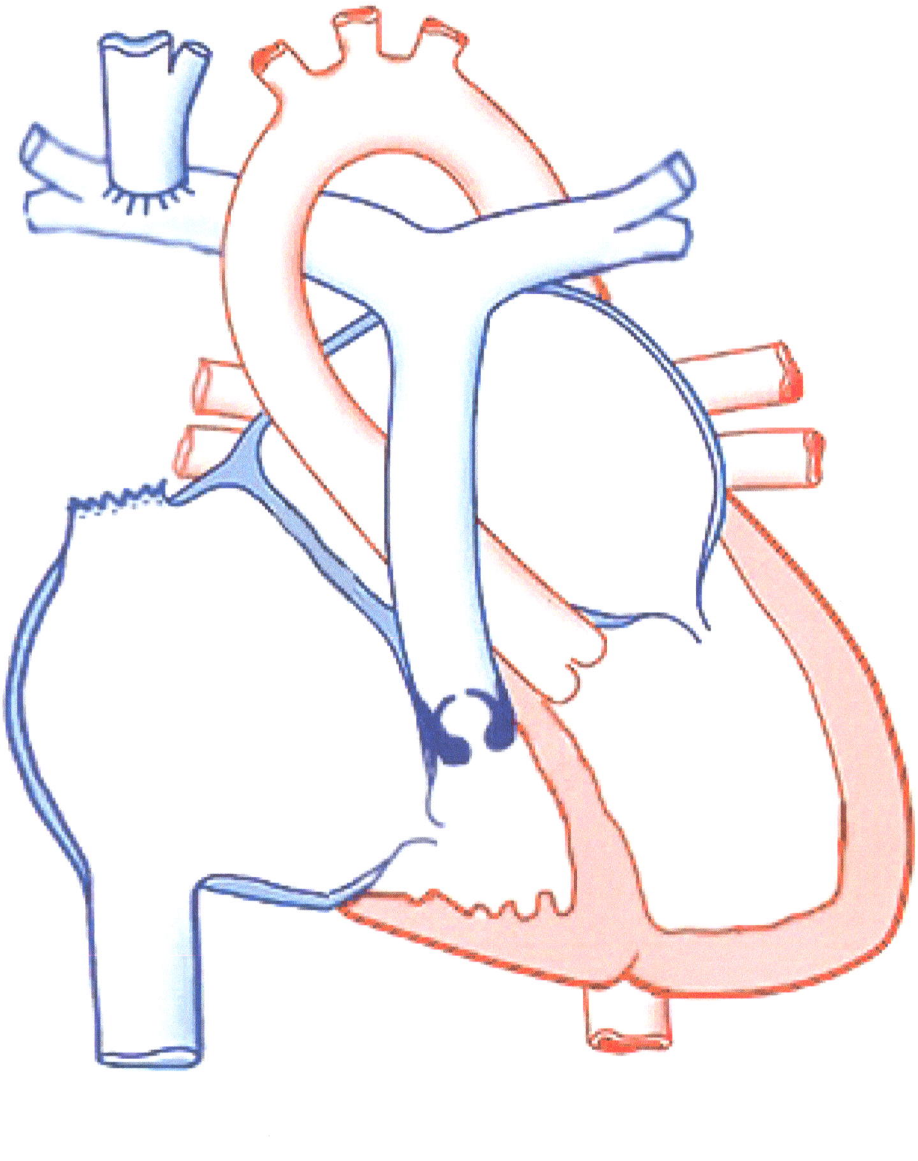

Figure 52: Bidirectional superior cavopulmonary (Glenn) anastomosis, severe pulmonary stenosis.

*Corresponding author Oran B: Medicana International Hospital, Department of Pediatric Cardiology, İzmir, Turkey
E-mail:boran@medicana.com.tr and bulentoran@hotmail.com

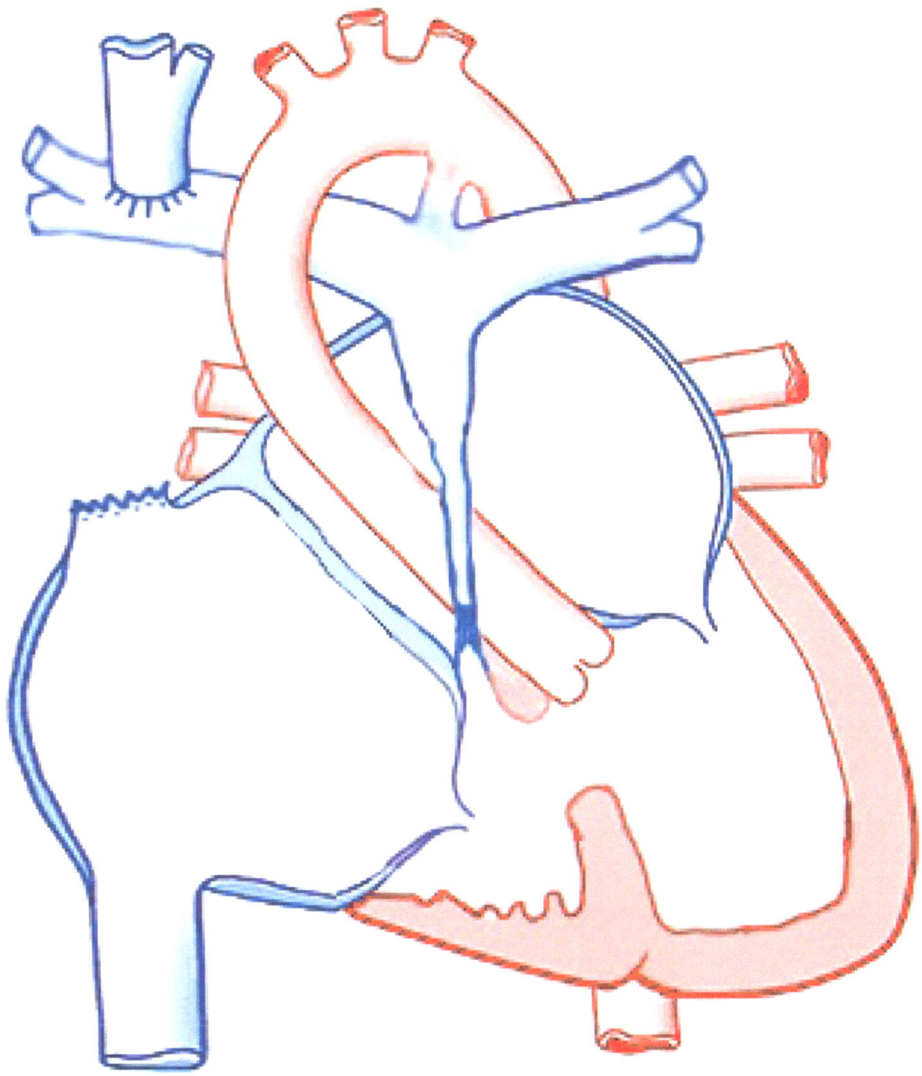

Figure 53: Bidirectional superior cavopulmonary (Glenn) anastomosis, pulmonary atresia, VSD.

*Corresponding author Oran B: Medicana International Hospital, Department of Pediatric Cardiology, İzmir, Turkey
E-mail:boran@medicana.com.tr and bulentoran@hotmail.com

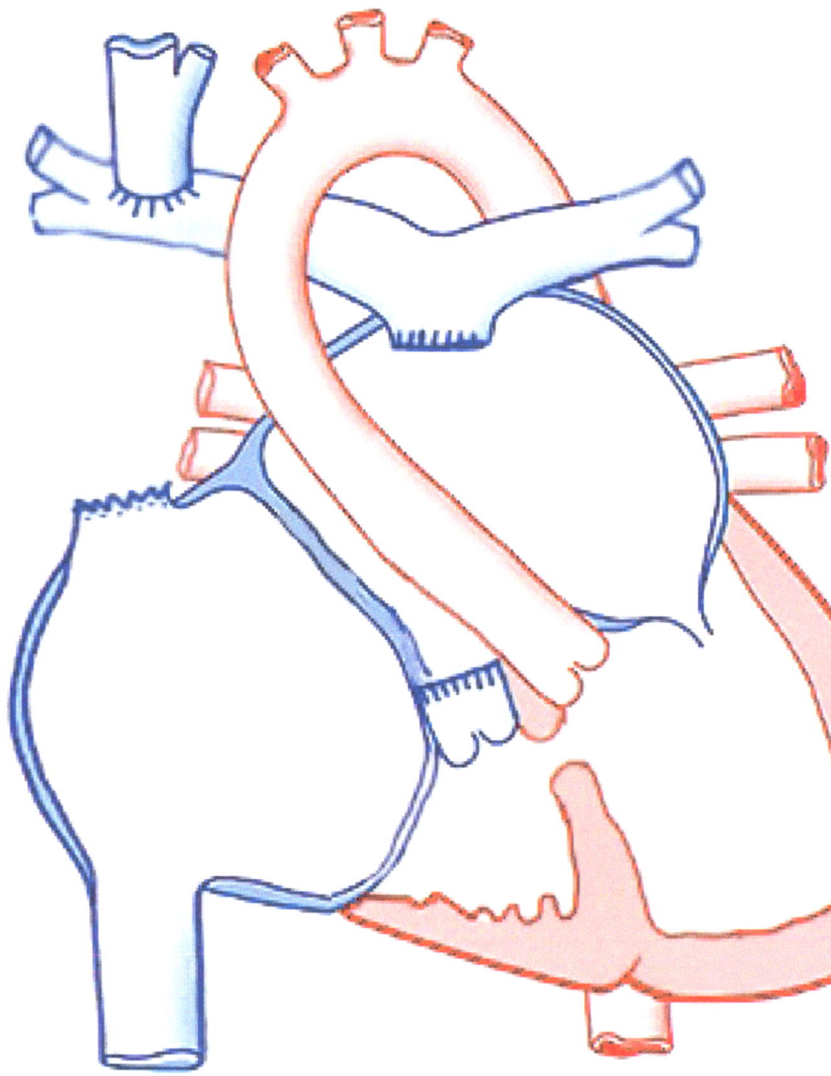

Figure 54: Bidirectional superior cavopulmonary (Glenn) anastomosis, tricuspide atresia, VSD.

*Corresponding author Oran B: Medicana International Hospital, Department of Pediatric Cardiology, İzmir, Turkey
E-mail:boran@medicana.com.tr and bulentoran@hotmail.com

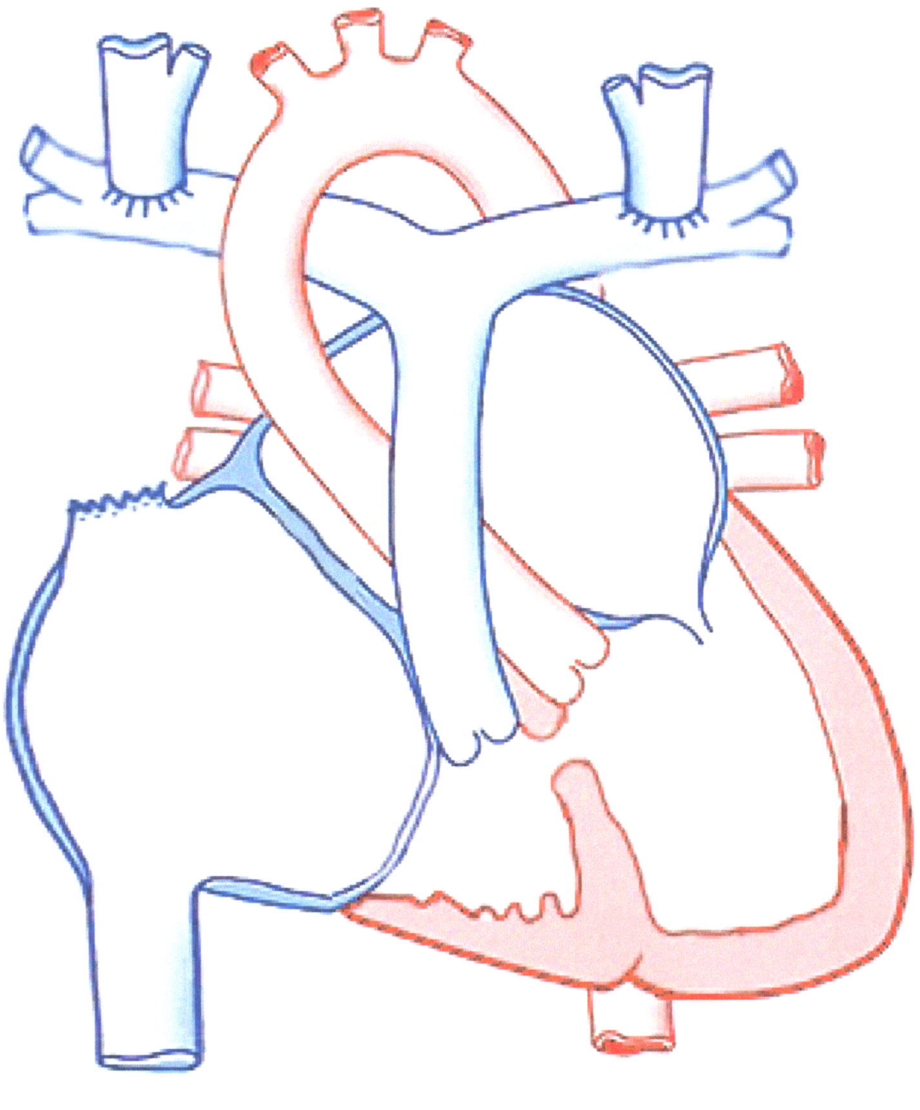

Figure 55: Bidirectional superior cavopulmonary (Glenn) anastomosis, tricuspide atresia, VSD with left persistant superior vena cava.

*Corresponding author Oran B: Medicana International Hospital, Department of Pediatric Cardiology, İzmir, Turkey
E-mail:boran@medicana.com.tr and bulentoran@hotmail.com

Fontan Procedures

Fontan operations and Fontan modifications are palliative therapies for patients with single ventricle defects who cannot undergo biventricular repair. These open-heart surgical procedures involve forwarding the systemic venous return to the pulmonary arterial bed, without passage through the ventricle. The pulmonary venous blood flow is pumped by a single ventricle to systemic arteries.

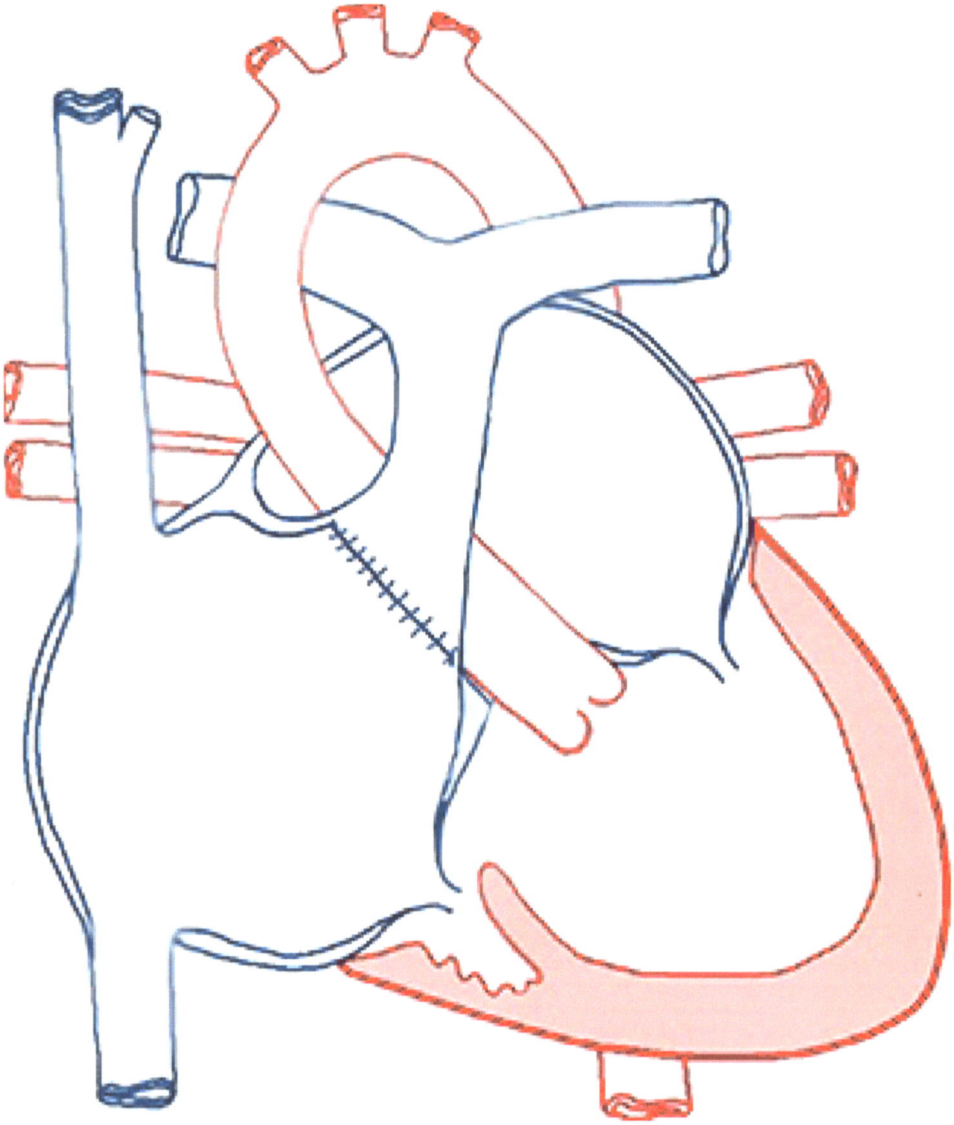

Figure 56: Fontan procedure with direct atrio-pulmonary anastomosis, RV hypoplasia.

*Corresponding author Oran B: Medicana International Hospital, Department of Pediatric Cardiology, İzmir, Turkey
E-mail:boran@medicana.com.tr and bulentoran@hotmail.com

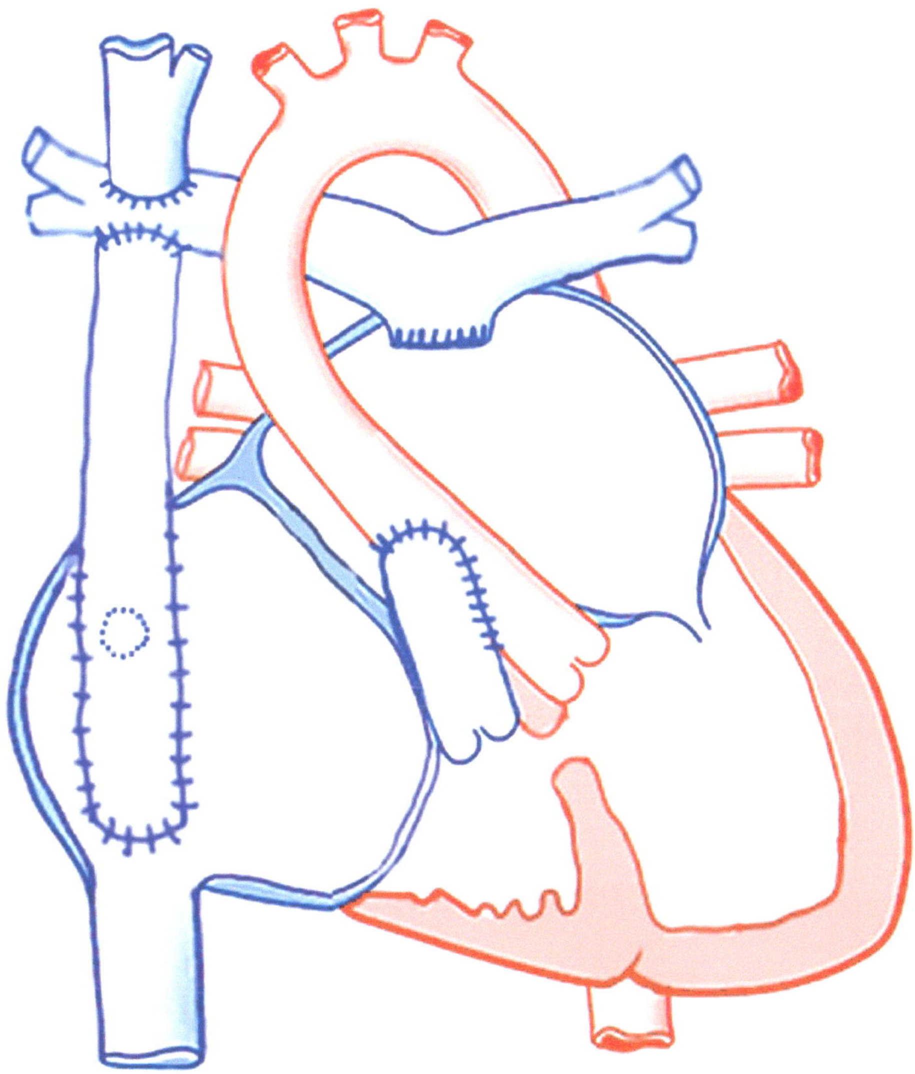

Figure 57: Total cavopulmonary conn (TCPC) with lateral atrial tunnel.

*Corresponding author Oran B: Medicana International Hospital, Department of Pediatric Cardiology, İzmir, Turkey
E-mail:boran@medicana.com.tr and bulentoran@hotmail.com

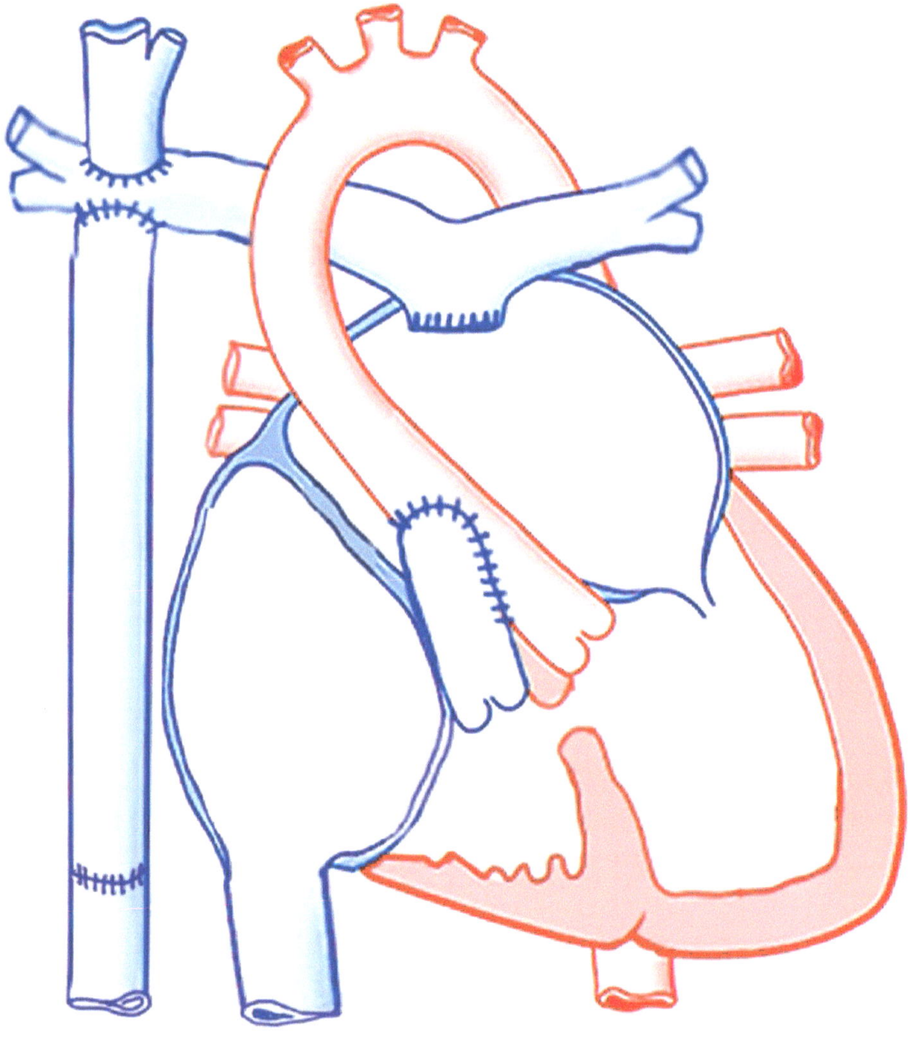

Figure 58: Total cavopulmonary conn (TCPC) using extracardiac IVC-PA conduit.

*Corresponding author Oran B: Medicana International Hospital, Department of Pediatric Cardiology, İzmir, Turkey
E-mail:boran@medicana.com.tr and bulentoran@hotmail.com

Ross Procedure

The Ross Procedure (aortic root replacement using a pulmonary autograft) is a surgical option for patients with severe aortic valve disease. This procedure involves aortic valve replacement using a pulmonary autograft. It is also known as homograft pulmonary valve replacement.

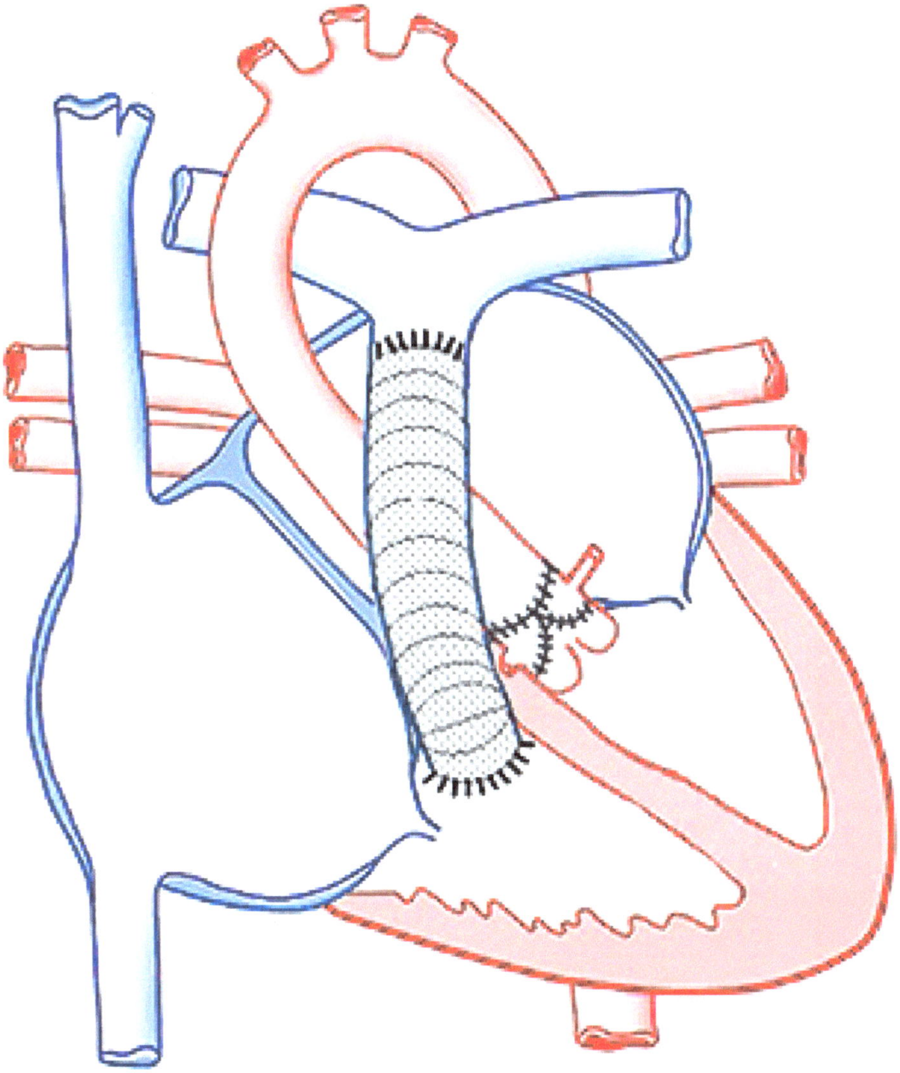

Figure 59: Ross procedure (Aortic root replacement with pulmonary autograft).

*Corresponding author Oran B: Medicana International Hospital, Department of Pediatric Cardiology, İzmir, Turkey
E-mail:boran@medicana.com.tr and bulentoran@hotmail.com

Damus-Kaye-Stensel Procedure

This procedure involves direct anastomosis of the main pulmonary artery to the aorta, thereby forming a single artery originating from the heart. Pulmonary circulation is supported by systemic circulation; the right and left branches of the pulmonary artery are linked with the aorta or its branches through a shunt or conduit pathway. The goal is to establish a wide corridor for the systemic ventricle and to provide functional single-ventricular circulation in patients with complex aortic stenosis, sub-aortic stenosis, or aortic hypoplasia.

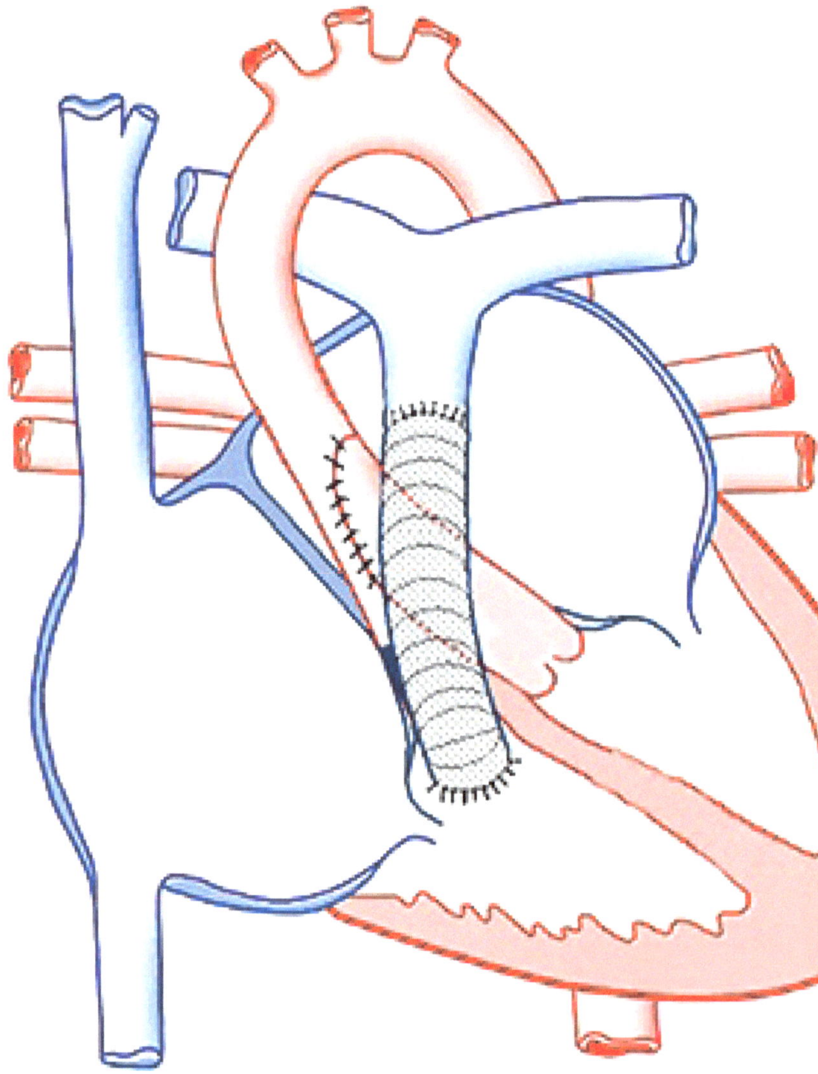

Figure 60: Damus-Kaye-Stansel type procedure: pulm trunk to aorta end/side anastomosis.

*Corresponding author Oran B: Medicana International Hospital, Department of Pediatric Cardiology, İzmir, Turkey
E-mail:boran@medicana.com.tr and bulentoran@hotmail.com

REFERENCES

[1] Anderson RH, Tretter JT, Spicer DE, et al. The Fate of the Outflow Tract Septal Complex in Relation to the Classification of Ventricular Septal Defects. J Cardiovasc Dev Dis 2019; 6: (1).

[2] Anderson RH. Terminology (2009), In: Pediatric Cardiology, (Eds.) Anderson RH, Macartney FJ,

Shinebourne EA, Tynan M., 1st ed., Churchill Livingston, p. 66-107, London.

[3] Baskar S, Gray SB, Del Grippo EL, et al. Cardiac Morphology for the Millennial Cardiology Fellow: Nomenclature and Advances in Morphologic Imaging. Congenit Heart Dis 2018; 13: (5), 808-810.

[4] Edwards WD (2001), Cardiac Anatomy and Examination of Cardiac Specimens. In: Moss and Adams, Heart disease in infant, children, and adolescents, (Eds.) Allen HD, Gutgesell HP, Clark EB, Driscoll DJ., 6th ed., Lippincott Williams & Wilkins, p. 80-142, Philadelphia.

[5] Franklin CG, Béland MJ, Anderson RH. et al. Nomenclature for Congenital and Paediatric Cardiac Disease: The International Paediatric and Congenital Cardiac Code (IPCCC) and the Eleventh Iteration of the International Classification of Diseases (ICD-11). Cardiol Young 2017; 27: (10), 1872-1938.

[6] Jacobs JP, Pasquali SK, Quintessenza JA. Heterotaxy: Lessons learned about patterns of practice and outcomes from the congenital heart surgery database of the Society of Thoracic Surgeons. World J Pediatr Congenit Heart Surg 2011; 2: (2), 278-86.

[7] Kearney DL, Titus JL (1998), Cardiovascular Anatomy. In: The Science and Practice of Pediatric Cardiology, (Eds.) Garson A, Bricker JT, Fischer DJ, Neish SR., 2nd ed., Lippincott Williams & Wilkins, p. 127-154, Baltimore.

[8] Lopez L, Houyel L, Anderson RH, et al. Classification of Ventricular Septal Defects for the Eleventh Iteration of the International Classification of Diseases-Striving for Consensus: A Report From the International Society for Nomenclature of Paediatric and Congenital Heart Disease. Ann Thorac Surg 2018; 106: (5), 1578-1589.

[9] Mullins CE, Mayer DC (1991), Congenital Heart Disease: A Diagrammatic Atlas, Wiley-Liss.

[10] Park MK (2014), Specific Congenital Heart Defects. In: Pediatric Cardiology for Practitioners. 6th (Eds.) Mosby inc. Missouri.

[11] Praagh RV, Praagh SV (2006), Morphologic Anatomy and Segmental Approach to Diagnosis. In: Nadas' Pediatric Cardiology, (Eds.) Keane, JF, Lock, JE, Fyler, DC. Saunders, Inc., 2nd ed., p. 27-46, Philadelphia.

[12] Tretter JT, Tran VH, Anderson RH, et al. Assessing the Criteria for Definition of Perimembranous Ventricular Septal Defects in Light of the Search for Consensus. Orphanet J Rare Dis 2019; 14: (1), 76.

*Corresponding author Oran B: Medicana International Hospital, Department of Pediatric Cardiology, İzmir, Turkey
E-mail:boran@medicana.com.tr and bulentoran@hotmail.com

*Corresponding author Oran B: Medicana International Hospital, Department of Pediatric Cardiology, İzmir, Turkey
E-mail:boran@medicana.com.tr and bulentoran@hotmail.com

*Corresponding author Oran B: Medicana International Hospital, Department of Pediatric Cardiology, İzmir, Turkey
E-mail:boran@medicana.com.tr and bulentoran@hotmail.com

www.ingramcontent.com/pod-product-compliance
Lightning Source LLC
LaVergne TN
LVHW070949210926
848482LV00002B/150

9781949872392